Perfection is always the goal [of Yoga], and, as we shall soon see, it is neither athletic nor hygenic perfection. Haṭha Yoga cannot and must not be confused with gymnastics.

Mircea Eliade, *Yoga: Immortality and Freedom* (1990: 228)

YOGA
IN
MODERN INDIA

The Body between Science and Philosophy

Yoga in Modern India engages the details of yoga philosophy and metaphysics. It brings out the transformation of yoga as a popular activity in the modern age, idolized for its health value. Alter explains through translations from Sanskrit sources how Yoga is based on modern ideas about science and medicine.

YOGA
IN
MODERN INDIA

The Body between Science and Philosophy

JOSEPH S. ALTER

New Age Books

ISBN: 978-81-7822-324-7

First Indian Edition: 2009

Published by Princeton University Press,
41 William Street, Princeton, New Jersey 08540

Published by
NEW AGE BOOKS
A-44 Naraina Phase-I
New Delhi-110 028 (INDIA)
Email: nab@vsnl.in
Website: www.newagebooksindia.com

For Sale in South Asia Only

Printed in India
at Shri Jainendra Press
A-45 Naraina Phase-I, New Delhi-110 028

Living in the house amidst wife and children, but being free from attachments to them, practicing Yoga in secrecy, a house-holder even finds marks of success. And thus, following this teaching of mine, he ever lives in blissful happiness.

Śivasaṃhitā V:212

For Peter and Nathaniel:
my children, and my attachment to the world;
my happiness, bliss notwithstanding.
My immortality if not my freedom.

CONTENTS

ILLUSTRATIONS

PREFACE

THIS IS A book about modern Yoga written from the vantage point of an anthropologist. Its purpose is to understand social change and change in some of the structures of meaning that have taken place in India as a result of colonialism and postcolonial transnationalism.

Insofar as it is concerned with embodied structures of meaning, *Yoga in Modern India* engages with many of the details that have come to constitute Yoga philosophy and metaphysics, and draws heavily on translations of and commentaries on a range of Sanskrit sources. It is, therefore, both similar to and very different from Gregory P. Fields's *Religious Therapeutics: Body and Health in Yoga, Āyurveda, and Tantra* (2001). Topically *Yoga in Modern India* is similar, to the extent that it is concerned with the body and various aspects of classical "Hindu" thought. But in focus and theoretical orientation it is very different. The rather sharp disjunction between topical similarity and difference in theoretical orientation requires brief comment. Apart from this, however, attention is drawn to *Religious Therapeutics* as it is a book that will have much greater appeal to practitioners of modern alternative traditional medicine than will *Yoga in Modern India*. *Religious Therapeutics* is also, in many ways, unique as an academic work. It ambiguously reflects many of the patterns of Yoga's textual—and "spiritual"—popularization and medicalization as both have developed over the past seventy-five years. Those who dislike the fundamental skepticism in *Yoga in Modern India* will find the holistic model of religious therapeutics much more appealing. However, it is the persuasive power of this model in the public sphere—and most dramatically in popular culture—that is also its academic Achilles' heel.

Fields is not particularly concerned with the history of classical thought's modernization. His book tends to uncritically blur the line between New Age perspectives on holistic health on the one hand and what classical texts have to say about biology and the nature of the body on the other. As a consequence, the meaning of "health" is usefully expanded—at least for those of us living in the holistic New Age—but also expanded to such an extent into the domain of religion and spirituality that one tends to lose sight of the profoundly materialist and empirically grounded structure of the body, as this structure is theorized in traditions—for lack of a better term—that stretch across space from Greece and North Africa through to Japan, and through time from the sixth century B.C.E. up to the present. When health is expanded to encompass something as ephemeral as spirituality, it is much too easy to exoticize and mystify—in the mode of a latter-day Orientalist—the practical, pragmatic, and very down-to-earth features of Tantra, Āyurveda, and Yoga. Most problematic, in this respect, is what Fields posits as a "model of religious therapeutics" derived from Āyurveda, Yoga, and Tantra. It is wrong to use religion as a frame of reference to understand the way in which Yoga defines the body and nature, particularly since so much that is important about Yoga is not only not religious, but dead set against many features of orthodox—and even unorthodox—religiosity. The same is true, for different but equally important reasons, with respect to Āyurveda and Tantra.

Regardless, attention is drawn to *Religious Therapeutics* in order to make—by way of contrast—a clear and unambiguous point that is at the heart of this project. The concept of culture is intimately linked to nationalism, and not just, or even primarily, the militant and fanatical kind. To analyze modern cultural constructs by contextualizing them with reference to regional intellectual history, standardized canonical archives, and the bounded authenticity of tradition—even while acknowledging their mutability—is to reproduce and reinforce nationalism, and to impose the logic of nationalism on history in general and on intellectual and social history in particular. This is all the more problematic when the scope of study is putatively global, cross-cultural, and comparative—as well as philosophically synthetic—since New Age export often adds the insult of modular packaging to the injury of reification. Nationalism and modernity artifactually reflect and refract each other, just as history and tradition do. Analysis must reflect this, although it means seriously taking into consideration the extent to which Yoga is—with apologies to A. L. Basham—not a unique product of Indian civilization or a New Age antidote to the evil that civilization as such has wrought. It is fundamentally a social product of the "wonder that is the world," as this is immortalized in a place called India, but also as it has developed in places within and between other places that have come to have different names: Afghanistan, Pakistan, Tibet, Nepal, and China, for example, to say nothing of England, Germany, and the United States.

Content notwithstanding, *Yoga in Modern India* should not be read as a study of Yoga philosophy or as a study of Yoga from the vantage point of a Sanskritist. Because the focus of analytic attention is on how Yoga has been made to make sense over the course of the past century, there is no sense in which this book seeks to define Yoga's authentic form or delimit its authoritative canon. The individuals and institutions who are analyzed and described in this book are not included because they speak with any more or less authority than anyone else. They have been selected because they provide a perspective on a kind of modern history—and a particular bracket of time within history—that is often regarded as insignificant. Insignificant, that is, in light of a much grander history of civilization that provides the usual context for understanding Yoga's past. The individuals and groups analyzed here have also been selected because they provide insight into the messiness of antiquity's convergence with modernity. As a consequence, this book may well grate on the intellectual nerves of purists, frustrate classically oriented Sanskritists, and ruffle the feathers of orthodox historians. This is not so much intentional as a function of the way in which the postmodern condition of the New Age requires a certain analytical orientation to the subject at hand.

Part of the problem has to do with the time frame. How does one adequately and accurately represent a system of thought and embodied practice that is several thousand years old when seeking to understand the modern interpretation of this system over the course of the past century? Add to this the problem that, in many ways, novel interpretations—if not misinterpretations as such—constitute the subject of study, and it can easily seem that this is a misguided book about misunderstanding based upon mistakes! In any event, it is a work of interpretation that seeks to be true to the significance of each specific case. Most of the cases in question straddle an awkward period of time somewhere between the ethnographic present and the historical past. At least from the vantage point of anthropology, it is difficult to know how to interpret events and social formations in the twentieth century, given the intimate connection between the present—as a decidedly future-oriented point in time—and things just past that have not had a chance to settle into history, so to speak.

Although the work of interpretation is ultimately inconclusive, it is, I think, the best way to approach what might be called the nonhistorical past. It is during this period when orthodoxy tends to take shape, as orthodoxy is dependent on the strategic—if not necessarily conscious or collusive—editing of events to produce coherence, logic, and a sense of systemic progress. Clearly strategic editing goes on in the present, and often it is events of ancient history that get edited—think, for example, of the so-called Aryan invasion or of the question of where on earth, and more specifically where in Ayodhya, Lord Ram was born. But it is in the just-past of the present—say, a period of one hundred years or so—where there is a high degree of looseness, flexibility, and slippage in the control of knowledge and meaning. Various individuals and groups have a powerful interest in constructing the meaning of events of this time in particular ways. Consider, as I have done in a previous book, what has been made of Mahatma Gandhi's life (Alter 2000a), and what you can make of it—and, more importantly, what can be made of things related to it that have been forgotten—if you look past both hagiography and the standard orthodox canons of colonialism, postcolonialism, and postcolonial nationalism: arenas within which there is intense editing, to be sure.

Essentially the present's just-past is a time frame of rapid remembering and forgetting, compounded by the transmission of knowledge from one generation to the next. In other words, the just-past of the present—which I take to be different from modern history, even though modern history seeks to deal with this period of time as a time period—is when facticity matters a great deal, but when individual memories produce competing and contradictory realities. The arguments about who was the first to popularize, modernize, and demystify Yoga may be relatively less significant than the question of whose sense of holiness defines the Holy Land, or how events transpired there in the aftermath of World War I—to choose a highly politicized and volatile example—but the dynamic is very much the same. Beyond this, however, there is, in the present's just-past, the seductive sense that someone is really right, and that with enough information the truth can be established.

In terms of more ancient history there is both more and less nervousness about the relationship between definitive truth and interpretation—consider what the famous *pāśupati* seal from the Indus civilization signifies with respect to the antiquity of Yoga. But also consider the whole question of whether the enigmatic, four-thousand-year-old seal signifies anything about Yoga at all, apart from a rather vague formal similarity between the body posture of the seated figure with horns on his head and descriptions of Haṭha Yoga postures that only took shape as such in the medieval period. Is the figure on the seal Lord Śiva seated in a Yoga *āsana,* or not? In any case, it is fundamentally wrong to answer questions such as this by making an argument about "what" is right. "What" is invariably a question of "who"—although the displacement of object-into-subject made possible by variable indeterminacy does have a way of masking the pronominalism of nationalism. Interpretation must show that in any scenario construed as a clear dichotomy, both perspectives are wrong. An interpretive study such as *Yoga in Modern India,* which is based on skepticism rather than on relativism, does not seek to provide a right answer to the question of what counts as Yoga and how and why modern Yoga came into being. As will be explained in Part 3, the goal here is to remain true to the meaninglessness of contextualization and to focus on the way in which wrong answers and mistakes—defined in relationship to one another, rather than as such from any privileged perspective on what is intrinsically or definitively right—produce history in the ethnographic past. *Yoga in Modern India* is designed to produce and understand this version of history.

Dealing with the just-past of the present is a problem that is compounded by the relationship between texts unto themselves and texts in relationship to what people say. Historically, both the theories and the methods of anthropology have been based on nontextual resources. Social and cultural anthropology in particular has focused on what people say rather than on what they have written. Participant observation is a methodology based on the authority of the spoken word and on what would otherwise be unrecorded—if not by any means unremembered—events. What, then, is the relationship between ethnography and formal, published texts? There are many ways to answer this. In some ways the question itself can simply be ignored, given the fluidity of disciplinary boundaries. But it is an important theoretical and methodological question. The approach taken here—which is simple, pragmatic, and straightforward rather than theoretically sophisticated—can best be explained by way of an analogy.

Conducting field research involves listening to numerous people say numerous things, and only arriving, after the fact—and after what is an inherently open-ended process of trying to make sense of what is going on—at an understanding of what is important and what is thought to be meaningful. To state the obvious, field notes are comprehensive and contain a great deal of detail about many different things, even when the research project is focused and methodologically well organized. Good field notes are indiscriminate and unkempt; they define a space in between speech and written language. Any given published resource is, in many respects—and Derrida notwithstanding—the antithesis of this. It discriminates knowledge, is selective, and is structured and highly formulaic with respect to representation and the production of meaning.

Over the course of the past century or century and a half, however, publishing has produced a curious phenomenon whereby books, pamphlets, magazines, brochures, printed notices, and countless other things are manufactured and then reproduced in massive numbers on a huge scale. As comprehensive cataloging—and the pedantic, compulsive obsessiveness of scholars—falls short, it becomes possible to engage with a body of literature almost as though it were a discursive field. To be sure, one can never engage with a collection of written texts in the same way as one can engage with an interlocutor. But provided one does engage with real live interlocutors—in the sense that is required in social and cultural anthropology—it is possible to deal with certain bodies of literature in the mode of a participant observer. This is also a strategic means by which to engage with the just-past of the present.

The analogy is simply this. The shelves in my office are full of over two thousand published items dealing with Yoga that date from about 1909 to the present. I have purchased, photocopied, or received as gifts anything I could get my hands on or that came my way. For example, after driving around Delhi for several hours and following several dead-end leads, I finally located the central office of the Bharatiya Yog Sansthan in a lower-middle-class neighborhood of Old Delhi. The BYS is an organization devoted simply to the promotion of Universal Brotherhood—coded in terms of modern, Hindu values and ideals—through the popularization of Yoga training. The president of the organization was expecting me, but being unexpectedly busy he asked me to wait before beginning our interview. Graciously he directed me to sit in a chair in one of the back rooms of the office, where a clerk was working on some files. The clerk and I got to talking and in the course of the conversation I realized that the organization published a quarterly magazine called *Yog Manjari.* Immediately I filled out and paid for a lifetime membership subscription. Without much hope of success I also asked if it was possible to purchase any back issues. To my surprise and delight, the clerk pulled out stack upon stack of old magazines dating to the late 1960s. This was the last available set, but since the person for whom it had been compiled had never sent the required bank draft for advance payment, the option to buy—as they say—was mine. It is not as though *Yog Manjari* is unique in its marginality, or unique in the way it has slipped past most of the systems set in place to codify, classify, regulate, and authorize writing. Archives are, after all, full of such things. What is somewhat unique is the way in which the sheer volume of this kind of topically specific material, dating from about 1920 to the present, can historicize the contemporary practice of Yoga. It can historicize the present.

The vast majority of the texts collected in the fashion described above are discriminately indiscriminate. If any one of the authors were to read what another had written, he or she would be as likely to disagree as agree with what is claimed. Many authors write as though they are the only person writing on the subject with any authority, and that what they are saying is new. Yet if there is one single thing that characterizes the literature on Yoga, it is repetition and redundancy in the guise of novelty and independent invention. It is interesting to imagine—given that each one has had a deeply vested interest in being right, where others have been wrong—how Yogi Ramacharaka in 1905 would have read, and have been read by, Deepak Chopra in 2004. Apart from the question of being right or wrong, both Ramacharaka and Deepak Chopra have produced numerous books, and this is characteristic of authors who write in the genre. As Sarah Strauss has pointed out, Swami Sivananda, who founded the Divine Life Society in 1932, established himself as an authority on the subject of Yoga at least in part through the production of a massive popular corpus of books and pamphlets. This corpus has helped to construct a "transnational community of practice" based on the articulation of both a structured routine of exercise and a broadly defined spiritual philosophy of everyday life (2000: 162–94). Sivananda was prolific, as was Ramacharaka. Deepak Chopra continues to be. Each of these men has articulated a version of the truth; and this truth, once publicized, is authorized and rendered meaningful and coherent—at least in the view of self-proclaimed disciples, if not a general audience—through publication and republication. My concern is less with the coherence of any single author's collected works than it is with the way in which the whole collection of collected works produces unstable knowledge.

Regardless of where and when they are published and printed, books, magazines, and pamphlets such as these are what might be called pulp nonfiction. Price and quality of print production is not so much what matters. Yogic pulp nonfiction can be defined as texts that put forth the idea that you can teach yourself Yoga by reading a book, even if one of the lessons is that you should stop reading and go and find a *guru*. For practical and logistical reasons alone, only a fraction of books such as these—ranging from anonymously authored pamphlets purchased from railway station vendors through Theos Bernard's beautifully illustrated *Haṭha Yoga: The Report of a Personal Experience* (1944) to B.K.S. Iyengar's magnificent *Light on Yoga* (1976)—are referenced in this study. In a very important way, however, they define, collectively, a discursive field that is "out there," and out there much in the same way as are the open-ended conversations that went on before, and continue well after, the momentary and infractively fragmentary event of participant observation.

The point is that this discursive field—as distinct from any given set of texts or any delineation of the texts as such—marks off a significant part of the ethnographic space of modern Yoga, and this space cross-cuts time, although it does not transcend it. Yogic pulp nonfiction is not completely different from other genres of "popular" literature. But it is significantly deep, rich, and idiosyncratic enough as to defy any sort of totalizing synthesis. This chronic open-endedness is exactly what brings it to life. And there is a certain ironic symmetry between this kind of virtually spoken textuality and the textuality of field notes that capture—but manage to keep alive—words once spoken.

Beyond this, the discursive field of yogic pulp nonfiction makes the whole problem of ethnographic representation much more complicated, since there is a pervasive—and highly exaggerated—tension in the field between the textuality of speech and the textuality of published texts. In a distinctly iconic sense, *gurus* literally embody and thereby speak the truth of Yoga, though always in the idiom of a secret. To write about and publicize that of which *gurus* secretly speak produces many contradictions and raises questions about truth, experience, and representation. To a significant extent this tension has opened a space for analysis where plastic understanding can intercede when the question of authoritative, hard, inflexible truth inevitably falls short as a consequence of dialectical disarticulation. This study is located in that space.

Yoga in Modern India is divided into three parts, encompassing seven chapters. Part 1 deals with the problem of making Yoga a subject of sociohistorical study, the main argument being that although it has been constructed as a timeless icon of Indian civilization, Yoga is, in fact, a very modern phenomenon. The second chapter in this part focuses on the way in which modern Yoga struggles with the relationship between metaphysics and the gross materiality of the body. Part 2 contains three chapters that deal with the historical development and contemporary practice of Yoga as medicine and its institutionalization as a form of public health. The first chapter in this section focuses on Swami Kuvalayananda, the chief architect of modern medicalized Yoga in India. The case of Swami Kuvalayananda shows how central the discourse and practice of science was to the institutionalization of Yoga research in pre-independence India. The second chapter is concerned with the legacy of Gandhi's advocacy for health reform, and the convergence of naturopathy and Yoga. The third chapter focuses on the oblique relationship between Yoga, health, and the culture of Hindu fundamentalism. Part 3 is a conclusion in the sense that it brings the discussion back to the key question of science, the body, and modernity by integrating theoretical points made in parts 1 and 2. The first chapter in this section shows how a simple yogic procedure—drinking one's own urine—has become popular in India as a consequence of the transnational exchange of knowledge during the colonial and early postcolonial period. Since Yoga is all about relativism—Self in relation to self, embodiment relative to transcendence—and the disillusion of opposites, the final chapter uses insights drawn from a history of modern Yoga to focus on the culture concept and the problem of cultural relativism in anthropological theory.

ACKNOWLEDGMENTS

IT IS DIFFICULT to identify the point in time when this study began. In some important respects Yoga has been lurking in the shadows of all my previous research.

It was there in my desire to return to the Himalayas in 1981 while working on my M.A. thesis and to locate, define, and reveal some sort of nonexotic, universal truth about cultural difference while simultaneously trying to maintain the aura and exotic mystery that characterizes the abode of yogis. It was most certainly there in the person of Dil Das, a true sage of the Himalayas, and a *pāśupati* in his own right (see Alter 2000c).

It was there, explicitly—but also in the shadow of a more grossly embodied form of practice—in my first encounter with Indian wrestling in 1977 (see Alter 1992). Dr. Shanti Prakash Atreya, onetime Uttar Pradesh state champion and son of the well-known early-twentieth-century Sanskritist and Yoga scholar B. L. Atreya, founded an *akhāṛā* (gymnasium) on the grounds of his father's academic retreat at Kuthalgate in the Himalayan foothills. The retreat was known as the Yoga Manovijñān Kendra, which—despite the ironic fact that *manovijñān* is most commonly glossed as anthropology—is translated as Research Center for Yoga Psychology. Just before his death in the mid-1990s, Dr. Atreya was working on a series of articles explaining the theoretical and embodied connection between Yoga and wrestling.

Yoga was there when I began to read, beyond the principle of *bhakti* and the apparent preeminence of the *Gītā* in the Mahatma's life, about Gandhi's more pervasive concern with embodied morality and the politics of health and fitness (see Alter 2000a). Gandhi corresponded with Swami Kuvalayananda, one of the principal founders of modern Yoga, and experimented with *āsana* and *prāṇāyāma,* although he was never convinced of their efficacy. In many ways, however, Gandhi's whole project can be thought of as an attempt to define the physiology of Karma Yoga—the Yoga of Action—and to devise an ethics of the body that is on par with the power manifest in Haṭha Yoga, but neither so inherently mystical and magical nor so easily perverted—and thereby rendered irrelevant to moral questions—as are *āsana, kriyā,* and *prāṇāyāma.*

Finally, Yoga has been lurking in the shadows of my analyses of celibacy, sexuality, and the desire for immortality (see Alter 1994a, 1999). This is not only because *brahamcarya* (celibacy) is the fourth of the five *yama* (restraint)—and thereby a linchpin in Yoga's *aṣṭāṅga* structure of progressive development—but because the physiology of sex is, as it turns out, at the very heart of Yoga.

All this said, however—and the extent of acknowledgment thereby spanning twenty-five years—it was while conducting research in India's National Archives and at the Nehru Memorial Library in New Delhi during the winter of 1993 that Yoga emerged from the shadows of my consciousness. I was, at the time, engaged in research on the history of embodied nonviolence in modern India. The research had taken me into the realm of physical education and alternative medicine. It was while reading this literature, in early 1994, that it struck me that Yoga might provide a clear and comprehensive framework for making sense of a series of related problems that I was having difficulty sorting out. However, in trying to sort through the intersection of physical fitness, medicine, nature cure, and sexuality it gradually became clear that Yoga was constituted by this intersection. It manifested the crux of the problem itself—the problematic location of the body in relation to knowledge in the context of modernity—rather than its ultimate solution through resolution. This book has emerged out of this realization.

Therefore I am indebted to the American Institute of Indian Studies for providing funding and support in 1993–94, before the study really began, and then again in 1999 when it was more clearly developed. In 1999 funding through the AIIS was made possible by a grant from the National Endowment for the Humanities. The National Science Foundation provided a grant that funded research in 1998 and 2000. In 2001 funding was provided by a grant from the Hewlett International Grant Program, administered by the University Center for International Studies, and a grant from the FAS Faculty Research Grant Program, both at the University of Pittsburgh.

In India I received help from a great number of people involved directly in Yoga practice—many of whom I met and spoke with only briefly—to whom I am deeply indebted. I would like to thank the late Dr. Shanti Prakash Atreya; Dr. Nair of the Bapu Nature Cure Hospital and Yogashram; Prakash Lal and Rishi Ram Sharma of the Bharatiya Yog Sansthan; Dr. Kumar Pal of the Yoga International Institute for Psycho-Physical Therapy; Dr. Brahmchari of the Central Council for Research on Yoga and Naturopathy; Dr. S. V. Karandikar of Sunderraj Yoga Darshan; the staff of the Yoga Kendra at Banaras Hindu University; and Dr. O. P. Tiwari, along with the librarians and staff in the publications division of Kaivalyadhama Yoga Ashram. Although I wish to acknowledge my debt to each of these individuals, I must point out that the views presented in this book are mine and mine alone. They do not necessarily reflect the views or opinions of these individuals or of others connected to the institutions noted above whose work is cited here.

I was invited by various individuals and groups to present academic papers that evolved into several of the chapters in this book. I attended a conference organized by Martha Selby under the auspices of the Asian Studies Center at the University of Texas, Austin, in 2001. In 2001 and 2002 I participated in a two-part conference at the University of Cambridge organized by Elizabeth De Michelis under the auspices of the Dharma Hinduja Indic Research Center. I was also invited to speak about my research at the University of British Columbia; the University of Illinois, Urbana/Champaign; and Syracuse University. I would like to express my gratitude and debt to all of these institutions and organizations, and to Martha Selby and Elizabeth De Michelis in particular.

Beyond this I would like to thank a number of anthropologists, sociologists, historians, and other academicians who have been kind enough to engage with me, at various points, on some of the material that has come together here, in particular Nancy Abelmann, Lawrence Cohen, Waltraud Ernst, Julius Lipner, Sarah Lamb, Mckim Marriott, Peter Schriener, Patricia Uberoi, Susan Wadley, Dominik Wujastyk, and Kenneth Zysk. As always, numerous students in various seminars—Shamanic Healing; Nationalism, Colonialism and the Body; Asian Medical Systems; Gender and Health—have provided vital input and inspired me to think about things much more broadly than would otherwise have been the case.

At the University of Pittsburgh I would like to thank my colleagues in the Department of Anthropology and the Asian Studies Center.

Finally, special and heartfelt thanks to Nicole Constable.

PART 1

INTRODUCTION AND ORIENTATION

To summarize, society is by no means the illogical and alogical, inconsistent and changeable being that people all too often like to imagine. Quite the contrary, the collective consciousness is the highest form of psychic life, for it is a consciousness of consciousness. Being outside and above individual and local contingencies, collective consciousness sees things only in their permanent and fundamental aspects, which it crystallizes in ideas that can be communicated. At the same time as it sees from above, it sees far ahead; at every moment it embraces all known reality; that is why it alone can furnish the intellect with frameworks that are applicable to the totality of beings and that enable us to build concepts about them. It does not create these frameworks artificially but finds them within itself, merely becoming conscious of them.

Emile Durkheim, *The Elementary Forms of Religious Life* (1995: 445)

1

HISTORICIZING YOGA: THE LIFE AND TIMES OF LIBERATED SOULS

> Nevertheless, there is a definite point where Yoga and shamanism meet. They meet in "emergence from time" and the abolition of history. The shaman's ecstasy recovers the primordial freedom and bliss of the ages in which, according to the myths, man could ascend to heaven and physically converse with the gods. For its part, Yoga results in the nonconditioned state of *samādhi* or of *sahaja,* in the perfect spontaneity of the *jīvan-mukta,* the man "liberated in this life." From one point of view, we may say that the *jīvan-mukta* has abolished time and history.
>
> Mircea Eliade, *Yoga: Immortality and Freedom* (1990: 339–40)

> The Hindu universe is a kind of four-dimensional Mobius strip, finite but unbounded, negatively curved. . . . In all of these [mythological] images we encounter the inversion of time as well as space. . . . The Mobius strip, then, is the shape of time and space in India. . . . If there *is* a final level, it is the level of the Godhead, *brahman,* the impersonal, transcendent continuum beyond even Rudra. This is the level of the universal soul, the source of all mental images that assume material form.
>
> Wendy Doniger O'Flaherty, *Dreams, Illusion, and Other Realities* (1984: 241–43)

Orientation toward the Subject

IT WOULD be extremely surprising if anyone reading this book had not at least heard of Yoga and developed some basic idea about what it is. On the one hand, it is one of the six main schools of classical South Asian philosophy, most explicitly articulated in Patañjali's *Yoga Sūtra.*[1] In this regard it is as central to the history of thought in South Asia as is the philosophy of Aristotle to the intellectual history of Europe. On the other hand, Yoga is a modern form of alternative medicine and physical fitness training. This book is concerned with the way Yoga can be these two things at once in modern India, and with the historical transmutation of philosophy into physical education, public health, and institutionalized medical practice.

Emerging out of South Asia, Yoga is a complex and comprehensive philosophy of transcendental consciousness that crystallized into a school of thought sometime between 150 and 500 C.E. (Whicher 1998: 42).[2] In essence Yoga holds that the world, as it is commonly perceived by the mind through self-consciousness, is an illusion based on ignorance. As Eliade puts it: "For Sāṃkhya and Yoga the world is *real* (not illusory—as it is, for example, for Vedānta). Nevertheless, if the world *exists* and *endures,* it is because of the 'ignorance' of spirit; the innumerable forms of the cosmos, as well as their processes of manifestation and development, exist only in the measure to which the Self (*puruṣa*) is ignorant of itself and, by reason of this metaphysical ignorance, suffers and is enslaved" (1990: 9). The practice of Yoga is designed to transform illusion into reality by transcending ignorance and training the embodied mind to experience Truth. The experience of Truth is *samādhi,* which can be translated as a transcendent condition of ecstatic union of subject and object.[3] Significantly, *samādhi* is both the technique for realizing this condition and the condition itself. The transcendental Self is *samādhi* as a condition of Ultimate Truth that is beyond time and space. In this regard Yoga can be understood as so profound as to make standard categories of thought such as religion, spirituality, metaphysics, and science—to name but the most standard—singularly imprecise and dubiously qualified to articulate Truth.

Although Yoga is one of the so-called six orthodox schools or *sad darśanas* and is almost two thousand years old, it is important, particularly in the context of this book, to appreciate the fact that there has been a long, if not by any means continuous or systematically developmental, history of Yoga scholarship and textual redaction. In other words, if one can say that Yoga as a school of thought was systematized by Patañjali around the second or third century of this era, ever since then there have been attempts to understand it, and make it understandable, on the basis of various degrees of both engaged practice and intellectual distance. Yoga philosophy has never existed as a fixed, primordial entity, even though the canonical status of a few primary texts gives this impression.

Taking the *Yoga Sūtra* as an object of study, analyses of Yoga in the form of commentaries and elaborations date back to the fifth century with Vyāsa's *Bhāṣya* (see Misra 1971). Subsequent works by Vācaspati Miśra in the ninth century (see Misra 1971) and by Bhoja Rāja (see Shastri 1930) and Vijñāna Bhikṣu (see Misra 1971) in the eleventh and sixteenth centuries indicate an ongoing tradition of scholarship, study, and practice. Although more research is needed to clarify the nature and extent of intellectual developments in the late classical and medieval periods, there is clearly a long history of intellectual engagement with Yoga that has produced an extensive primary literature.

Ian Whicher provides a succinct and up-to-date overview of this literature, pointing out that "with some exceptions, the secondary literature on classical Yoga can tend to be dry and repetitive, which underlines the notion that Yoga, in its authentic context, has always been an esoteric discipline taught mainly through oral tradition" (1998: 320–22). This point is of tremendous significance—often noted by a range of scholar practitioners, such as Georg Feuerstein (1989: 176)—and must always be kept in mind. There is, in other words, a history of Yoga that is not circumscribed by the hegemony of "dry" textual redaction. Most importantly this oral tradition, manifest in the practice-based teaching of *guru*s to their disciples, enables an appreciation for the relevance of a history of Yoga that picks up at that moment in time when it is possible to find texts that comment directly on the form and content of this oral tradition, rather than simply—and "dryly"—on other, older texts. As yet it is not possible to fix a date for this shift, since further study of the classical and medieval literature—including, perhaps most significantly, the early Persian sources—may reveal critical commentaries.

By the end of the nineteenth century, however, there seems to have been a paradigmatic shift away from commentary and textual redaction to critical analysis and a search for the most authentic oral tradition manifest in practice.[4] Ironically the valorization of the oral tradition fractures the continuity of history by producing texts that purport to reveal, to us moderns, the most ancient of ancient truths. This is ironic, since, in many ways, the shift is closely associated with modernity, the idea of historical continuity, and an essentialized, primordialist view of Indian civilization. In any event this history, as well as the intellectual tradition of commentary and redaction found in the secondary literature—ranging from the earliest commentaries up to Barbara Stoler Miller's recent translation (1996)—must be understood as having made Yoga what it is, rather than as having simply revealed yogic truth as a predefined entity. One could argue that, in this era of constructionist and deconstructionist scholarship, this point should go without saying. The problem, however, is that Yoga, even more so than religion and science—respectively its much "older" and much "younger" intellectual siblings—is constructed as both timeless and beyond time. And so it is all the more important to situate it in history as a product of human imagination.

Apart from the key issue of trying to write an oral tradition of practice, a close reading of Yoga's literary history of commentary and redaction shows how it has been subject to the inevitable process of interpretation, a process that is distinct from the obvious features of intellectual refinement and clarification, if not exclusively so. Whicher points out that the

Yoga Bhāṣya of Vyāsa (see Misra 1971), written in the fifth or sixth century, is the oldest commentary on the *Yoga Sūtra,* and the one upon which almost all subsequent commentaries are based. Following on late classical and early medieval works by Bhoja Rāja (see Shastri 1930) and Mādhavācārya (1882) , probably the second most important commentary is by Vijñāna Bhikṣu, who was "a renowned scholar and yogin who interpreted Yoga from a Vedāntic point of view. One of his main contributions is his attempt to establish points of unity between the dualistic perspective of Sāṃkhya and theistic/nondualistic thought in Vedānta" (Whicher 1998: 321). Bhikṣu's disciples, Bhāvāgaṇeśa and Nāgojī Bhaṭṭa, provide a further redaction of their *guru*'s Vedāntic perspective on Vyāsa (see Shastri 1930), but another seventeenth- or eighteenth-century work by Nārāyaṇ Tīrtha (see Bhatta 1911), which is devotional in orientation, is based directly on Patañjali's *Yoga Sūtra* independent of either Vyāsa's or Bhikṣu's works. Although it would be fascinating to study the literature in the late pre-Mogul and Mogul period so as to gain an understanding of when and how the first critical studies of Yoga developed—as more or less distinct from direct commentaries, which continued to be written up to twentieth century—it seems clear that it was not until the late nineteenth and early twentieth centuries that a well-defined "tertiary" and synthetic literature came into being. Here, again, however, early Persian sources such as al-Biruni's translation of a now lost version of the *Yoga Sūtra* (Pines and Gelblum 1966; Ritter 1956) warrant close examination based on the assumption that the authors of these works were engaged in both literary *and* "cross-cultural" translation. In any case, Sadāśivendra Sarasvatī's eighteenth-century *Yoga-Sudhā-Ākara* (see Shastri 1930) and Ananta-deva Pandit's nineteenth-century *Padacandrikā* (see Shastri 1930) are, arguably, the last articulations of a kind of scholarship reflecting *ṭīkā* glosses and commentaries as well as the *vṛtti* style of nonargumentative redaction that was characteristic of the preceding centuries.

Orientalist studies of Yoga as philosophy, as distinct from indigenous commentaries on Yoga as Truth, are exemplified in the scholarship of Richard Garbe (1894, 1917), J. Ghose (1930), N. C. Paul (1851, 1888), Paul Deussen (1920), A. B. Keith (1925), and Sir John Woodroffe (1927) among numerous others. In this context Surendranath Dasgupta's scholarship (1920, 1924, 1930) is seminal. In many ways his intellectual influence on Mircea Eliade defines a critical nexus in the development of Yoga research and analysis. As a leading Bengali intellectual directly involved in a complex process of modernization, whereby "Eastern and Western" traditions were, to various degrees and on various levels, being creatively synthesized, Dasgupta became Eliade's teacher and *guru.* This produced a critical link between "modernity and tradition," East and West.[5] As a

European scholar, Eliade was able to extend this link and, with obvious intellectual insights of his own, translate the ferment of modern ideas in Bengal and other parts of India—most notably Rishikesh (Strauss 1997, 2000: 172)—into a tome of classic significance in the genre of Western comparative religious studies. His *Yoga: Immortality and Freedom* (1990) is a work of definitive, late-Orientalist scholarship.[6]

In many respects the well-known Orientalist literature on Yoga—in particular Eliade's study, which extends beyond the *Yoga Sūtra,* and Sir John Woodroffe's *The Serpent Power* (1931; see also1927)—provides a critical backdrop against which this book is written, and in relation to which it must be read. In part this is because the Orientalist literature tends to ignore the way in which modern history in India has defined the intellectual context and climate within which "ancient" Yoga is understood. Eliade studied with Dasgupta at the University of Calcutta from 1928 to 1931, and resided in an *āśram* in Rishikesh for six months. The book he wrote based on these experiences makes no reference to colonialism and the profound changes that were taking place in the practice of Yoga at this time. It is precisely with these changes that this book is directly concerned.

But there is also a specific reason for "writing against" the legacy of Orientalism. Even though yogic literature is concerned with the body, it is clear that Orientalist scholars were almost exclusively concerned with philosophy, mysticism, magic, religion, and metaphysics. They were not particularly concerned with the mundane physics of physical fitness and physiology. There is a great deal of rich detail about the body and yogic physiology in Eliade's book, but fundamentally it is about the mind, the limits of consciousness, and the freedom of transcendence. Similarly Woodroffe's book is full of detail concerning the physiology of Yoga, but in his analysis what is important is not the body as such but its mystical, esoteric, and inherently symbolic value as a good medium through which to think, and—with apologies to Lévi-Strauss—to get beyond thinking. Metaphysics and a preoccupation with the occult prevented almost all Orientalist scholars from trying to understand the value of the body in terms of what might be called elemental yogic materialism.

During the heyday of early-twentieth-century Orientalist scholarship there were a number of people—mostly if not exclusively men living in northern and western India—who sought to revive Yoga in practice, dissociate it from magic and arcane mysticism, and focus attention directly on the body. As we shall see, however, they focused on the physical aspects of Yoga with some ambivalence about the implications of what they were doing. In any event, these men were not nearly as well known as the key players in the Yoga renaissance, namely Sri Aurobindo and Vivekananda. The approach that the "antimystics" took to the body was in terms of physical fitness, applied medical research, and pragmatic populism rather than arcane philosophy and spiritualism. Although somewhat in the shadow of Vivekananda and Aurobindo—both then and now—these men have, in fact, had a profound effect on the history of Yoga. Even casual awareness of what is going on in the global marketplace of alternative medicine and self-help therapy shows that over the past century the body has become ever more central to the practice of Yoga. The fact that it has can be traced directly back to events in western central India in the years just before 1920.

In the context of modern practice since then, the body has come to be understood in ever more pragmatic, rational, and empirical terms, just as the final goal of Yoga—*samādhi*—has come to be understood as more and more abstract. In conjunction with this, it is important to note that, in contrast to the profound intellectualism of Orientalist scholarship, the main trajectory of Yoga's modern development is populist and plebeian. Anyone can publish a book describing how to reach enlightenment, and anyone anywhere can open a school to teach *āsana*s, breathing exercises, and self-realization. Many, many people have, in India and elsewhere. So many people have, in fact, that it would be impossible to do justice to the global scope of modern practice in a single publication. Therefore this book is, somewhat narrowly, a book about Yoga in India. And to put it that way—narrowly in India!—provides a clear appreciation of the ironic discontinuity between discourses of origin and the brute fact of transnationalism, each of which defines "narrowness" in a radically different way. As signs, pamphlets, and bookshops in countless small towns, bus stops, and railway stations attest, Yoga, a profoundly antisocial form of self-discipline, one that is structured in opposition to human nature—if Eliade is right—occupies an important place, and defines an explicitly public space, in the modern world of medicine, self-help therapy, and public health.

Using the insights and methods of historical anthropology, this book is an intellectual history of modern Yoga's embodied practice. It is a modest effort to force Yoga out of classical texts and locate its history in the body of practice, as the body of practice is a fact of everyday life, rather than as a means to achieve transcendental consciousness. It is a critical analysis—and critique—of the legacy of Orientalism and the myths of continuity, intellectualism, and High Culture that all scholarship, even scholarship on culture with a small "c," produces and reproduces. In this respect it is guided not so much by theories of cultural critique and deconstruction, as by a kind of neo-sociology that directs attention away from agency, meaning, and culture as such so as to provide analytical focus on the contingent history of social facts, in this case the social facticity of Yoga. This social facticity is not at all the same as, and not directly dependent on, either Yoga's goal of final liberation or on claims made about its use, value, and significance by those who engage in its practice.

First brought to the "consciousness" of the American reading public by Henry David Thoreau, who was inspired to think about meditation in an Oriental mode (De Michelis n.d.: 2), and then brought to the United States and Europe by an array of *gurus* in the early 1900s (see Narayan 1993), some elements of Yoga are now taught in the physical education curriculum of many American universities. Other elements are used in weight-loss programs, to reform and relax incarcerated prisoners, to energize executives, and to help rehabilitate drug addicts. As Gerald Larson blithely points out, the "ecumenical possibilities" of Yoga are almost endless, including everything from Patañjali to the YMCA (1978; quoted in Whicher 1998: 6). Invoking a shudder of dismay—or perhaps a sigh of relief—I. K. Taimni, a chemistry professor at Allahabad University who produced one the of the first "popular" commentaries on the *Yoga Sūtra,* puts it this way: "There is no subject which is so much wrapped up in mystery and on which one can write whatever one likes without any risk of being proved wrong" (1961: v).

In the world today, one can "learn" Yoga by taking lessons from an established school, or teach it to oneself by reading one of approximately ten thousand popular books on the subject. Alternatively one can study it by logging on to one of the numerous websites on the Internet. Dick's Sporting Goods, a U.S.-based athletics equipment retailer, now markets a line of Yoga workout clothing and exercise equipment, and both the Discovery Store and Whole Foods carry a line of Yoga self-help videos as well as various accessories for practice, such as mats and "bricks" to enhance the effectiveness of specific *āsana*s or postures.[7] But lest one be seduced by the ultra-modernity of the Discovery Store display of mass-produced videos and mats, it should be pointed out that outlets in India have, for many years, produced and sold hundred-count packets of waxed-cord catheters for *sūtra neti* (sinus cleansing), as well as copper and plastic *jal neti* pots for "nasal purification." As early as 1930, Swami Kuvalayananda was "mass producing" Yoga instructors so as to transform the physical education curriculum of public education in India.

Over the course of the past century not only has Yoga been radically transformed; the very radical nature of this transformation has influenced the way in which "classical" Yoga is understood. In turn this understanding has directly influenced the way in which Indian culture is thought to be linked—at least in the popular imagination—almost exclusively to the transcendental nature of "classical" Yoga, whereas "modernized" physical Yoga is thought to be a product of Western "misunderstanding." In other words, the very idea of Indian spirituality and contemplative mysticism—its Orientalist albatross, one might say—is, in some sense, a derivative of the way in which Yoga as "physical culture" is thought to be the product of Western "perversion" and misunderstanding. In fact, as this book is designed to show, things are much more complicated and interesting than this.

Yoga in all of its manifestations is directly linked to Indian modernity. It was in India that Yoga was modernized, medicalized, and transformed into a system of physical culture. Significantly this happened in tandem with, and is closely linked to, the modern development of Yoga philosophy as a so-called science of higher consciousness distinct from embodied forms of experience and practice. It is extremely difficult—and wrong headed—to make a clear and unambiguous distinction between so-called physical and so-called contemplative Yoga, and yet the history of Yoga is characterized by the seductively modern and simplistic allure of this problematic distinction. In this light the medicalization and "gross embodiment" of Yoga provides an interesting perspective on postcolonialism and global modernity insofar as the power/knowledge configuration involved cannot be neatly assimilated into the standard binarism of modernity/tradition, East/West, colonizer/colonized, or science/religion, any more than it can be assimilated into the distinction between gross and subtle domains of experience.

Objective: The Object as Such

In and of itself the word "Yoga" means union. Technically it is the union of the individual self with the universal, cosmic Self and the transcendence of all things, although obviously it is not as simple as that. Recognizing the full range of possible meaning, and explicitly concerned with placing it in "its proper historical and philosophical context," Whicher defines Yoga as "South Asian Indian paths of spiritual emancipation, or self-transcendence, that bring about a transmutation of consciousness culminating in liberation from the confines of egoic identity or worldly existence" (1998: 6). Quite apart from its inherent metaphysical complexity—discussed and analyzed by Dasgupta (1924) and more recently by Whicher (1998)—Yoga has come to be regarded by many as so mystically profound as to defy comprehension. Comprehension, by virtue of being rooted in the senses and located in the intellect, is precisely that which Yoga seeks to transcend. Many adepts have said that Yoga cannot be understood. It can only be experienced as such. What it is only becomes clear from a perspective wherein self and cosmic Self are one. Thus it cannot be understood until true understanding is achieved. This is a situation in which the tautology of gnosis confounds the logic of knowledge.

In fact Yoga is the full range of practices that lead to this paradoxical end, including intellectual training, meditation, strict standards of moral and ethical behavior, along with rigorous physical training. In any case, it is in the enormous gaps between experience, knowledge, and embodied practice, as well as in the multiplicity of forms that Yoga can take—as a profound aphorism on the one hand or a more grounded but somewhat less profound quest for weight loss or sexual potency on the other (Neelam 1993; Sharma and Sharma 1991)—that one must confront the meaning of Yoga as nontranscendental and both derived from and relevant to the world of grounded human experience.

In this comprehensive light, *Bhargava's Standard Illustrated Dictionary: Hindi-English* defines Yoga as follows.

> Yoga: *n. mas.* One of the six schools of Hindu philosophy, a union with the Universal Soul by means of contemplation, means of salvation, the 27th part of a circle, a sum *(arith)*, total, profound meditation to earn and enhance wealth, unity, conjunction, union, combination, mixture, contact, fitness, property, an auspicious moment, plan, device, opportunity, recipe, connection, love, trick, deception, as a suffix used in the sense of "capable, fit for."

Idiosyncrasies in punctuation notwithstanding, it is important to keep the full—polysemic, ambiguous, and ironic—spectrum of meanings in mind: Yoga as a world-class philosophical system, no question; Yoga as profound meditation, to be sure. But how is this reconciled with the connotations of "trick" and "deception"? And "Yoga as profound meditation to earn and enhance wealth?" What? Impossible! Is *this* a trick? A deception? Wealth and the accumulation of wealth are the antithesis of Yoga, are they not? How are these levels of meaning—if that is what they are—to be explained? Is there one Truth or many truths? Dictionaries are designed to reflect the objective truth, but they do this inclusively, not exclusively. They are not prescriptive. They are not analytic. They are not speculative. They are concerned with the direct connection between words and the objects those words signify. In this regard they can be, as Samuel Johnson knew before Bhargava, blithely cynical and critically tuned to the vagaries of cultural pretense and a whole range of attempts to control and regulate meaning.

What I take to be Bhargava's blithe cynicism and skeptical sarcasm directed against the modern industry of Yoga—by giving a much too literal and late-capitalist interpretation to the magical reference in *Yoga Sūtra* II, 37, where "all jewels come to him" who masters the discipline of *asteya* (not-stealing)—reflects an important analytical perspective taken in this book. As an anthropologist trained to understand difference, and to apply the rigorous principles of cultural relativism in order to understand difference on its own terms, I would be expected to employ sympathetic appreciation and empathy rather than "wield the sword" of sarcasm. After all, is it not the golden rule of anthropology to gain an insider's perspective and to analytically represent culture, no matter how fluid and multivocal, as a system of meaning that justifies people's belief, even their belief in the fact that they are so categorically right and others so categorically wrong as to "justify" violence against them? To a degree, yes. But Yoga, like other cultural categories of human experience—religion, "free trade," nationalism, democracy, the state—has become so reified as a thing unto itself as to mask, distort, and ultimately undervalue the human creativity that went into its production. Beyond this there is also the more serious problem of conscious human creativity being reified in the ideathing of culture. On these terms culture has increasingly come to stand in as a proxy category for social facts, even though social facts are epiphenominal to meaning as such.

Anthropology is not alone in confusing things made—including, most certainly, cognitive things—with the makers of things. But the tendency in anthropology to suspend belief and take an insider's view of the world plays directly into the hand of human self-deception—the idea, to employ a cliché, that God created Man rather than the other way around. By dealing with texts and representations, rather than with people, philosophers, historians, literary critics, and religious studies scholars are able to maintain, if they wish, a degree of distance from the moral, ethical, and methodological problems this creates. By virtue of the first-person pronominal methodology that defines the discipline of anthropology, as well as a tendency to identify research expertise with "a people"—however loose, open, and global that identification has become—ethnography must confront the intractability with which real people, in making sense of themselves, forget their complicity in the production and reproduction of culture, and then vehemently defend their absolute cultural right to do so. On some level, as anthropology, this study must be a study of those people who practice Yoga, and it is precisely the ambiguous relationship among Yoga as a thing, the cultural construction of Yoga, and the claims made about Yoga as a thing by practitioners that create a profound analytical problem.

In part the problem emerges from the very concept of culture. No matter how "constructed" it is imagined to be, the act of constructing culture constantly displaces agency. Cultural production is thought to be meaningful, thereby enabling people to produce quintessentially meaningful things—which then take on a life of their own. Recall Taimni's comment about Yoga quoted above: "There is no subject which is so much wrapped up in mystery and on which one can write whatever one likes without any risk of being proved wrong" (1961: v). This neatly captures the reification of *both* culture *and* cultural construction in relation to Yoga as an essentialized category of experience. One can say anything about Yoga, and yet, somehow, it does not matter what one says because Yoga will never change. This logical slippage from the agency of practice to the displaced attribution of agency to things—which is not restricted to the domain of Yoga—has directed anthropological attention to culture and cultural construction and, ironically, away from the condition of being human. We have made both Yoga as such and the possibility that it can be anything—and thereby that it is, as such, nothing—and it is this possibility that is obscured by the construction of culture and by the concept of culture as a term that denotes human experience within the limited context of meaning. A focus on the condition of being human beyond what is contextually meaningful certainly runs the risk of unconsciously universalizing particular experience and prioritizing specific values. But this risk is worth taking if it can unmask the pretense of magnanimous things, dislocate firmly located cultural beliefs, and do all of this while maintaining a sense of value in the infinitely multiplex sociality that constitutes being human through time, as against the divisiveness of difference and the study of difference as a time-bound thing unto itself. To think globally about difference in analytically useful terms is to act historically.

The invocation of religion to help define the problem of reification manifest in the concept of culture is not accidental. Yoga is a metaphysical philosophy of transcendence that is distinct from, but clearly linked to, a range of teachings which find expression in Sāṃkhya philosophy and in Vedic, post-Vedic, and preclassical religious texts, most notably the *Bhagavad Gītā*. Technically, however, Yoga is not a religious system. It does entail a kind of provisional, strategic faith in God, but God as "created," not as creator. Thus in a very important sense, Yoga is a step beyond religion in terms of soteriological conceptualization. Although the past century has witnessed the dramatic "secularization" of Yoga on the one hand and its articulation as a kind of universalist, nonsectarian "spirituality" on the other, in many ways Yoga has become the functional equivalent of a distinct religion. Practitioners of Yoga will, of course, argue this point. But in doing so they underscore the nature and complexity of the problem. Yoga has become something you believe in. But, unlike religion, the Truth of Yoga is thought to be transcendent and beyond belief. It entails rigorous practice and self-discipline, but does not require either faith or ritual. The scholarly and analytical problem, then, is that, unlike religion—of which there are many and apart from which there must be belief in atheism—a critique of the cultural form of Yoga cannot even begin from a clearly defined point of sacrilegious disbelief and iconoclastic faithlessness. Not only is there no ontological basis for knowing anything about Yoga apart from Yoga, there is no way to develop a critique of it in modern practice, since there is nothing external to it, such as God in religion and Natural Law in physics.

Added to this is the extent to which Yoga and the practice of transcendence is thought to be embodied. Transcendence of the self notwithstanding, embodiment makes the practice of Yoga a very personal and personally meaningful endeavor. To deconstruct Yoga is not simply to challenge the ontology of belief, but to deconstruct the body of those who practice it. The reaction to this can be a kind of visceral fundamentalism. If this fundamentalism is confronted and radically questioned—in the manner of an atheist questioning the logic of the Holy Trinity—what you are left with, in terms of culture, is not very much at all. At least an atheist does not have to question the ontology of culture upon which religious faith is based. But that is exactly what is involved in the critique of Yoga—it is all or nothing: either a transcendental critique of culture as such, or the recognition that our organic humanity is the beginning and end of what counts as real. As a consequence of this kind of "positive negativism" about the form, structure, and meaning of embodied culture, one is able to gain—in the spirit, if not in the mode, of both Durkheim and Weber—a much clearer perspective on the sociological basis of being human than is afforded by a demystification of religion as social fact and of religious beliefs as such. To hold this view one must, of course, believe not so much in humanism as in both the limits and possibilities of life itself: that everything in human experience is a human construction and that there is no experience—nothing real—beyond the limits of sensory experience. I take this to be the basis of both knowledge and experience. Since the concept of culture and cultural construction intrude into consciousness as what might be called proxy bases for knowledge and experience, and bring with them figments and fragments of reality that are not really real, they get in the way of understanding. In any event, this book is bound to alienate both those who embody Yoga and those who embody a faith in culture, as the two are intimately intertwined.

Themes

There is probably no tradition that has been construed as more timeless, more intrinsically authentic, more inherently Indian than Yoga. It has become a kind of pristine cultural icon linking together, in a seemingly unbroken line, the past glory of the Indus civilization with the present and future possibility of modern, postcolonial India. My purpose in this book is to question some of the most fundamental assumptions about Yoga and, by extension, to question assumptions about civilization, modernity, and nationalism. I start with the simple assumption that Yoga, in all its profound complexity, is fundamentally an ingenious human construct. Like everything else it is incidentally social and cultural, not transcendental. But, precisely because it is constructed as both meaningful and transcendental, a critique of Yoga also provides a way of thinking about the limits of culture as an analytic framework. This perspective is taken not in order to challenge Yoga's legitimacy, but to unravel its mystique, and, by extension, to unravel the mystique of culture that has played a strong hand in the construction of Yoga. My purpose is not to uncover the truth behind Yoga—much less experience Truth. Nor is it my purpose to delineate what is good Yoga from what is bad, what is authentic and what is not. My purpose is to illustrate the genius of transnational imaginations, grounded in India, making and remaking the body, society, and the world. But my purpose is also to define the limits of genius, as those limits are defined not by human potential—collective or individual—but by the historical configuration of social relations that are not configured logically or bounded by time and space. Hence this book is not so much about the cultural heritage of India as it is about the convergence of human ideas and practices in colonial and postcolonial India. The perspective taken may seem, at times, overly skeptical and sarcastic—in the non-Barthian sense—with regard to the practice and beliefs of specific groups and individuals. However, it is a perspective that must take this risk in order to relocate the foundational sociality of human nature in a body of practice, a body of practice that, by conflating person, self, and cosmic soul, seems to have extended itself beyond the limits of a Nietzschean critique of God and humanism, a Durkheimian critique of religion, and a Marxist critique of ideology. To critique Yoga along these lines and in these terms—though not simply in the same way—is, in some sense, to do what is fundamental in all social analyses: to gain an understanding of human experience without letting any particular human experience define what counts as understanding.

An example. In the late 1990s the organization built around the cult of Maharishi Mahesh Yogi had an all-day broadcast on Indian television called Veda Vision, designed to disseminate the teachings of the master. In 1999 I was in Lucknow trying to make contact with various Yoga hospitals and was flipping through the channels on the hotel television when I suddenly stopped, mesmerized. On the screen was a group of about fifteen men and women, all dressed in white, sitting in *padmāsana,* one of the most common *āsana*s for yogic meditation. But they were not just sitting; they were doing something called "yogic flying," derived, I think, from the long-held belief that adept practitioners of Yoga can levitate and fly through the air.[8] The group was in a smallish room, on the floor of which was a soft, rubberized gymnastic-type mat. In unison they were "flying" from one end to the other, taking short hops of about two feet at a time.[9] I was fascinated because this intensely physical, dramatically modern kind of Yoga, sandwiched in between World Cup Cricket on ESPN and Ricky Martin belting out "Living a Vida Loca" on MTV, was precisely what I had been studying for the previous five years.

In and of itself this vision of "yogic flying"was phenomenal, but the voice-over, with occasional shots of the suited Dutch commentator surrounded by charts and graphs, was truly amazing in light of the fact that I had also been studying the way in which Yoga and science—social, political, biological, and medical science—had converged over the course of the past century and a half. For almost half an hour the commentator described, graphically illustrated, and "statistically proved" how the "Maharishi Effect," produced directly through "yogic flying," could, essentially and without equivocation, save the world. This was not a religious appeal per se. Nor was it ideological, in the sense that the commentator was not trying to convince viewers that they should change their beliefs. The appeal was, simply, a mechanical instruction: get down into a *padmāsana* and "fly" to resolve all social, moral, physical, and political problems in the world. For example, the commentator said—and here I am quoting from field notes I had never expected to be writing, since I had been in search of some light entertainment—that if 1 percent or even "the square root of 1 percent" of the population practiced yogic flying, it would reduce crime, reduce "national strife," and resolve international and global conflict. And there it was, charted out on a bar graph: crime decreasing steadily as the percentage of "flyers" increased. He also said that if enough people in India practiced "yogic flying" the Maharishi Effect would produce a "Rashtriya Kavac," a National Shield, that would protect the country from aggression. To this end he advocated the establishment of a "preventative wing of yogic flyers" to stop international warfare before it started.[10]

Soon after the events of September 11, 2001, when two planes were crashed into the World Trade Towers and a third into the Pentagon, there was a full-page advertisement published in the *New York Times* calling for the establishment of immediate and comprehensive world peace through the practice of yogic flying. I can think of nothing that so clearly reflects the absolute absurdity of cultural belief. But also nothing that provides such a visionary glimpse of being human, wherein "being" subjunctively extends beyond the limits of located, meaningful, cultural experience. In point of fact yogic flying could bring about world peace. Not by means of the embodiment of magical power and transcendental consciousness, but as a somewhat inadvertent consequence of the profound sociality of collective human action. The square root of 1 percent of the population notwithstanding, if everyone in the world collectively sat in *padmāsana* and bounced through time and space, it would produce a global culture that could inhibit many things, including, perhaps, violence.

It would be easy to say, from the vantage point of a "true adept," or from the perspective of one seeking the Truth, that yogic flying is either the answer to everything or the most ridiculous thing ever imagined. In other words, those who do not believe what the Maharishi teaches can say that yogic flying is an absurd perversion of true Yoga. But the question then is what is "true Yoga" and where do you draw the line. Do you draw it above or below the Yoga of B.K.S. Iyengar, probably the world's most famous teacher, who learned from Krishnamacharya, a turn-of-the-century Yoga teacher who invented a new kind of Yoga based on a synthesis of *āsana*s with Western gymnastics (Sjoman 1996)? Do you draw it above or below Ramananda Maharishi, locked up in an air-tight box, being studied by scientists (Anand, Chhina, and Singh 1961)? Do you draw it above or below the practice of members of the Bharatiya Yoga Sansthan, assembled at their annual convention, collectively performing *śavāsana*, the corpse pose, to relieve their own and the country's "nervous tension" (Alter 1997)? Do you draw it above or below the Yoga of Swami Sivananda, a medical doctor turned spiritual *guru* who founded the Divine Life Society?[11] Above or below the Yoga of Swami Kuvalayananda, a research scientist, who, in 1924, measured the "Madhavdas Vacuum" by inserting a pressure gauge into the rectum of an adept performing *nauli* (abdominal rotation)? Do you draw it above or below the performance of "Bharatiyam," mass-drill Yoga *āsana*s performed by schoolchildren on Republic Day and at international events such as the Asian Games? And does Dr. K. N. Udupa's research on the neurological effect of Yoga on rats count, since the rats were forced into test tubes and inverted into the Yoga posture *śirṣāsana*? Or, as probably most people would want to have it, is the only real Yoga performed and taught by some unknown sage lost to the world in the high Himalayas? That, everyone would probably agree, is where the truth about Truth ultimately lies, at least in the confined, contained, and contingent realm of sensory, worldly consciousness.

The sage lost to the world in the Himalayas is an extremely powerful reference point in the search for authentic Yoga, and it is a reference point that has played an important role in the development of modern Yoga (see Brunton 1939; Carpenter 1911; Haanel 1937).[12] This is not because the sage-lost-to-the-world has been found, but because men like Swami Rama (1978), Shri Yogendra (Rodrigues 1982), Swami Sivananda, Swami Yogeshwaranand, and Theos Bernard (1939, 1944), among countless others, have all gone in search of the sage.[13] Most significantly, they have returned, and through religious reform movements, research centers, clinics, and retreats such as the Divine Life Society, the Himalayan Institute, Yoga Niketan Trust, and the Yoga Institute, they have defined modern Yoga. Along similar but scaled down lines, whenever I spoke with a modern practitioner of Yoga—such as the research officer at the Central Institute for Yoga Research in New Delhi, the Yoga research officer at the Yoga Center at Banaras Hindu University, and a middle-aged woman who teaches Yoga classes in her living room in Pune—I was told that he or she had a "real *guru*" who was a "true adept" and that if I wanted to know anything about Yoga I should talk to a person of that caliber and stature.

The perspective taken in this study is that there are no real *gurus* and no true adepts. You can find a sage in the Himalayas, but what he is doing is no different from what anyone else is doing—seeking knowledge, searching for a master, and looking for something to call Truth. In this sense Yoga is, as many people claim, a science. It is based on direct experience rather than on revelation or the interpretation of inspired teaching. It is also primarily epistemological rather than ontological, in the sense that Yoga is defined by procedural methods for realizing Truth that can otherwise only be inferred. In the case of Yoga, however, there is an even greater problem than in science concerning the way in which its philosophical assumptions, theoretical principles, and methodology define Truth and Reality in terms that are exclusive. No matter how spiritualized or scientized, Yoga is fundamentally more Sāṃkhyan than Cartesian. In any case, all forms of Yoga must be considered alike—at least as a point of analytical departure—insofar as they are linked together by a common history of development and practice. In terms of culture, and the culture of practice, Dr. Udupa's headstanding rats, Swami Rama's "New Age" psychology, and Swami Sivananda's Divine Life Society may seem to belong to different worlds altogether, but they are simply variations on a common theme. What all practitioners of Yoga are trying to do is move beyond the world of direct, particulated experience and thereby improve themselves and others in various ways—through the stimulation of the autonomic nervous system, through the Maharishi Effect, through "toning up" the liver and spleen, through simple relaxation, or through its profound corollary, the realization of the *ātman* (individual, self, or soul) in the *paramātman* (universal, transcendent self, or soul) and the attainment of *jīvanmukti* (embodied transcendence, the living sage lost-to-the-world) or *mokṣa* (final liberation).

One might well ask, however, whether or not the classical texts dealing with Yoga provide a "gold standard" that can be used to measure the relative authenticity of various kinds of practice. As pointed out above with reference to the *Yoga Sūtra*, this is certainly the assumption in all Orientalist scholarship, and is the logical rationale for a great deal of ongoing research. Looking beyond the *Yoga Sūtra*, however, the question is this:

What else counts as an authoritative text, and on what basis are different texts ranked in terms of relative importance? How are they to be compared one with another if your point of reference is not the corpus itself but modern practice? The most obvious answer to these questions is to be somewhat restrictive and judiciously limit the scope to what are regarded as the primary texts—the *Yoga Sūtra,* the *Yoga Upaniṣad*s (see Ayyangar 1952), the *Bhagavad Gītā* (see van Buitenen 1981), and the three main Haṭha Yoga texts of more recent, medieval antiquity, the *Haṭhayogapradīpikā* (see Sinh 1997), the *Śivasaṃhitā* (see Vasu 1996a), and the *Gheraṇḍasaṃhitā* (see Vasu 1996b). But this presents problems, since in these texts Yoga blurs into Sāṃkhya, Tantra, and the "cult of Kṛṣṇa" among other forms of practice, systems of religious thought, and philosophical reasoning. Quite apart from the problematic convergence of ignorance and faith in God that occurs when reading the *Gītā* in light of the *Yoga Sūtra* there is, throughout the canon, the whole question of the body and its subtle physiology in relation to knowledge, consciousness, and many other conceptual and relatively—but by no means ontologically—immaterial things.

As Paul Deussen noted as early as 1906, it is possible to trace references to *āsana, prāṇāyāma, pratyāhāra,* and *dhyāna* through the middle-period *Upaniṣad*s (1906: 387–95). Sāṃkhya philosophy—the oldest of the orthodox schools of thought—provides a theory of perpetual elemental "creation" for Yoga's systematically experimental and step-by-step "regressive" concern with single-pointed concentration and liberation.[14] This is based on the relationship between knowledge, ignorance, and suffering common to both Sāṃkhya and Yoga. As Eliade points out, however, although the same in most other ways, Sāṃkhya and Yoga differ significantly in terms of methodology and, therefore, in terms of how the body is involved in practice:

> Sāṃkhya seeks to obtain liberation solely by *gnosis,* whereas for Yoga an *ascesis* and a *technique of meditation* are indispensable. In both *darśana*s human suffering is rooted in illusion, for man believes that his psychomental life—activity of the senses, feelings, thoughts and volitions—is identical with Spirit, with the Self. He thus confuses two wholly autonomous and opposed realities, between which there is no real connection but only an illusory relation, for psychomental experience does not belong to Spirit, it belongs to nature (*prakṛti*); states of consciousness are the refined products of the same substance that is at the base of the physical world and the world of life. (1990: 14–15)

Samādhi, the ultimate experience that is beyond experience in Yoga, is, in some respects, the embodiment of pure, pre-elemental, timeless consciousness reflected in the principle of *puruṣa* that is expounded in Sāṃkhya.

In many respects tantric literature, which chronologically follows closely on the "classical" literature and predates almost all of the commentaries on the *Yoga Sūtra*, provides a theory of *nāḍī* physiology upon which yogic *prāṇāyāma* is based. As Eliade points out,

> the human body acquires an importance it had never before attained in the spiritual history of India. To be sure, health and strength, interest in physiology homologizable with the cosmos and implicitly sanctified, are Vedic, if not pre-Vedic, values. But tantrism carries to its furthest consequences the conception that sanctity can be realized in a "divine body." . . . And since liberation can be gained even in this life, the body must be preserved as long as possible, and in perfect condition, precisely as an aid to meditation. (1990: 227)

Both the primary and the secondary literatures on Sāṃkhya and Tantra are vast in scale and scope. When trying to discern the relevance of texts to contemporary practice—if not also unto themselves—it is necessary to make a somewhat arbitrary distinction about what can be counted as a textual commentary on themes of yogic significance from within this corpus. Since many aspects of Tantra and Sāṃkhya are relevant to Yoga practice, any analysis of modern Yoga that also seeks to be historically contextual can easily spiral outward in any number of different directions until it is no longer an analysis of Yoga as such.

But the problem of the body is magnified even in the context of the Yoga literature strictly defined. What appears to be most cerebral—*citta*, consciousness or mind—in the *Yoga Sūtra* is, by virtue of being sensory, a quasi-material embodied thing, making control of the mind a physiological problem in much the same way as is control of breathing and control of the autonomic nervous system. In yogic terms knowledge and cognition—and by extension the whole world of ideas—fall into the inclusive domain of transmutable materialism. This is a critical point to keep in mind, since it signals a key question about the relationship between philosophy and physiology that will be taken up in the chapters that follow.

While this perspective on reality as a kind of materialist illusion, or sensory misidentification, links the most philosophical with the most physiological yogic texts—and the most mystical with the most magical ones—on the level of practice there is a significant degree of disarticulation between mind and body. On the one hand, the *Yoga Sūtra* has very little to say about *āsana*s and, on the other, the *Haṭhayogapradīpikā* is about *āsana*s and *prāṇāyāma* and very little else. The late medieval period, between the thirteenth and fifteenth centuries, is very important to understanding modern Yoga in general and the ambiguous disarticulation of mind and body in particular. It is at this time that one can begin to link up the development of Yoga with various concrete aspects of political, economic, and social history, albeit tenuously (Briggs 1938; M. Singh 1937; D. White 1996). Any meaningful commentary on this period is well beyond the scope of this book, but it is important to note that the Nātha Yogis who refined, expanded, and perfected Haṭha Yoga also engaged directly with the intellectual problem of representing the truth of embodied practice. In many respects a further analysis of fourteenth- and fifteenth-century documents could provide the earliest example of embodied Yoga's struggle with textual reification on the one hand and the mystification of both text and body on the other.[15]

At the other end of the historical spectrum, the late nineteenth and early twentieth centuries are interesting in that one is able to find texts that emerge directly out of documented practice. This is precisely the period to which Sjoman (1996) directs his critical attention.[16] Almost all turn-of-the-century texts claim to be authentic and authoritative. In and of themselves of course they are. But all of the ones I have collected claim to be based on the teaching of "true adepts" or derived from the "classical literature." And yet each of these texts explicitly or implicitly combines, in various ways and to various degrees, gymnastics, physical training, and hygiene with *āsana, kriyā,* and *prāṇāyāma*. In point of fact this is not altogether different from what the Nātha Yogis were doing in the ninth century by combining aspects of Tantra, Siddha alchemy, and yogic purification in their quest for immortality and embodied perfection as a "total experience of life." Granted the "global influences" at this earlier time may have been from what is now China, but the Nātha Yogis strategically "confused" materialism and magic in a way that anticipates the New Age. In any case, when studying the numerous examples of conscious and unconscious modern mimesis, it is necessary to read Eliade's famous dictum about bodily perfection across the plane of its singular Orientalist meaning: "Perfection is always the goal [of Yoga], and, as we shall soon see, it is neither athletic nor hygienic perfection. Haṭha Yoga cannot and must not be confused with gymnastics" (1990: 228).[17] Prescriptive injunctions aside, it is precisely this "confusion"—extending from the ninth through the twentieth centuries—that has made Yoga what it is.

In many respects the literature on Haṭha Yoga—the *Haṭhayogapradīpikā* (1350 C.E.) and two significantly later but very similar texts, the *Gheraṇḍasaṃhitā* (1650 C.E.) and the *Śivasaṃhitā* (1750 C.E.)—can be regarded as most directly relevant for this study. Each of these texts describes *āsana* procedures, *prāṇāyāma,* and techniques of purification, though cryptically and without much commentary. Beyond this, however, the Haṭha Yoga literature emerges out of a context of practice where the central problem was not physical fitness, at least in any simple, physiological sense. Rather, what concerned the Nātha Yogis was the embodiment of immortality and the materialization of magic. As Eliade points out:

> One of the essential points of this new "revelation" [the integration and synthesis of Sahajīyā tantrism, Nāgārjuna and Carpaṭi's alchemy and Gorkhnāth's Haṭha Yoga, among others] was that it finally completed the synthesis among the elements of Vajrayāna and Śivaist tantrism, magic and alchemy and Haṭha Yoga. In a way, it was a continuation of the tantric synthesis. But a number of the Nāthas and Siddhas put more emphasis than their predecessors had done upon the value of magic and Yoga as inestimable means for a conquest of freedom and immortality. (1990: 304–5)

It is both the emphasis on embodied, materialized magic and what appears to be the "populist appeal" of Haṭha Yoga in the medieval period—Eliade situates his discussion within the context of "aboriginal" India and folklore—that seem to anticipate many aspects of modern practice. Significantly, however, it is important to note that modern Yoga in practice does not, in any sense, emerge directly from these texts, but rather from an elaborate oral tradition. Apart from this, even though the three texts are intensely physical, in their focus on magical power and conquering death they are, in many ways, more abstract, mystical, and explicitly oriented toward the occult than the *Yoga Sūtra*. This is not surprising. But from the perspective of modern Yoga—which is radically antimystical and self-consciously rational and pragmatic—it is difficult to know how to make sense of the relationship articulated in these texts between magic and the physical body. What does it mean—in terms of embodied experience based on precisely defined procedures—to be able to fly, to be clairvoyant and invisible, and to conquer death and destroy sickness? And how—beyond simple analogy—does this meaning relate to more modest claims, such as being healthy and physically fit?

Beyond this, the description of *āsana*s given in the *Haṭhayogapradīpikā* and the other texts is very imprecise and incomplete, perhaps because the foundational basis of practice in Yoga was not the textual relationship between word and object but the far more primary relationship between *guru* and *celā,* or disciple.[18] In all probability the descriptions are designed as mnemonic aids, although they do not take the highly condensed aphoristic form of *sūtra*s. In any case it is clear that these descriptions are not the basis for a tradition in practice, and the texts are not anything like self-help manuals. It is best to conceptualize the texts in a dialectical relationship to practice, since they constantly reiterate the importance of practice. Certainly most of the initial modern publications and translations with commentary (Ayyangar 1893; Brahmananda 1889; Sinh 1997; Vasaka 1877; Vasu 1895) appear to predate the earliest developments of practice-based modern Yoga—at least as documented in modern texts—by about fifteen years. But then, by the late 1920s and early 1930s, various people who were engaged in practice—and the modern textual representation of practice—used the *Haṭhayogapradīpikā,* the *Śivasaṁhitā,* and the *Gheraṇḍasaṁhitā* to authenticate a broad spectrum of modern techniques and styles. Thus the texts tend to be used to authenticate the tradition as a whole by virtue of being "ancient" and authored by semi-divine sages—and to connect modern, medieval, and ancient practice into homogenized historical continuity—but their currency as practical reference books is not very great.

Another problem with using the Haṭha Yoga literature as a gold standard is that one would have to discount a significant percentage of what counts for Yoga today, including a common procedure known as *sūrya namaskār* (salutation to the sun), which is not mentioned as a physical exercise in any of the standard texts published or printed earlier than the nineteenth century. What appears to be a headstand is mentioned in the *Yogatattva Upaniṣad* (see Ayyangar 1952) as well as later Haṭha Yoga texts, but it is also mentioned in the *Mallapurāṇa,* a sixteenth-century text, as one of the exercises in the regimen of medieval wrestlers. This presents a further problem as to what counts as Yoga, and whether or not all headstands can or should be counted as the same thing in fact. In other words, the well-recognized problem that Yoga has multiple meanings is magnified considerably when dealing with different elements of practice—where do you draw the line between deep breathing, *prāṇāyāma,* and certain kinds of rhythmic prayer?[19] Here as well there is the problem of what counts as "classical" texts delineating a timeless, coherent tradition, and other texts that bring that tradition into a more delineated but multivectoral historical framework. Does the *Mallapurāṇa* count, for example? As N. E. Sjoman notes, it is possible to trace the history of ideas about Yoga philosophy through time, and possible to follow the development of *prāṇāyāma* from puranic times up to the present, but there is virtually nothing that allows for the construction of a history of *āsana* practice. Clearly this signals the need for ongoing research. Sjoman's analysis (1996) of the *Śrītattvanidhi* and *Mallapurāṇa* texts in relation to some of the earliest efforts at Yoga revival manifest in the *Vyāyāmdīpikā* (Bhardwaj 1896) and the *Yogamakaranda* (Krishnamachariya 1935) is directly relevant. But the paucity of any clear history of practice in the eighteenth and nineteenth centuries should raise a red flag of sorts concerning the putative antiquity of everything that is now counted as Haṭha Yoga.

It is also important to keep in mind that—apart from practice—the Haṭha Yoga literature can be, and perhaps should be, read in conjunction with the *Yoga Sūtra* and other classical texts. Certainly there is a strong tendency among some who engage in "physical" Yoga to link it directly and unambiguously to the metaphysics of liberation. In part this is done to counteract the modern tendency to categorically distinguish between mind and body, and to see the body as relatively unimportant as concerns higher consciousness. In other words, the relative antiquity of Haṭha Yoga—and all that is associated with ancient esoteric wisdom—makes it possible to "read" metaphysics into modern practice, and read Yoga *darśana* into the nitty-gritty of medieval *sādhana,* regardless of the extent to which practitioners of that vintage were concerned with the relationship of their practice to Patañjali's text, or to the texts that were being produced on so-called Rāja Yoga in the fourteenth, seventeenth, and eighteenth centuries. In any case, given the fact that texts and textual knowledge crosscut time and space, the emergence of Rāja Yoga as such has meant that Haṭha Yoga can never suffer the fate of gymnastics, sports, and athleticism. These very physical activities were integral to classical philosophy in Greece, and thereby integral to the European Renaissance, but—barring the discovery of a late classical Greek text on wrestling that picks up where Plato left off—they have long since come to be regarded as profoundly anti-intellectual. Whereas it is virtually inconceivable that a modern Greco-Roman wrestler might embody platonic idealism, even the crudest form of modern Yoga can lay claim—and, in fact, lays claim despite itself—to the idea that time can be escaped and immortality embodied.

Beginning in the 1930s, and then with support and encouragement from Yehudi Menuin in the late 1950s, B.K.S. Iyengar transformed *āsana* and *prāṇāyāma* into what has come to be known, around the world, as a kind of full bodied, prop-assisted, performative Yoga gymnastics.[20] Although very much like other forms of practice dating to the 1920s, Iyengar's method involves a great deal of effort of the kind more often associated with aerobic physical fitness.[21] Given the etymology of *haṭha* as "violent effort," one might say that Iyengar put the "force" back into "forceful" Yoga, and even that he has reestablished the violence of control as central to practice; in yogic terms, the "violent" union of sun and moon is integral to a perfect mastery of the body (Eliade 1990: 228–29). In any event, Iyengar's style of Yoga has a fairly short history, and emerges out of a career devoted primarily to the physical dimension of practice rather than to metaphysics, meditation, and liberation (Sjoman 1996). But significantly, the short history of Iyengar's Yoga is linked not only to the power of physical transubstantiation found in the medieval texts, but also to the ancient history of ultimate liberation and freedom. Iyengar's translation of and commentary on the *Yoga Sūtra* (1993) is amazingly detailed and precise, and perfectly authentic in its own right. But it is a commentary that has grown out of a kind of yogic practice that is intensely physical and very unique. *Light on Yoga* (1976), probably the most important and widely read modern text on Yoga, is, in many ways, an elaboration and extended commentary on the Haṭha Yoga literature.

As they appear in *Light on Yoga,* the descriptions of how to perform *āsanas* are incredibly detailed and exact, whereas the descriptions in the *Haṭhayogapradīpikā* are rather vague and cryptic. With regard to *śavāsana* (corpse pose) Iyengar gives us almost two pages, with careful anatomical reference and measurements, phenomenal concern with the details of body-plane and ground-plane interface, and a complex calculus of geometric positioning that is virtually poetic. The *Haṭhayogapradīpikā* hardly says more than "lie flat on your back like a corpse," the homology with embodied death—and by extension enstasy—being rather obvious. In Iyengar's elaboration the homology is refined, and the corpse pose becomes both more physical and more metaphysical. His genius is in making the arcane nature of medieval practice explicit, clear, and unambiguous. In Iyengar Yoga, as in medieval Haṭha Yoga, the body becomes the materialization of magic. But whereas Haṭha Yoga of the fourteenth century was alchemical—and also purely allegorical and metaphoric since it, too, shifted out of situated practice and into texts—Iyengar Yoga is dependent on the magical transmutation of quantum physics: the real possibility of the impossible. To manipulate the body is not to reflect reality, but to transform it.

Thus in an important way, and with reference to contemporary practice, the classical literature is no more or less authentic and authoritative than the putative sage-lost-to-the-world in the Himalāyas. If we are to take Dr. Udupa, Swami Kuvalayananda, and "yogic flying" seriously—and I believe we must if we are to appreciate the genius of transcultural innovation rooted in modern India—then it cannot be otherwise. Unless Yoga itself is recognized as a historical construct that has no meaning as a thing apart from the contingency of human experience, and unless everyone who claims to practice it is taken seriously—including B.K.S. Iyengar and those who teach themselves by reading *Yoga for Dummies* (Feuerstein and Payne 1999)—everyone other than the sage himself ends up looking like a fool, and anything other than the "standard canon" has to be read as pulp fiction.

Scope and Focus

Although this book is fairly comprehensive, attempting to deal with as much of the Yoga literature as possible and focusing on a broad spectrum of practice, it is oriented to the subject in a particular way and carries with it, therefore, a certain obvious bias. Historically, the time frame is the modern era and the focus is on twentieth-century texts and late-twentieth-century practice. However, reference is made to the classical and medieval literature to the extent that this literature is strategically incorporated into modern discourse and practice. Topically, the focus here is on physiology and physical fitness rather than on metaphysics, meditation, and soteriology. There is a whole body of nineteenth-century literature that deals with what was referred to as Yoga's occult or mystical aspect. In this study I deal with that literature only to the extent that many of the first advocates for "Yoga physical education" were explicitly antimystical and critical of the occult tradition. Finally, this study is concerned mainly with the way in which Yoga is conceived of as a science, and the way in which discourses and practices of science have given shape to modern Yoga.

Although historically, topically, and theoretically thus circumscribed, this study seeks to show that Yoga is an example of the extreme degree to which the truth of historically situated social life is obscured by powerful cultural beliefs about the nature of human experience. These beliefs are on a par with but in some ways more powerful than religious beliefs by virtue of being embodied by the self of direct experience. Beyond this, a critical analysis of Yoga's history will show that it is a product of the colonial era, a product of a particular concern with health and morality, and a product of science and scientific practice. At the same time, however, Yoga will be shown to "chip away" at the edifice of the empire, redefine what is meant by health in modern India, and problematize and creatively expand the practice of science.

In delineating the parameters of this study it is necessary to define what follows with reference to the two chief architects of the Yoga renaissance, Swami Vivekananda and Sri Aurobindo.[22] At the end of the nineteenth century, Vivekananda, an upper-middle-class Bengali disciple of the mystic sage Ramakrishna, revolutionized Hinduism by advocating a kind of no-nonsense, self-confident, muscular—and, therefore, masculinized—spiritualism. As is well known, he did this, most dramatically, in 1893 on the stage of the World Parliament of Religions in Chicago, and thus almost single-handedly both popularized and globalized Hinduism. On the national stage Vivekananda's "clarion call" for the revival of a Hinduism-to-be-proud-of defined a new kind of patriotism at the turn of the century—a kind of patriotism that was religious, but extended easily into other areas of cultural life. Among other things, Vivekananda articulated a kind of spirituality based on Vedānta, but expressed in terms of what he called Rāja Yoga.[23] Most significantly he was critical of asceticism and world renunciation and advocated a kind of "Yoga theology" linked to the world of direct experience.

At about the same time, Aurobindo Ghose, another upper-middle-class Bengali, educated in London, was active in the Indian National Congress and directly involved in the Freedom Movement. Gradually, however, he withdrew from active participation and began to pursue spiritual goals and live the life of an ascetic. Although at first involved in direct teaching, he had his greatest influence through the publication of books on Yoga philosophy, cosmology, and metaphysics. As with Vivekananda, Aurobindo's interpretation of spiritualism was proactive, one of the key features being the idea that through a synthesis of Yoga humankind could evolve to a higher state of what he called supramental consciousness.

Although there are interesting, and very important, physiological features to both Aurobindo's and Vivekananda's teachings—the former has quite a bit to say about physical education and hygiene (Aurobindo n.d., 1949; Bhattacarya 1952, 1968; "The Mother" 1979; Purani 1950) and the latter about football and muscle building—the influence of both men has been almost exclusively on the plane of institutionalized religion, spiritualism, and philosophy. They created a new climate for the critical study of Hinduism and Indian philosophy as well as for a less critical adherence to tradition. Certainly the influence of both men is profound in the intellectual history of modern India.

It is somewhat surprising, therefore, that there is little, if any, mention made of either Vivekananda or Aurobindo by those men who were responsible for the revival-cum-reinvention of yogic *āsana*s, *kriyā*s, and *prāṇāyāma* in the early part of this century. Perhaps this is because their influence was so great as to not require comment. However, the two main characters in the history of modern Yoga as it is linked to health and fitness—Sri Yogendra (1930, 1936, 1991) and Swami Kuvalayananda (1924a)—claim to have been taught and inspired by a relatively unknown, Bengali, ex-civil servant known as Madhavdas, who renounced the world and practiced Yoga in the latter part of the nineteenth century while wandering in the Himalayas. Although Swami Kuvalayananda was also influenced by Aurobindo, who taught for some time in Gujarat, he was much more heavily influenced by Rajratan Manikrao's advocacy for physical fitness, indigenous exercise, and mass-drill physical training. For his part, Sri Yogendra was a wrestler and exercise buff before becoming a practitioner of Yoga.[24]

There can be no doubt that Vivekananda and Aurobindo—and to a lesser degree, and in a much more oblique sense, Mahatma Gandhi[25]—defined the broader intellectual context within which there was a renaissance in the practice of Yoga *āsana*s, *kriyā*s, and *prāṇāyāma*. But the history of this renaissance seems to "slip past" these men, since there is a much more direct link between innovative Indian experimentation in the

1920s and transnational ideas about health, strength, and physical fitness all over the world in the mid- to late nineteenth century and early in the twentieth. At the risk of sounding heretical, I think Eugene Sandow, the father of modern body building, has had a greater influence on the form and practice of modern Yoga—and most certainly modern Haṭha Yoga—than either Aurobindo or Vivekananda. In fact, given this history it would be possible to undertake a revisionist study of Vivekanand's "muscular Hinduism." Perhaps even Aurobindo's seemingly abstract philosophy of evolved consciousness needs to be rethought on the basis of what he and "The Mother" had to say about the importance of physical fitness and physical education: "Physical culture is the best way of developing the consciousness of the body, and the more the body is conscious, the more it is capable of receiving the divine forces that are at work to transform it and give birth to the new race" (1979: 205). In other words, with regard to the present state of knowledge—which tends to be bound by the narrow framework of institutionalized religion and nationalistic philosophy—Vivekananda and Aurobindo could be considered marginal to the historical development of modern Yoga in India. However iconoclastic it may seem, the history of Yoga slips past spirituality and intellectual philosophy. It is unambiguously linked to rules that apply to nature and the body.

Science and Yoga: The Merging of Myths

If there is a single word associated with the development of Yoga in the twentieth century it is the English word "science," as well as that word's numerous, and exceedingly ambiguous, sanskritic synonyms. Indeed, the English word science is just as ambiguous, and has been used to mean so many different things by different people that, when dealing with translations, and translations of translations, it is almost impossible to know what, exactly, is signified by this slippery, polysemic field of signifiers. With respect to the English word, however—and much of the early-twentieth-century Indian literature on Yoga is in English—it is clear that one of the connotations of science is authority, legitimacy, and power. Moreover, the concept of science seems to have defined a particular perspective on gaining knowledge, a perspective that is meticulous and comprehensive rather than speculative. To an extent, science opens up the body—as well as many other things such as the environment, geography, and population—for both examination and, significantly, translation.

One of the problems in a study like this one is to avoid the reflex tendency—at least it is a reflex tendency of someone born in the Himalayas who went in search of sages in the United States—to regard science as a transcultural, atemporal, purely objective system of knowledge. The term as such tends to conjure up images of white-coated teams of lab technicians under the supervision of senior scientists working with precise theories to test and retest hypotheses in order to discover some unknown fact, prove something as true, or invent something new. And the tendency is to regard this image of science as more or less the same regardless of where in the world it is transplanted. In other words, science as a mode of knowledge and a means of producing knowledge is probably one of the most powerful hegemonic forces of this and the previous two centuries, intimately linked to politics and political power, academia and intellectual authority, as well as to economies and the political economies of socialism, communism, and capitalism. In a sociological sense, science is the religion of modernity.

Over the course of the past twenty years, the work of Bruno Latour and Steve Woolgar (1979) among many others—including, of course, Thomas Kuhn's earlier revolutionary study (1970)—has both demystified and complicated the meaning and significance of the conceptual basis, practical application, and philosophy of science. Over the years feminism has provided a particularly effective critique of science, and this critique has become increasingly focused on the various ways in which power/knowledge is configured in scientific discourse. All of this has led to increasingly well stated and firmly grounded questions about the legitimacy and limits of science as a distinct way of knowing and way of controlling knowledge.

Although it is not really possible to speak of a crisis in science comparable to the crisis in social science brought on by the so-called interpretive turn, work in quantum physics has clearly blurred the lines between philosophy and science. Most significantly, this "blurring" is not just on the level of theory; it is part of laboratory research. In an important way ontological questions about the nature of time, space, and matter posed in terms of theoretical physics can be seen as posing challenges to the structural basis of science. Obviously science as such cannot be said to have "responded" to sociological and philosophical critiques—the power and beauty of science is in its structural conformity to so-called Natural Laws—but it is interesting to note that changes in the seemingly unchangeable laws of nature have made it possible to extend the sociological critique beyond practice as such to the very theoretical basis of science.

Added to this is the way in which history provides an important perspective on the changing nature of science and, therefore, on the contingency of its claim to represent reality. As research in the history of science continues to show—but also as common sense would suggest—one cannot assume that what is meant by science in the year 2000 is what was meant by science in 1900 or even 1950. In other words, taking into account all of these critiques, it has become increasingly possible to "chip away" at the hegemonic structure of science by using the tools of deconstruction—critical, "ethnographic" phenomenology on the one hand, and, on the other, critical history. The end result is a scaled-down, fragmented image of science that is much more realistic and true to the world of human experience.

A problem in this, however, is that Swami Kuvalayananda, for all his nominal world renunciation, did not limit himself and his search for Truth to the simple technology described in the *Haṭhayogapradīpikā* or to what was taught to him by his *guru* Madhavdas. He did not practice Yoga as a yogi. As we shall see, he wore a white lab coat, built a laboratory and clinic, imported X-ray machines and electrocardiographs. To a significant extent he modeled himself and his study of Yoga on the hegemonic image of science, as that hegemonic image—which is just as nominal as world renunciation—was emerging in the early part of the twentieth century. But Kuvalayananda, among many others, did not just co-opt the trappings of science, the *materia scientica* that is, in many ways, the materialization of technocentric modernity. He engaged with science as a way of knowing, as a philosophy of knowledge. In this regard he set about testing specific aspects of Yoga practice. But in this project, Yoga as a theory of psychic function came to hold a status very similar to that of evolutionary theory in biology. Although regarded as a theory, and therefore in principle still subject to questions of proof, for all practical purposes a yogic theory of psychic function functioned more ontologically than epistemologically in the structure and logic of experimental reasoning.

Laboratory experimentation and "field research" on Yoga were meant to provide an increasingly refined, empirical understanding of the material manifestation of a cosmic principle, as this cosmic principle was understood as a "theory" of absolute freedom. In this regard one might say that whereas religion holds science at arm's length—since faith and reason are fundamentally incompatible—the underlying materialism of Yoga, its *prakṛtic* structure, seductively draws science in. In its own way Yoga is based on a Cosmic Principle that is comparable to the Natural Law of physics. But whereas this makes Yoga and science analogous—and is the basis for a whole history of interaction—Yoga takes control of science, as science is understood as knowledge that must be transcended. It is comparable—but only that—to a physicist whose research on the relationship between time, energy, and matter changes the nature of reality as we know it—but not, of course, reality as such—including the reality of the idea of "proof" as a time-dependent entity.

What is being dealt with in this study is, therefore, the complex intersection of at least two powerful myths—the metaphysics of Yoga, and yogic physiology in particular, and the methods of science and scientific knowledge. The purpose of this book is not to untangle this intersection so much as to reflect on its implications. To do so will provide a better and more complex understanding of some aspects of Indian intellectual history and a better understanding of the place of the body in the history of India's present. Although this study is built around the work of Swami Kuvalayananda, whose direct and indirect influence on modern Yoga is profound, it is a study that spirals outward from Kuvalayananda's research in Lonavala and moves backward and forward through time and around and about through the space of colonial and postcolonial India. It is a meditation on the nature of social history and an argument for the primacy of the "social" in social science—provided social facts are regarded as thoroughly infused with magic, as the epigraph from Durkheim's classic work would suggest. In this sense this study is engaged with the unreality of culture. It is focused on the historicity of human experience, as this historicity undermines culture and the idea of meaningful continuity upon which the reality of social life is thought to be based. In this sense it is, in essence, yogic—but with an orientation to the present and the past, not the future and any sort of final liberation. As a published work of scholarship it does, however, have a certain immortality and freedom.

2

YOGA AND THE SUPRAMENTAL BEING: MATERIALISM, METAPHYSICS, AND SOCIAL REALITY

> A new world beckons to us unmistakably, a happy and harmonious world, a creative world inspired and illumined by a new light, a world where Science and Spirituality walk together, hand in hand, like a newly wed couple. And Ancient Yoga joins hands with Modern Science in helping mental man to grow further and transform gradually into a Supramental Being.
>
> T. R. Anantharaman, *Ancient Yoga and Modern Science* (1996: 92–93)

> Blasphemy has always seemed to require taking things very seriously. . . . Blasphemy protects one from the moral majority within, while still insisting on the need for community. . . . Irony is about contradictions that do not resolve into larger wholes, even dialectically, about the tension of holding incompatible things together because both or all are necessary and true. . . . At the center of my ironic faith, my blasphemy, is the image of the cyborg. . . . A cyborg is a cybernetic organism, a hybrid of machine and organism, a creature of social reality as well as a creature of science fiction.
>
> Donna Haraway, *Simians, Cyborgs, and Women: The Reinvention of Nature* (1991: 149)

The Science of Science

IN THE VOLUMINOUS literature on Yoga in India—technical, academic, and popular—Yoga is often referred to as a science. As a precise and special way of knowing, however, the ultimate goal of Yoga is to transcend knowledge and realize absolute truth through direct experience. In this sense the justification and rationale for calling Yoga a science is far from clear, since the definitive, but fundamentally limited, goal of science is to produce knowledge in order to understand and explain reality, rather than to experience truth as the truth. Since, in many ways, Yoga's premise about the nature of Reality and Truth is problematically limited and restricted even by the terminology of philosophy and metaphysics, to say nothing of theology, it is difficult to know what value there is in further limiting its significance to the domain of science, no matter how broadly defined. At the same time the question of abstract value is somewhat moot here, since the term "science" is an eminently modern concept that is saturated with power implications and linked as much to a hierarchy of knowledge as it is simply to the rational techniques and procedures of knowing, and the nature of reality so known.

Because religion is a murky category tainted with blind faith, ritualism, and theology, and philosophy too intellectual and therefore "out of touch" with the body, for Yoga to rank as a way of knowing about the substantial and transubstantial nature of the universe, and for it to claim authority in the domain of culture, it must distance itself from belief, ritualism, and metaphysical speculation and define itself as a science par excellence. If this were not the case then it would make sense—and perhaps reflect a step forward in the advancement of knowledge—to turn the tables and argue that science is Yoga par excellence. That this does not "make sense" says more about modern configurations of power/knowledge than it does about the nature of reality, truth, or anything else. The word "science" applied to Yoga in modern India reflects a sustained engagement with this field of power/knowledge, an open-ended, historically structured—and therefore impersonal—engagement with what counts as real.

Most of this book is devoted to an analysis of Yoga that has an unambiguous physical component, not just in theory—which is the case for all Yoga—but directly in practice. The focus here is on what is commonly called Haṭha Yoga. As will be discussed at length in subsequent chapters, the physical component of Yoga is understood as "scientific" and has also been subject to extensive and exhaustive scientific study. It is important to note, however, that the discourse and practice of science is not restricted to the domain of *āsana*s alone but extends, by way of *prāṇāyāma,* into the mind and the material traces of consciousness in the psyche. It is of critical importance to realize that all psychic phenomena, ranging from basic cognitive thought to direct perception of the Self, are profoundly material and theorized in terms of a materialist philosophy of life. Hence this second introductory chapter focuses on the way in which a specific discourse of modern science has come to define and problematically construct the relationship of the mind to the body in Yoga, broadly defined.

The meaning of the term "science" as it is used in the context of Yoga is specific and precise as well as broad and general. Specifically it means, simply, that Yoga is not a doctrine or set of speculative beliefs but rather an objective technique for training the body and mind so as to comprehend ultimate reality. More generally, however, there is the sense—and it is, as we will see, a very problematic sense—in which the term "science" refers to the very precise, modern methods of experimentation, verification, and rational, positivist investigation. This "sense" of science has everything to do with translation: the specific translation of various Sanskrit terms as meaning "science," and the translation of general ways of knowing into the very specific way of knowing which is modern science.

As a way of knowing—perhaps the most highly developed way of knowing—Yoga is regarded by many people as inherently self-explanatory, if by that one can mean something quintessentially profound rather than something tautologically simplistic and obvious. It is not something that needs to be understood as such, since it is the means by which to understand what is beyond normal consciousness as well as to "understand"—in a transcognitive sense—what is beyond consciousness as such.

Although Yoga is regarded by many as a transcendental science, it has become the subject of philosophical speculation and more general academic study. More recently it has become the object of mundane scientific research and investigation. Over the course of the past eighty years, objective, rational, empirical research has been done on the techniques of Yoga to test its truth value and discover how and why it works. The first experiments, conducted by Swami Kuvalayananda in 1924, focused on such things as changes in blood pressure, intra-esophageal air pressure, and heart rate during and after the performance of various *āsana*s and *prāṇāyāma* exercises. With government grants from the Central Council for Research on Yoga and Naturopathy, similar studies are now being conducted at numerous centers, clinics, āsrams and universities throughout India. It is important to note that as this book goes to press, the *Yoga Journal*—a glossy, high-end New Age magazine published in the United States—contains an article entitled "Western Science vs. Eastern Wisdom," which, in spite of what its title might suggest, is about "science in the East," namely the study of Yoga by means of science in contemporary India. As a highlighted section of the text makes clear, the idea of relentless and inevitable progress underlies the characterization of this particular history of science: "The methodology of older Indian studies has been criticized. But contemporary researchers are getting much more sophisticated. Control groups, randomization of subject, and other hallmarks of Western investigative science have become standard" (McCall 2003: 93).

Experimental studies on the physiological effects and medical benefits of Yoga are clearly thought of as scientific in the modern sense of the term. In *Ancient Yoga and Modern Science* T. R. Anantharaman, a prominent professor of metallurgy at Banaras Hindu University and researcher of rapidly solidified alloys and metallic glass, puts it this way: "Modern (i.e. post-sixteenth century) Science. . . . has come to be characterized by some special features and may well be considered as distinct in its assumptions, procedures, goals and methods from the earlier sciences of Europe and from the traditional sciences of India and China. The most important hallmark of this Modern Science is a special and subtle combination of reason and experiment, theory and observation, mathematics and measurement, individual imaginative creativity and publicly repeated verification" (1996: 14). Although seeming to distinguish the special features of Modern Science from other ways of knowing, Anantharaman's book—which contains a fascinating chapter entitled "Meditation as a Monotectoid Reaction"—seeks to explain classical Yoga in terms of Modern Science.

There is a world of difference in thinking, first, of Yoga as a science unto itself, and then making it the object of scientific study and explanation. In the first instance, Yoga's orientation is toward the experiential realization of something transempirical, immeasurable, unquantifiable, and ultimately beyond knowledge and consciousness. In the second, however, it is objectified: Ultimate Truth is broken down into forms of embodied practice that are then subject to rational, empirical, objective study. Problems emerge when these two sciences intersect, as they inevitably do, since empirical science would seem to raise critical questions about the nature of Yoga as science. Problems also emerge since there is significant ambiguity in the meaning ascribed to each of these sciences, in the kind of knowledge they produce, and, most significantly, in the way in which they authorize, in the broadest ideological sense of the term, different conceptions about what Yoga is, where it fits in the mix of Indian culture, and what its relationship is, or should be, to questions of national identity.

This chapter seeks to understand the powerful and profound consequence of a monumental mistake. I use the term "mistake" purposefully and strategically to convey a sense of accidental confusion in meaning. But I use the term nonpejoratively to define the structural contingency of an impersonal historical process rather than to cast aspersions on the goal-oriented actions and ambitions of specific individuals or groups. It is a mistake, ultimately, in translation.

The ambiguous, imprecise, and flexible meaning of the words "science" and "scientific knowledge" has made it possible to look for, if not find, an aspect of absolute truth in the neurochemistry of laboratory rats placed in test tubes and inverted such that they "perform" yogic headstands. It has made it possible to conduct experiments on *samādhi:* to look for, if not find, the truth about yogic power by burying adepts in the ground and measuring the length of time they can enstatically survive without breathing. It has made it possible to look for, if not find, the proof of enlightenment in *prāṇic* physiology and the congruence therein of subtle *nāḍīs* and the gross but somewhat metaphysical function of the brain and nervous system. It is also a mistake that has led, progressively, to the ever more precise embodiment of Yoga and an ever-increasing concern with the body as such, including the extreme extent to which modern scholarship on Yoga has come to regard the body as profoundly problematic and a thing to be overcome and transcended.

Far from being a clear case of the degradation of tradition, or a simple case of how something profound can be turned into a cultural parody of itself, the argument here is that the confusion of one kind of science with other kinds of knowledge and experience has created a kind of hybrid trajectory of knowledge that is neither subjective nor objective, physical or metaphysical. Nevertheless it is concretely embodied in a comprehensive sense and directly experienced. In other words, the confusion of two realities—or, depending on your perspective, two partial truths—has created a powerful fiction, in the fully creative, open-ended, imaginative sense of the term. On the simplest level what this means is that a purely subtle element such as *prāṇa,* the vital life force, in the metaphysics of Yoga physiology is given agency in the gross anatomy of health, and in experimental research on the treatment of various diseases. A subtle element whose very conceptual basis is cosmological and transubstantial in terms of one "science" is embodied through the action of another. This kind of mistake has made Yoga what it is today—a tremendously popular, eminently public, self-disciplinary regimen that produces good health and well-being, while always holding out the promise of final liberation. In looking ever more deeply into the body, a discourse of science has fused and confused the embodied knowledge of transcendence, and the practice based on that knowledge, with the transcendence of knowledge. In essence this is a mistake that has allowed Yoga to have its cake and eat it too: to claim that Ultimate Truth can only be experienced and never understood, while all the while seeking to explain, so as to understand, the nature of Truth, and to locate Truth in the body.

Although focused on the writing of four individuals—Rajarshi Muni, Swami Yogeshwaranand, Swami Sivananda, and Dr. K. N. Udupa—the analytical approach in this chapter is based on an ethnographically indiscriminate reading of as much of the modern literature on Yoga in as much detail as possible. By "indiscriminate" I mean that no qualitative distinction is made between apparently authoritative accounts and those that are apparently less authoritative. Clearly Ian Whicher's *The Integrity of the Yoga Darśana: A Reconsideration of Classical Yoga* (1998) provides a comprehensive and detailed discussion of the metaphysics of Yoga from a philosophical perspective. As such Whicher's study is the most recent in a long line of classical scholarship, ranging from Surendranath Dasgupta's *A Study of Patanjali* (1920) up through Georg Feuerstein's

The Philosophy of Classical Yoga (1980). Needless to say, an overarching philosophical perspective gleaned from this literature could be used to "correct" many of the misperceptions of Yoga as science, and "correct" many of the perspectives on Yoga metaphysics that are informed by a discourse of modern science. Rather than do this, however, Whicher's study, along with works by Dasgupta, Eliade, Feuerstein, and others, is used here to provide a critical frame of reference for an ethnographic reading of more popular—but no less serious—texts that are based, primarily, on experience itself rather than on textual interpretation.

Overall what is employed in the context of an ethnographic reading of contemporary texts is a method of analysis that might be called radical skepticism. As such it is informed not so much by the scientific methods of sociology and anthropology as by the philosophy upon which sociology in the broadest sense—including anthropology—is conceived, namely that all expressions of culture are social facts. These facts appear to be real unto themselves as things apart, whereas in fact they are socially constructed. Sociology is inherently skeptical about claims that are made about the facticity of anything in human experience other than social facts. However, social facts as such are only contingently factual, since they emerge out of the inherently magical calculus that social life is real and meaningful, but also greater than the sum of its various parts and therefore real in a way that cannot be reduced down to direct experience. Speaking of the manifest tension between society as a reified thing and the fetishization of society as God in Durkheim's conceptualization of social facts, Michael Taussig underscores the significance of this: "Reification-and-fetishism—*res* and *deus*—was a powerful mode of reckoning in modern society, nowhere more so than when applied to 'society' itself, and Durkheim was correct in problematizing—to the degree of fanaticism—the invisible presence, the intangibility, the literally unspeakable but begging to be spoken nature of society" (1993a: 229). It is Durkheim's "fanaticism" that can point the way toward a radical problematization of culture as both tangible and intangible at the same time.

Skepticism allows for a kind of methodological self-deception—translated, through writing, into what one hopes are perceptive insights—whereby one shifts back and forth between two seemingly contradictory perspectives: deep empathy and close identification with what a single person believes and teaches, and the critical location of that person's point of view not just within its own cultural context—in this case Yoga—but in a context that is fundamentally critical of circumscribed cultural contexts and the self-legitimizing discourses of contextualization. This is self-deception, because in order to have the necessary degree of deep empathy, one must, at least momentarily, believe what any given person believes—however unorthodox and idiosyncratic it may be—

without becoming a believer. One must be able to take headstanding rats seriously. Only then can one raise the question about what is going on—and not what is going on in the mind of the scientist who designed the experiment, but what is going on at many different levels and trajectories of history that intersect in the laboratory. After all, it is in scientific laboratories that rats have had a very long career of doing many very serious things. And so it is with reference to this "context"—a contingent condition where blasphemy entails seriousness, as Donna Haraway puts it (1991: 149)—that inverted, furry mamalian bodies will serve as a leitmotif for this book.

It is on this level, and only on this level, that one may speak of modern scientific Yoga as a mistake, but not one that is at all unique. And it is from this perspective that the critique of Yoga-subject-to-science can tack back toward a critique of modern Modern Science.

Radical skepticism not only gives one a better, more comprehensive and subtle understanding of why people believe what they believe. It is also a method of analysis that avoids the serious pitfalls of many cultural studies that tend to jump into the game of making sense at an indiscriminate level of generality—this or that school of Yoga, this or that body of literature, this or that social group. To be sure, radical skepticism has its drawbacks, and it should never be regarded as the endpoint of an analysis. It is simply a strategic method of gaining insight into what people say and do so as to be able to make general statements about a domain of human experience without presuming—either implicitly or explicitly—what the dimensions, limits, form, structure, and purpose of that domain are.

The Pyrotechnics of the Subtle Body: Science, Pseudoscience, and Cyborgs

> While Western science is still struggling to find explanations for such phenomenon as acupuncture meridians, *kuṇḍalinī* awakenings, and Kirlian photography, yogins continue to explore and enjoy the pyrotechnics of the subtle body, as they have done for hundreds of generations.
>
> Georg Feuerstein, *The Yoga Tradition* (2001: 351)

In many ways Yoga as science and the scientific study of Yoga both fall into the category of pseudoscience. At least this is the case within the framework of a history and philosophy of science where there is a great deal of interest in trying to determine the difference between science and other ways of knowing and in theorizing about the relationship between science and truth on many different levels. A full integration of the literature on the philosophy of science is well beyond the scope of this study, as well as beyond my anthropological expertise. Nevertheless, the perspective taken here reflects—following the "proof" of ethnographic research—a version of what is commonly referred to as epistemological relativism. As John Ziman puts it: "Scientific knowledge is essentially *underdetermined:* in principle, there are any number of possible interpretations of a finite set of observations. For this reason it is impossible to demonstrate that all scientific knowledge must eventually converge on a coherent body of 'objective truth' about the natural world" (1984: 104). Without going into all the implications of this, the essentially underdetermined nature of scientific knowledge certainly makes the problem of distinguishing between true science and pseudoscience much more interesting and complicated.[1] Furthermore, if the underdetermined nature of scientific knowledge is placed into a context that takes seriously the profound range of cultural differences in worldview reflected around the globe—and it is also acknowledged that science gets put into practice in these contexts—then the arguments made by those who advocate the so-called strong program in the sociology of knowledge are significantly strengthened.

In the purview of the history and philosophy of science, pseudoscience includes such things as astrology, alchemy, phrenology, ESP, telekinesis, UFO studies, and creationism, as well as a range of alternative medical practices such as homeopathy, naturopathy, and healing touch, to name but a few. One issue, perhaps the most vexing, is that no one can agree on a clear and definitive line between real and fake science, either historically or in the present (Weyant, Hanen, and Osler 1980). Consider psychiatry and sociobiology, for example. Problematically, there is a tendency in the history and philosophy of science to include non-Western medical systems such as Āyurveda and Traditional Chinese Medicine into the category of pseudoscience, even though this clearly reflects—at least in part—the ethnocentric bias of Western scholarship (Wilson 2002). Beyond this, the category of pseudoscience is conceptually problematic, since it tends to include those forms of knowledge that claim to be alternative to science as well as those kinds of experience that confound the methods of Modern Science. In the latter case the problem is compounded by the desire to subject said experiences to modern scientific study to prove their truth value, and—quite apart from the quality of the scientific research—by the way in which the methods of Modern Science transform the nature of the experience and the kind of truth to which it is linked. In any case, as Marx W. Wartofsky points out in the introduction to *Science, Pseudo-Science, and Society,* "Pseudoscience is not merely what is not science proper. . . . [I]t is what either appears *as* science, or represents itself *as* science. Or else it is what science proper—the scientific establishment or the scientific inquisition—marks off as heretical: not simply alternative, or alien, or other but a clear violation of the true faith. What is dialectical about such a formulation is that pseudo-science cannot be determined as such without at the same time determining what is properly scientific" (1980: 4).

When Modern Science, in the form of empirical, positivist experiments, is conducted on Yoga, the dialectic of science and pseudoscience is ratcheted up, so to speak, in the sense that the closer one gets to the embodiment of transcendence, the more Modern Science must be concerned with the precision of its own distinct theoretical foundation and methodology. The dialectic takes you deeper and deeper into the problem of locating Truth, and what appears as a trajectory of convergence can just as easily be seen as divergence. It is this ambiguity that animates both science and so-called pseudoscience. Consider, on the other end of the spectrum, the kind of excitement and enthusiasm generated, in some quarters, by the apparent convergence of quantum physics and various kinds of mysticism. This has produced a New Age figuration of Universal Science (Boyle 1983), much to the dismay of many hard-nosed physicists. As Frederick Aicken puts it in his introductory book on the nature of science, referring to Werner Heisenberg's Principle of Uncertainty: "It introduces the possibility that bits of atoms can literally appear from nowhere, or exist in two places at once; that the atom itself, not the model, may be a figment of our imagination; that the real world is one of millions of co-existing worlds each impossible to visit from another; that we, as observers, actually create the world as we contemplate it. Small wonder that physics, to some minds, has acquired the mystical aura that used to be associated with the religions of the Far East" (1984: 108). In this regard it is worth noting what the philosopher of science Simon Altmann says: "Normative principles are required in order to organize experience, and they are meta-physical because although they have become a part of our mental structure through a learning process based on experience, they cannot be *derived* from experience. Metaphysics, instead, adds to and is beyond experience. The problem is that meta-physical and metaphysical propositions can very easily be mixed up" (2002: 32–33).

But Yoga introduces another problem into the mix, one that is anticipated by alchemy. Alchemy, which was metaphysically inspirational if not meta-physically integral to the development of Newtonian physics (Westfall 1998), at least in its medieval European permutation, was, in its South Asian form, directly related to the development of Haṭha Yoga. It has also had a significant influence on the theoretical structure of Āyurveda (D. White 1996; Alter 1999). To state it simply, Yoga is the embodiment of alchemical theory and experimental method on the premise that immortality can be achieved by doing to the body what is done to base metals in the process of transmuting them into gold. In this sense Yoga is different from other so-called pseudosciences—except perhaps psychiatry—in that it is self-oriented rather than concerned with external objects or phenomena—UFOs, bent spoons, Vilikovskian planets, and Lysenkosian plants. It is different even from psychiatry in the very important sense that it is a science of the self, by the self, for the self, so to speak, while also being a science of Universal Truth. In other words, the practitioner of Yoga transforms him- or herself by the science he or she practices, and this fetishization of the body—rather than of objects external to it, such as spoons, alien spacecraft, planetary signs, and homeopathic drugs, for example—further ratchets up the dialectic of science and pseudoscience (see Alter n.d.b.).

It is possible to gain a critically skeptical perspective on the positivist scientific appropriation of the yogic science of consciousness—and Yoga's appropriation of Modern Science—by thinking of contemporary Yoga in terms of cybernetics, and what the historian of science Donna Haraway calls cyborg hybridity. Fundamentally a cyborg is difficult to classify in terms of the standard dualities of nature and culture, organic and inorganic, animal and machine, truth and fiction. It is also, I think, a creature that takes the relationship between science and pseudoscience beyond a dialectical configuration. This is precisely the basis of its power, significance, and analytic utility. It is an unstable whole made up of two categorically different "halves," and thus strains against the idea of integrated holism and organic continuity. As Haraway points out, it is possible and necessary to think about being human in cyborg terms because of three conditions of postmodern reality: "[1] the boundary between human and animal is thoroughly breached. . . . [2] machines have made thoroughly ambiguous the difference between natural and artificial, mind and body, self-developing and externally designed" and "[3] the boundary between physical and non-physical is very imprecise" (1991: 151–53).

There are many different dimensions to Haraway's argument, the most primary being a concern with power, politics, and the development of radical feminism. Underlying these concerns—which are extremely important but beyond the scope of the discussion here—is a particular kind of knowledge, and a specific form of consciousness that emerges out of the ambiguities inherent in cyborg being. As Haraway puts it,

> The cyborg is our ontology; it gives us our politics. The cyborg is a condensed image of both imagination and material reality, the two joined centers structuring any possibility of historical transformation. In the traditions of "Western" science and politics—the tradition of racist male-dominant

> capitalism; the tradition of progress; the tradition of the appropriation of nature as resource for the productions of culture; the tradition of reproduction of the self from the reflections of the other—the relation between organism and machine has been a border war. (1991: 150)

The cyborg ontology out of which politics can emerge is inherently unstable, confused, mutated, and, significantly, never completely under control. As a result it is creatively and constructively destructive, not simply of the traditions of Western Science and politics as such but also of the entrenched forms of opposition to these traditions. In a sense cyborg ontology is not based on the principle of original inception and final conclusion. It is all process, "a kind of disassembled and reassembled, postmodern collective and personal self" (1991: 163) oriented toward justice rather than truth; justice that is located not so much in revolution—for that brings things around, and to conclusion—as in the realization of social reality as science fiction. Because there is no Truth, justice must be the condition of being human. It is in this sense that "cyborg being" provides an important perspective by bringing into focus the inherently magical structure of the relationship between social facts, social relations, and concepts of self.

The embodiment of Yoga through practice is a kind of cybernetic transmutation of self into cyborg, wherein the crucial boundary that is blurred is that between organism and cosmos. Here the physical and the metaphysical are combined to produce what Anantharaman, echoing Sri Aurobindo, calls a Supramental Being.[2] In yogic terms this "blurring"—a kind of forced union—may be understood as enlightenment. But Yoga, like technoscience, does not control that to which it gives rise, and so the modern practitioner of Yoga, like a postmodern cyborg, incarnates irony. The body of the adept is both material and immaterial at the same time, and it is exactly this kind of contradiction that allows for a blasphemous understanding of the relationship between fictions of science and social reality.

Terminology : Mimesis and Meaning

In the foreword to Anantharaman's book, a "pleased and somewhat embarrassed" D. P. Chattopadhyaya points out that "the meaning of words like science, philosophy, *jñāna, vijñāna, śāstra, vidyā,* and *avidyā* are not very definite or univocal. Over the ages and in different contexts of use these have undergone notable changes" (1996: ix). Added to this is the problem of translation. Exactly what "indefinite and multivocal" Sanskrit term should be glossed as "science," as distinct from philosophy or system of knowledge? What is meant by science in that context? The gist of Chattopadhyaya's preamble to Anantharaman's book is that the fairly precise distinction that tends to be made between science and other modes of knowing is a relatively recent development. To transpose this distinction onto the intellectual history of South Asia is extremely problematic.

With Chattopadhyaya's qualifications clearly in mind, the term most often translated as science is *vidyā,* which also means learning, scholarship, and philosophy. Thus *vidyā* is best understood as science in a sense that is very general rather than specific. In any case it is fairly imprecise. Terminology and translation can become somewhat more precise when considering the distinction between *jñāna* and *vijñāna.* If *vijñāna* is understood as science, in the sense of a "system of knowledge concerned with distinguishing, discerning, understanding and comprehending the truth," it is a kind of science that is focused exclusively on secular knowledge. *Vijñāna* is concerned with "the detailed discursive and rational knowledge of the principles of existence" (Chattopadhyaya 1996: xi). As etymology would suggest, *vijñāna* is related to but different from *jñāna. Jñāna* means wisdom and knowledge of spiritual enlightenment. Whicher, Eliade, and most other scholars translate *jñāna* as knowledge. But as R. H. Singh, the director of the Center for Yoga at Banaras Hindu University points out by quoting from the *Gītā Sankar* (6:8, 19:1), there is an important epistemological difference between *jñāna* and *vijñāna* that undermines the purely binary structure of their etymological relationship. "[Indian philosophers] always made a distinction between the knowledge or *jñāna* and the realization or *vijñāna.* Shankaracharya himself while clarifying the distinction between *jñāna* and *vijñāna* has stated that *jñāna* or knowledge refers to procuring knowledge of an object with the help of literature and from authoritative scholars. *Vijñāna* or realization means to realize the so known object in the same form and reality" (1991: 2–3). As this suggests, *jñāna* and *vijñāna* are not categorically different. Georg Feuerstein points out, in some cases *vijñāna* can "denote the ultimate liberating gnosis" just as *jñāna* is occasionally "equated with the ultimate Reality itself" (1990: 158, 392; see also 2001: 31).[3] It is possible to comprehend this apparent paradox by turning to the ontological premise common to both *jñāna* and *vijñāna.* This is expressed by Chattopadhyaya in his foreword to Anantharaman's book: "The empirical is both rooted and ends up in the transcendental. The supreme reality in its manifest (*vyakta*) form, manifest to sense-experience and analytic intellect, is the subject of scientific study. Its unmanifest (*avyakta*) or seminal (*vijakar*) form is available or realizable only in *jñāna* or wisdom. Under one of its aspects, the Supreme Reality, God or Absolute, Isvara or Brahman, is material; under another aspect, the same reality is spiritual" (1996: xi).

Thinking of empirical reality as rooted in the transcendental, and of manifest and unmanifest things as ontologically the same, provides a somewhat different and more mimetic perspective on the relationship between *puruṣa* (transcendental self) and *prakṛti* (elemental nature) than is allowed for by straightforward dualism, where there is little or no room for materialism in any sense. As in the case of *jñāna* and *vijñāna,* it is important to understand the way in which dualism in Yoga is mimetic rather than dialectical. As a consequence of this mimetic duality, material reality is configured as a fetish rather than as the baseline of what is really not real. In this sense the illusion of self-consciousness is in thinking dualistically—and seeking truth in the elimination of falsehood—whereas what is required is an experiential sense of mimesis. As Whicher points out, summarizing the most general conclusion of his exhaustive study of the *Yoga Sūtra* and its associated literature: "Patanjali's Yoga, defined as *cittavṛttinirodha,* need not imply the extinction or evaporation of our 'personhood' along with the objective, material world. Rather it seems more accurate to assert that Yoga culminates in the eradication of spiritual ignorance (*avidyā*)—the root cause of our misidentification with, and attachment to worldly (and otherworldly!) existence" (1998: 305–6).

A convincing case can be made that the eradication of spiritual ignorance involves a kind of mimetic embodiment. Most significantly *avidyā* is fundamentally material, sensory, and cognitive in nature, and therefore physiological. In fact *avidyā* is constituted of the eight *tattvas*—unmanifest *prakṛti,* intellect, sense of self, and the five subtle senses—which are the elemental principles of the body. But the eradication of *avidyā* does not mean the extinction of the body; it means the realization of a perfect relationship between *puruṣa* and *prakṛti* as against the fundamentally mistaken relationship that is our experience This realization entails embodiment, albeit a kind of embodiment that is transcendental and transubstantial. The modern science of Yoga is concerned with an empirical, rational understanding of this realization. From a sociological perspective this produces a condition of blasphemous irony—the ultimate fiction of science and penultimate science fiction: a fetishization of *samādhi* and the Supramental Being.

The remainder of this chapter is concerned with specific examples that illustrate the intellectual mechanics of fetishization in the mimetic interstices of Modern Science and Yoga.

Scientific Yoga, Materialism, and the Problem of Reality

Sri Yashvantsinha D. Jadeja was born in 1931. After earning his B.A. from Bombay University, he got an M.A. in sociology from Poona University and was "an active student and prize-winning athlete in several sports" (Amin 1995: xx). From 1954 until 1970 he was in government service, serving primarily as deputy director in charge of training executive officers. In 1969 he became deputy director of research under Dr. I. P. Desai, former director of the London School of Economics and Political Science. While in college Jadeja had begun to practice Yoga, and continued to do so throughout his government career. In the same year that he became deputy director, he met Swami Kripalvanandji, who initiated him into the practice of "spontaneous" Yoga. In early 1971, at the age of forty, Jadeja resigned his post, renounced the world, and became a *sannyāsi,* taking the name Rajarshi Muni—Royal Sage.

As Nanubhai Amin, a well-known and highly regarded Gujarati scientist, conservationist, and industrialist—with degrees in electrical engineering from MIT and Cornell—writes,

> Rajarshi Muni has written several books, mostly in Gujarati, that succinctly express and explain the philosophy of Yoga as revealed by the ancient scriptures and his own intensive Yoga Sādhana. In these books he vividly describes Yoga exercises and experiences in a scientific manner. . . .
>
> While humble, he is also confident about what his experience, research and insight communicate to him as the Truth. Though possessed of a highly scientific mind, he is not interested in watering down or softening the Higher Truths of Yoga because they might be hard to swallow or do not necessarily meet the empirical requirements of modern Physical Sciences. . . .
>
> Scientific knowledge of the physical world is discovered through the means of the mind, five senses, and manufactured instruments. The fully liberated sages, or Siddhas, who composed the ancient scriptures, possessed supersensory powers which enabled them to perceive the workings of both the physical and non-physical worlds, and beyond. (1995: xxi)

This commentary appears in the introduction to Swami Rajarshi Muni's 184-page book *Yoga: The Ultimate Attainment—The Philosophy and Psychology of "Spontaneous Yoga"* (1995). In fourteen chapters and two lengthy appendices, the book contains a clear, concise, and down-to-earth discussion of what most people would call Hindu philosophy and metaphysics. For instance, chapter 7 is entitled "Theory of Rebirth"; chapter 9, "Doctrine of Karma"; chapter 11, "Human Life and Its Purpose"; chapter 13, "Modifications of Consciousness and Yoga." Chapter 4 explicitly locates "spontaneous" Yoga within the framework of Indian philosophy by showing the similarities and differences between each of the six primary schools of thought: Yoga, Sāṃkhya, Mīṃāṃsā, Vedānta, Vaiśeṣika, and Nyāya. Similarly, chapter 5 deals with what the author refers to as Yoga metaphysics, and contains a detailed discussion of the relationship between the cosmic principles of *puruṣa* and *prakṛti,* the three psychodynamic *guṇa* attributes—*sattva, rajas,* and *tamas*—and their relative balance, the distinction between subtle and gross elements, the functioning of *nāḍī* conduits and the agency of *prāṇa* in the universe and within the body, among many other things. In light of this, Rajarshi Muni makes the following statement:

> These doctrines are not mere dogmas, but are scientific truths, and those who have experimented with them have invariably borne witness to their transformative power.
>
> This means that Yoga is not merely theoretical philosophy, but a practical discipline based on an unfailingly recurrent pattern of spiritual experiences. It is an ancient yet timeless science of spiritual self-development, based on laws governing the natural forces and their relation to the Supreme Essence; a science that is as perfect as it is exact in its methodology and techniques. (1995: 3)

Before trying to unpack what is meant by this, let us consider another example.

Sri Yogeshwaranand Parmahans was born around the turn of the nineteenth century. In his autobiography he recounts how, against his parents' will, he pursued the life of a yogi, practicing austerities, studying the scriptures, and going in pursuit of a true master, whom he found near the source of the Ganga in the Himalayas. Under the guidance of his master Yogeshwaranand was initiated into the practice of higher Yoga. Based out of an *āśram* in Rishikesh, he traveled and taught extensively throughout the 1950s, 1960s, and 1970s. Before his death in the early 1980s he had conducted three world tours and had founded the Yoga Niketan Trust.

Under the auspices of the Trust, Yogeshwaranand wrote a number of books. Five have similar titles: *Science of Soul* (1997), *Science of Divinity* (1983), *Science of Divine Light* (1983), *Science of Vital Forces* (1978), and *Science of Divine Sound* (1984). The description of the first book, published originally in Hindi in 1959, is "[a] Practical Exposition of Realization of Soul with 30 multi-coloured pictures." In this book, translated into English in 1964 and republished for the sixth time in 1997, it is clear that the author used "science" to mean *vidyā* and *vijñāna,* since all three of these words evoke the idea of truth in and through knowledge.

Significantly, however, one cannot find the "right" translation of *vidyā* and *vijñāna* and thereby escape into the comfort of sanskritic tradition to make sense of Yogeshwaranand's teaching. *Science of the Soul* exists in translation, even in its original Hindi. It is ambiguously and ingeniously empirical, rational, and mystical. The truth it articulates is located somewhere between the meaning of science and the meaning of *vijñāna*. In other words it articulates truth mimetically. It draws directly and explicitly on the language of Modern Science to show how *parmātman* is embodied. As such it produces a fabulous image of a cosmic cyborg. Needless to say, Yogeshwaranand's image of embodied *parmātman* was not the first of its kind, and it most certainly was not the last. But it is one of the most detailed, spectacular, and well known.

To understand Yogeshwaranand's discussion of the science of the soul, it is necessary to begin with the idea that the perceived body is one dimension of a larger, more subtle and complex reality that is characterized by the *pañca kośa* (five sheaths) (see also Majumdar 1999: 584–88).[4] In general terms the physical body is said to be made up of the *annamaya kośa* (food sheath) and *prāṇamaya kośa* (vital breath sheath). Together these "offer gross service to the *jīvātman* [nescient, embodied soul]." The strength of the physical body is derived from the *sūkṣma śarīra* (subtle body), "which is devoid of nerves, veins, arteries or flesh and bones; it is made up of extremely subtle vapour-like element, it is even devoid of limbs, but pervades the whole physical body" (1997: 15). The subtle body is composed of the *manomaya kośa* (mind sheath) and the *vijñānamaya kośa* (intellect sheath), the root *vijñāna* here taking on a slightly, but significantly, different meaning from either knowledge in general—beyond the intellect—or science in particular. Thus, in essence, Yogeshwaranand subdivides four of the sheaths into two subsets, one relatively gross and the other relatively subtle.

Animating both the gross and the subtle body from within there is what Yogeshwaranand refers to as another, undifferentiated, causal body: *kārana śarīra*. The vitality of this body is located in the *ānandamaya kośa* (bliss sheath). Summing up the interrelationship of these bodies, their sheaths, and the sheaths' different properties, Yogeshwaranand makes the following statement about what he refers to as the "castle of the body."

> *Citta* is the knowledge predominating part of the *Ānandamaya Kośa*. *Ahamkāra* or ego, which is the action predominating part of the Bliss Sheath, spreads both types of energy and brings them out of the *Ānandamaya Kośa* in the form of *Sūkṣma Prāṇa* or subtle vital force. This force enters the astral [subtle] body with a jerk or push. The astral body becomes alive by this life force and in turn makes the physical body alive and active. This process continues throughout the life of an individual.
>
> The method by which one enters into this castle of the body and gains knowledge of conscious spirit (soul), veiled by unconscious matter, is known

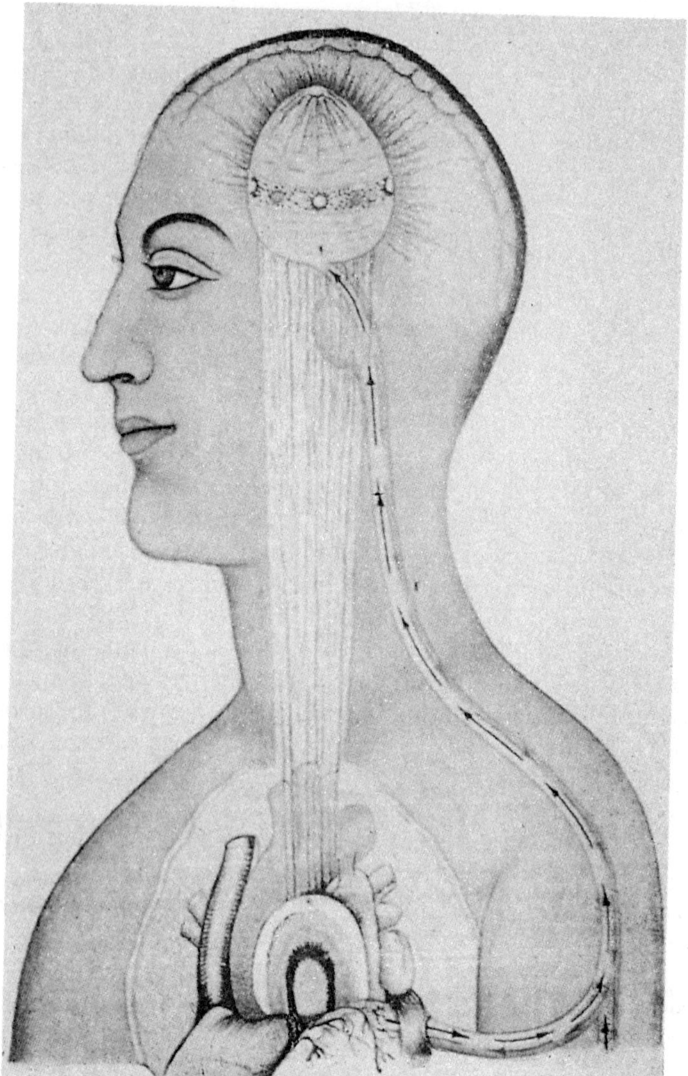

1. "The fourfold *Aṇṭaḥkaraṇa* and mutual relationship." *Source:* Yogeshwaranand Parmahans, *Science of Soul,* 5th ed. (New Delhi: Yoga Niketan Trust, 1997), illus. no. 12. Reproduced with permission from the Yoga Niketan Trust.

as *Ātma Vijñāna,* the science of soul, or self-realization. The present book gives a detailed exposition of this science. (1997: 16–17)

It is not very surprising that in his discussion of the physical body's food sheath Yogeshwaranand provides a detailed discussion of gross anatomy, with separate sections on the skeletal, muscular, digestive, and circulatory systems.[5] It is, however, highly significant that he moves, systematically in this section, from a discussion of the nervous system in general and the brain and spinal column in particular, through to the glandular system and the reproductive organs specifically. After a brief discussion of sleep, he concludes with a lengthy discussion of the *nāḍī* conduits and *cakra* centers through which the awakened power of *kuṇḍalinī* flows.

How you get from the nerves and organs of sense to *nāḍī*s and *cakra*s is a critical facet of the story which follows. It is critical to understanding the link between Yoga as science and the scientific study of Yoga.

As with almost all other writers on the subject, Yogeshwaranand makes a direct and explicit correlation between the spinal cord and the axial, *suṣumṇā nāḍī* through which the practice of Yoga is designed to channel the latent energy of *kuṇḍalinī.* The two other primary channels, *iḍā* and *piṅgalā,* intersect the *suṣumṇā* at the eight *cakra* centers and, along with all of the other *nāḍī,* carry the vital energy of *prāṇa* throughout the body as a whole. Although referring to the *cakra*s as "sensory motor nerves" which "pervade the entire body to rejuvenate it with life force in the form of knowledge and action" Yogeshwaranand goes on to say that "some modern writers have identified these channels as the spinal cord with the sympathetic nervous chains, and the *cakra*s as the nervous centers (plexi) of the body. This is incorrect, *as these structures are not perceived without special meditation,* nor can their activity be equated with their gross structure. It is rather like the filaments of an electric lamp which establishes a gross circuit, but light does not shine until electricity flows" (1997: 69, emphasis added). There is, in other words, a point at which the gross body shades into the subtle body, but it requires heightened insight to see this point. As Georg Feuerstein puts it: "The organs of the subtle vehicle are thought to be as real as the organs of the physical body. Hence they are visible to clairvoyant sight" (2001: 350).

In some sense, as with all of the other numerous books on the subject of embodied transcendence, Yogeshwaranand's *Science of the Soul* is a lengthy discourse on that illusive point and its possible discovery. As a scientific treatise of many different kinds, the text as a whole is designed to make visible what remains invisible and misunderstood without proper meditation. If, metaphorically speaking, meditation flips the switch, science provides a lasting image once the light goes out. Most significantly, it provides a graphic image for those who have never seen the light. But, as an image, what is its relationship to reality?

Yogeshwaranand's discourse is clearly transcendental, but it is also grounded in what must be regarded as the materiality of the lived body. As a systematic survey of the multiple bodies and sheaths that constitute a person, *Science of the Soul* is—somewhat ambivalently—about the illusive cybernetic structure of *cittavṛttinirodha,* wherein the controlled mind perfectly reflects Truth.[6] Yogeshwaranand takes his readers into the structure.

> Having entered into the orb of the heart, one sees before one's vision a wheel of luminous wires, resembling hair-springs. Associated with this is a hollow place like a shadow. Inside this is a brilliant light, white in colour. When the divine enters this the light spreads. In the centre of this circle shines a luminous particle like a diamond. On the external margin of the orb of *Citta,* vast luminous waves of golden colour are seen. This is the circle of *Rajoguṇa.* Having gone across this, just below it. (1997: 282)

In this light it is important to keep in mind that the word *vijñāna,* as in the Hindi title of Yogeshwaranand's book, *Ātma-Vijñāna,* carries with it the strong connotation of visualized knowledge. This is conveyed in the English subtitle: "A practical exposition of ancient method of visualization of Soul." The point is that Yogeshwaranand's book is not so much about supernatural visions of *Citta* or other things, as about being able to move from the skin, muscle, and bone of the food sheath through to the causal body, in order to see through the bliss sheath to the soul. The procedure for doing this is scientific. Whether intentionally or not, the scientific procedure of anatomical reference and physiological function—as well as the more straightforward use of knowledge based on language to describe an indescribable experience—leads to a rather "gross" characterization of that which is, in the end, most subtle.

> It is in this heart that the *Liṅga śarīra* or Bliss Sheath resides. If the heart is dissected longitudinally into two parts, you will find an oval-shaped hollow similar to a small seedless grape: the Bliss Sheath pervades the space. The heart is the center of blood purification. . . . With the circulation of the blood, the functions of knowledge and action also pervade the entire body. . . .
>
> This is shown in Illustration No. 1 in the chapter of Food Sheath. It can be seen by divine vision that this human body . . . contains the heart, of the size of a pear, or like a lotus bud drooping downwards. Inside this heart is a hollow of the size of a small seedless grape. Inside this hollow is the Bliss Sheath, luminous like a golden egg. This Bliss Sheath is an aggregate of six luminous orbs. It is very pleasant to see and appears like an oval mass of light.

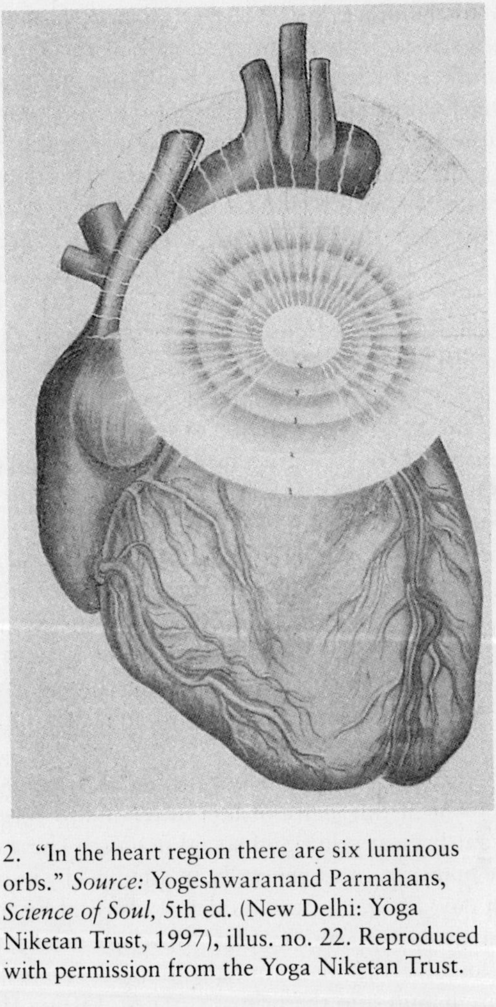

2. "In the heart region there are six luminous orbs." *Source:* Yogeshwaranand Parmahans, *Science of Soul*, 5th ed. (New Delhi: Yoga Niketan Trust, 1997), illus. no. 22. Reproduced with permission from the Yoga Niketan Trust.

> The outermost circle or orb, called the orb of Brahman, the Absolute, is all-pervading and interpenetrating; thus it may seem absurd to locate *Brahman* in a circle, yet it is not so ridiculous. (1997: 258, 259)

Science, Spirituality, and Embodied Power

In their orientation toward Yoga both Rajarshi Muni and Yogeshwaranand fall more into the camp of spirituality than into the camp of science. Although the body is integral to their respective sciences of spirituality, and ultimately to the practice of Yoga—no matter how cerebral—their textual discourses are oriented toward something metaphysical. As such Yogeshwaranand's and Rajarshi Muni's books are not at all unique. Although concerned with embodiment, they fit into what might be called a genre of literature that is primarily concerned with transcendence, liberation, and the realization of higher consciousness. This modern genre has historical precedent in the Orientalist literature on the occult (Abhedananda 1902; Atkinson 1934; Bosc 1893, 1913; De Laurence 1909; de Sarak [1902] 1990; Dvivedi [1885]1992; T.C.R. Iyengar 1908; Kadir 1909; Levi [1922] 1969; Pilai and De Laurence 1910; Ramacharaka 1904, 1911; Richardson and Hensoldt 1911; Sankaracarya 1888; Sarkar 1902; Spalding [1924] 1955; Wood 1927), as well as a precedent in the literature produced by the Theosophical Society in particular (Besant 1907, 1913; Blavatsky 1931; I. Harris 1919; Olcott 1885).[7] In an important sense the historical referent for this literature is found directly in the work of Vivekananda.[8] Vivekananda's *Raja Yoga* is replete with references to the physiology of *prāṇic* enlightenment. In *Nervous System in Yoga and Tantra*, Ashok Majumdar quotes Vivekananda as follows: "Why should not the mind send news without any wire? We see this done in nature. The Yogi says, if you can do that, you can get rid of the bondage of matter. How to do it? If you can make the current pass through the *Suṣumṇā*, the canal in the middle of the spinal column, you have solved the problem. The mind has made this network of the nervous system, and has to break it" (1999: 556).

In taking a broad view of the modern history of Yoga, it is possible to see the development of this genre of literature, and to classify it as such on the basis of fairly clear criteria of social practice. These criteria of social practice are manifest, most generally, in attempts by individuals to establish modern-day *āśrams* on the model of classical hermitages where adept *gurus* instructed aspiring disciples. More specifically, the criteria of social practice involve the institutionalization of "ethical" and moral practices that are manifest in the primary stages of *yama* and *niyama* restraint—truthfulness, chastity, nonviolence, a lack of desire for material wealth, asceticism, and devotion to God. Although concerned, primarily, with the problem of embodiment, another feature that characterizes this genre is the institutionalization and structured teaching of the highest stages of meditation and what is sometimes called Raja Yoga.

By referring to a body of literature that may be regarded as concerned with the esoteric embodiment of spirituality and transcendence, I do not wish to suggest that it is easy or necessary to fit all works on Yoga exclusively into this genre or into some other. For example, Ashok Majumdar's *Nervous System in Yoga and Tantra* (1999) begins with a detailed discussion of *Aṣṭāṅga* Yoga and then engages with philosophical issues in the *Yoga Sūtra* and various tantric texts before concluding with a discussion of the physiology and pathology of *tridoṣa* theory in Āyurveda. It is, nevertheless, useful to think about a large body of literature in terms that seem to identify important themes and shared orientations to common problems. More specifically, it is important to understand the way in which the literature on Haṭha Yoga is linked to the literature on meditation and higher consciousness via the medium of the body and the problematic "materialism" of embodiment. One of the most important books that defines the parameters of this genre—though not, by any means, all or even most of the modern, *āśram*-based social criteria of practice—is Gopi Krishna's book *Kundalini: Path to Higher Consciousness* (1992). What is characteristic of this book is the way in which it is concerned with the most mundane aspects of embodied experience as well as the most metaphysical aspects of embodied experience—with the biographical and phenomenological self as well as with the universal, cosmic Self—and how the body can be described as having changed completely and yet as having not changed at all.

Gopi Krishna did not establish an *āśram* or even affect the persona of an enlightened sage. There are many who have, and it is from within the institutionalized framework of modern-day *āśram*s that much of the literature on supramental embodiment was, and continues to be, produced. Some of the literature on modern Haṭha Yoga that will be discussed in detail in the following chapters also emerged, and continues to emerge, from these *āśram*s. But it is in the very nature of *āśram*s to be concerned with Yoga as science in ways that extend beyond the scientific study of the physiology and health value of *āsana* and *prāṇāyāma*. For example, Swami Sivananda of the Divine Life Society has written numerous books on the science of Yoga and *prāṇāyāma,* and his teaching is suffused with the discourse of science as well as a discourse of divine life (1935a, b, 1944, 1950, 1955a, b, 1961, 1962a, b, 1981; Sivananda and Venkatesananda 1986). The Bihar School of Yoga, founded by Swami Satyananda Saraswati, a disciple of Sivananda's, is both a research institute for the scientific study of Yoga and yogic health and a spiritual retreat for the study of Yoga as science (see Satyananda Saraswati 1966, 1973a, b, 1975, 1984). Among other things, the Bihar School of Yoga has established training courses for people who wish to renounce the world and experience enlightenment. Swami Rama's books on Yoga reflect his own experience of enlightenment (1978), while the literature produced by him and others under the rubric of the Himalayan Institute is heavily influenced by psychology and the scientific study of the mind and cognitive function (1972, 1976, 1986; Rama and Ajaya 1976; Rama and Ballentine 1976). Much of the literature is oriented toward mental and physical health as well as spiritual well-being. There are, of course, numerous other examples: Shri Surath's *Scientific Yoga for the Man of Today* (1979), Yogi Pranavananda's *Pure Yoga* (1992), Swami Krishnananda's *Yoga as a Universal Science* (1997), Swami Atmananda's *The Four Yogas* (1991), I. K. Taimni's commentary—informed, at least in part, by his training in chemistry—on the *Yoga Sūtra* in *The Science of Yoga* (1961), and Narendra Nath Kaul's *Seven Steps for Simple Samadhi* (1989), to name but a few (see also Abhedananda 1946; Chakravarti 1985; Giri and Pattnaik 1981; Murty 1979; Mathur 1998; Varadachari 1969) A key theme in works such as these is perhaps best summed up in *Practical Lessons in Yoga*, the most well known and popular of Swami Sivananda's three- hundred-plus books:

> Yoga and Science are inseparable. Science and Religion are inseparable. Science is part of Religion. Science and Religion are necessary correlatives. Scientists are also monists in one sense. They also emphatically declare that there is only one thing viz., Matter or energy. A Yogi tries to control the mental forces, a scientist the physical forces. This is all the difference between a Yogi and scïentist. A scientist is also an unconscious Raja-Yogi, but his mind works in external groves. (1997a: 203)

Supramental Bodies: The Internal Groves of Physical Force

Turning away from specific individuals, what follows is a detailed analysis of the key elements of Yoga physiology as outlined in works of yogic science that, at first glance, appear to be purely metaphysical and therefore not concerned with the body at all. This is not so much an analysis which focuses on the structure and function of this physiology—although that may certainly be derived from it—as a meta-analysis: a study of the studies and an analysis of the analyses. The basic argument is that supramental beings, if not constituted of flesh and blood as such, are nevertheless produced by and take embodied shape in a fusion of the cosmic Self and the individual self. This fusion is enabled by a discourse of science on the one hand and the ontological materialism of consciousness on the other. In a sense, supramental beings incarnate the irony and contorted dialects of cyborgs—creatures produced by the contrived unification of organic and inorganic elements. Unlike cyborgs, however, supramental beings are, at least without concern for the accuracy of neat division, made from the elemental unification of the physical and the metaphysical. Half human, half cosmos, they embody universal holism.

In its basic structure Yoga physiology and metaphysics has a great deal in common with the anatomical principles and metamorphology of Āyurvedic medicine, since both are closely aligned with the principles of

Sāṃkhya philosophy (see Larson and Bhattacharya 1987). In this light, the key elements of Yoga physiology—and of the whole material world, for that matter—are *puruṣa* and *prakṛti*. *Puruṣa* is usually translated as the individual soul or animating principle, whereas as *prakṛti* is said to be inanimate nature.[9] Life as we know it is the consequence of *puruṣa* becoming "embodied in the subtle and gross elements of Prakṛti due to primal ignorance (*Avidyā*), and is thereby bound to the cycle of births and deaths" (Rajarshi Muni 1995: 52). Creation is understood as a kind of devolution of *prakṛti*, as *prakṛti* is animated by *puruṣa*.[10] But all things that are *prakṛtic* by nature lose sight of and misunderstand *puruṣa* as a consequence of being thus animated.[11] Thus the structure, function, and form of all organic matter, both subtle and gross, is regarded as the by-product of a cosmic error.[12] Yoga may be understood as the means by which to undo this error, by working backward through gross and subtle physiology to disembody the soul. It is important to keep in mind, in this regard, that although "primal ignorance" is a good translation of *avidyā*, the term can also mean antiknowledge or antiscience.[13]

On its own, *prakṛti* is often conceived of as "the primordial metaphysical principle that has the potential to manifest into the enormous empirical universe" (Rajarshi Muni 1995: 56). In this state it is made up of the three principal attributes of nature—*guṇa*—balanced in a perfect state of equilibrium known as *sāmyāvasthā*.[14] Once disturbed the relative imbalance of the *guṇa* attributes gives form to the "enormous empirical universe," the natural world, and the human body. The initial unbalancing of the three *guṇas* sets in motion an endless process of combination and recombination which is the process of life.[15] It is important to keep in mind that this process is understood as a "devolvement" or an "involution" rather than as something intrinsically and inherently positive. On an ontological level it is a movement down and backward, not up and forward as in the popular perception of developmental, progressive change.

In and of themselves the three *guṇa*—*sattva, rajas,* and *tamas*—have neither positive nor negative qualities as such. Nevertheless, as attributes of nature, they have different properties, and *sattva* is regarded as more noble or virtuous than *rajas* and *tamas*. For example, as "mental conditions" a predominance of *sattva* creates "peace," a predominance of *rajas*, "restlessness," and *tamas*, "dullness." As "phenomenal radiations of visible light" *sattva* is white luminosity, *rajas* dull redness, and *tamas* dark blackness. In most general terms sattvickness is closest to godliness. As a "psychological modifier" it is described as "steadiness; intellectual growth; heightened understanding; simplicity; spiritual fervor; health; happiness; goodness; humility; love; compassion; charity; truthfulness; forgiveness; fortitude; tenacity; contentment; enthusiasm; cheerfulness; fearlessness; gentleness; self-restraint; moderation; etc." (Rajarshi Muni

1995: 59). Significantly, *sattva* is regarded as synonymous with *citta* in the *Yoga Sūtra* because *sattva* predominates in pure consciousness. On this basis Patañjali makes a distinction between *aindriya,* immaterial reality, and *bhautika,* material reality. What must not be forgotten, however, is that both realities are not categorically different, but only relatively so. Both are *prakṛtic* in nature and thus meta-material. Therefore, however much the attributes of sattvick *citta* may sound positive, in the scheme of yogic physiology they are more means than ends, in the sense that a person seeks to embody them in order to transcend the involution of matter.

The primordial disturbance of the *guṇa*s gave rise first to *jīvātman* (soul in bondage) and *citta* (individual consciousness) and subsequently to the twenty-three *tattva* categories: *buddhi* (intellect), *ahamkāra* (ego), *manas* (mind), *jñānendriyas* (five senses), *karmendriyas* (five actions), *tanmātras* (five subtle elements), and *mahābhūtas* (five gross elements).[16] In classical Sāṃkhya the number of *tattva* is twenty-four, including *prakṛti.* Together, individual consciousness, intellect, ego, and mind constitute the *aṇṭaḥkaraṇa* (internal instrument) and the five senses, actions, subtle and gross elements constitute the twenty-part *bāhyakaraṇa* (external instrument). Rajarshi Muni describes this process as "vibrational densification" by means of which the soul is encased in ever more gross matter and ever more illusory experience. He uses the following analogy to describe the process

> Hydrogen and oxygen are already present in the atmosphere as gases. Through the influence of natural forces such as heat and gravity, etc., these two elements combine to form H_20 vapor. Through cooling this vapor condenses into water. With further cooling the water becomes ice.
>
> The state in which hydrogen and oxygen are existing as separate elements corresponds to *Prakṛti* in its state as Unmanifested Nature. The formation of vapor corresponds to the creation of the first *Tattva* and the causal body. The condensation of water and freezing into ice represents the formation of the subtle and gross bodies respectively, through the continued densyfying influence of the *Guṇas.* (1995: 71)

The whole structure of yogic physiology, starting with pure *puruṣa* and going all the way down to earth, the grossest of gross elements, is rigidly hierarchical and sequentially derivative. That which is subtle gives rise to that which is gross. This logic allows for movement back through all the various sheaths and layers of bodies, composed of the twenty-three *tattva,* right into the soul. This movement—a kind of return to the state of proto-creation—is best described as the embodiment of ever more subtle attributes (see, for example, Atmananda 1991: 104; Surath 1979: 19).

In the chapters that follow there will be occasion to focus on the relatively subtle aspects of the unambiguously gross body. In the context of the supramental being, however, it is important to briefly consider the meta-material nature of *citta* consciousness. As Whicher puts it, "the Sāṃkhyan dualism that Yoga utilizes is quite distinct from the Cartesian dualism that bifurcates reality into mental and material aspects" (1998: 90). *Citta* is, fundamentally, part of *prakṛti,* though it is pervasive rather than restricted to a singular ontic category. In some sense *citta* is that which is as a consequence of transcendental, cosmic consciousness being implicated in the perception of objects (see Whicher 1998: 92), even though, as pointed out, the direct perception of objects as objects is a product of *avidyā* In this regard Feuerstein notes that

> the *citta* is thought to be suffused with countless "subliminal activators" (*saṃskāra*) combining into what are called the "traits" (*vāsanā*). These are responsible for the production of the various psychomental phenomenon, in particular the set of five fluctuations (*vṛtti*). In aphorism IV:24 [of the *Yoga Sūtra*] the *citta* is declared to be ultimately geared toward the liberation of human beings. Upon the realization of the Self, consciousness (which is really a material phenomenon) is dissolved because Self-realization presupposes the "involution" (*pratiprasava*) of the primary constituents or "qualities" (*guṇa*) of Nature. (1990: 79)

Given that *citta* is a meta-material phenomenon, its direct relationship to the body as such raises questions. A number of different commentaries present views on whether or not *citta* is restricted to the body or is a meta-material phenomenon that is all pervasive. In many respects this is the same question as to whether or not *citta* is a specific evolute of *prakṛti.* There appears to be some consensus on its being all pervasive and only restricted to the body with respect to the five fluctuations. This is, of course, germane to the question of how a supramental being takes shape, as well as the nature of its consciousness. It would seem, at least in part, that Vyāsa, Vācaspatimiśra, and other classical scholars as well as contemporary authors like Yogeshwaranand, Sivananda, and Rajarshi Muni are vexed by the way in which consciousness and the body are linked together ontologically.[17]

Most books on the subject refer to the eight limbs of Yoga: *yama* (abstinence, rules of conduct), *niyama* (observances, rules for self-purification), *āsana* (postures, exercises), *prāṇāyāma* (breath control), *pratyāhāra* (withdrawal of the senses), *dhāraṇā* (concentration), *dhyāna* (meditation), and *samādhi* (superconsciousness). All practitioners of Yoga must start at the beginning, and although those who reach the higher, more subtle levels of experience enter into realms such as those described by Yogeshwaranand, most people spend a lifetime grappling with the gross and subtle bodies of direct, conscious experience manifest in the first four stages. That is to say, even though the rules of conduct and self-purification are preliminary, they are of critical importance and require significant effort. In fact, a number of books point out that the term "*haṭha*" in Haṭha Yoga—the branch which focuses on the practice of the first four limbs—means force or exertion.

The eight limbs of Yoga correspond, roughly, to the layers of relative subtlety within the body. But *prāṇa,* and the agency of *prāṇa,* is of critical importance in understanding both the structure of supramental physiology and the body's manipulation through practice. *Prāṇa,* as vital force, is considered by some to be a kind of pre- *prakṛtic* wild card if you will, since it is an element that, quite literally, cuts through the body and can influence both that which is subtle and that which is gross. In this sense, unlike everything else within the body, it is not a derivative of creation but is, rather, thought to be transubstantial and stands alone as a monadic, pure force in an otherwise dualistic, destabalized, devolved world order. According to most scholars, *prāṇa* is, in fact, an evolute of *prakṛti* and is synonymous with *mahat* or *buddhi,* the first and most pure products of creation. But whether it is considered an evolute or not, *prāṇa* is the material essence of absolute subtlety, if not Reality itself. What is significant about this is that as such it can have two meanings, one rather mundane and the other profound; and in essence these two meanings are the same—*prāṇa* is the force of all life and the vital life force.

All sources do not agree on this, but since *prāṇa* is considered the very essence of action it is often said to be the motive force of creation—the first consequence of the union of *puruṣa* and *prakṛti.* Even though *prāṇa* is the force behind mundane activities such as walking, talking, and eating, and is subdivided into five specific categories which vitalize the five cognitive senses—hearing, touch, sight, taste, and smell—and the five actions—speech, action, locomotion, excretion, and reproduction—there is an important sense in which *prāṇa* is understood as a holistic element that pervades the body. Rajarshi Muni puts it this way:

> Although the *Prāṇas* (vital energies) sustain and energize each component of the microcosm, and transfer data between the linked components, they are not mentioned in most classical texts with the hierarchical categories that evolve from *Prakṛti.* . . .
>
> The first and most important vital air, the ascending vital air (*Prāṇa*), derives its name from the generic *Prāṇa,* and has its seat in the chest region. . . .
>
> These five Prāṇas are often wrongly interpreted as the air that we breath[e], which is the unrefined form of the these five vital airs. The Prāṇas radiate directly from the central source of life-energy that manifests in the human body, namely the *Puruṣa* (Soul). (1995: 65–66)

While it is clear that in the view of most writers *prāṇa* is regarded as an extremely pure, subtle force, what is significant is that in many peoples' conception the difference between *prāṇa* and the air we breathe is relatively less than the difference between the gross and the subtle attributes of the body.[18] There is a sense in which "breath" and "soul" are synonymous. Even though they can be said to be very different, as words they are the same. Their ambiguous synonymousness—and also the ironic fact that in the *Yoga Sūtra* the word *prāṇa* is used to signify breath and breath alone (I:34)—allows for a subtle translation between two scientific languages. For instance, even though all of the five *prāṇa*s can be said to "radiate" from the soul, Yogeshwaranand describes each in very concrete, functional terms.

> *Apāna* is that which throws out the impurities in a special way and creates strength. The field of *Apāna* is from navel to the soles of the feet.
>
> Because of the predominance of the earth element, it is characterized by heaviness and, therefore, it moves downwards. It draws urea from the kidneys, and brings it to the bladder, then it expels urine from the bladder; at the time of copulation it causes the flow of semen and of menses. (1995: 107)

In the context of the five vital airs, *prāṇa,* as distinct from *Prāṇa*—but only to a degree, and that is what is important here—is described in terms where the difference between it and the air we breathe is so subtle as to be almost imperceptible.

> That which bestows strength on the entire body and draws vital force from the air is known as *Prāṇa Vāta* or the *Prāṇa* Air. Ever engaged in activities, the energy that is being lost through inhalation and exhalation is recouped by this *Prāṇa Vāta* that draws special energy from the atmosphere and fills the body with this energy in the form of breath. (1995: 107)

This becomes clearer through a consideration of the way in which *prāṇa* is thought to move through the body. As pure, vital energy of life, *prāṇa* can be thought of as a luminous aura that pervades the body. But many books, when dealing with the specifics of controlling *prāṇa* and moving it through the various bodies and sheaths, refer to *nāḍī* conduits. These conduits are, significantly, embodied on a plane that seems to cross-cut gross and subtle domains, even though they are clearly located in the subtle body. Although there are hundreds of thousands of *nāḍī* which pervade the body, much like nerves or capillaries, the three primary ones are those mentioned above—*suṣumṇā, iḍā,* and *piṅgalā*—which intersect to form the six *cakra* centers, a seventh being outside the body.

The *cakras* are located along the axis of the spinal column but are said to be "seated" or situated at specific points of gross anatomy. The typical order of the *cakras* is from bottom to top with the *mūlādhāra* cakra at the anus, *svādhiṣṭhāna* the abdomen, *maṇipūra* the navel, *anāhata* the heart, *viśuddha* the throat, *ājñā* the forehead and *sahasrāra* the brain. Clearly this is a hierarchical order, since the first five *cakras* are associated with the five elements, five organs of sense, and the five organs of action, in ascending sequence through the range of relative subtlety. Thus the *mūlādhāra cakra* is associated with earth, smell, the nose, and the anus. The *svādhiṣṭhāna cakra* is associated with water, taste, tongue, and the organ of procreation. Each of the *cakras* has numerous other attributes, many of which would appear to be purely symbolic. This is particularly so for the "higher" *cakras*, which are not associated with any of the base attributes at all. For example, each of the *cakras* is associated with a color, but the *sahasrāra* is said to be colorless. Moving beyond the realm of the five subtle elements, the *ājñā cakra* is said to have the attributes of *mahat tattva* (elemental consciousness) and the *sahasrāra* to be *tattva tit* (without any elemental attributes). Regardless of the apparently symbolic or metaphysical attributes of the higher *cakras*, it is clear from Yogeshwaranand's description that they have concrete physiological features (see also Majumdar 1999: 507–15):

> *Ājñā Cakra:* This *cakra* is located between the eyebrows in the region of the frontal sinus and ethmoid bone in the skull. Here are two glands like brown coloured sand particles. Surgeons consider them useless, but they are wrong because they do not know the actual function of these glands. They are bodies with electrical charges, one positive and one negative. (1997: 91–92)

In the case of each of the *cakras* there is a direct and important link between it and the particular features of the gross body with which it is associated. For example, "[The *svādhiṣṭhāna cakra*] shines in the area of the seminal vesicle like liquid in a golden cup. In *sattvik* state, it appears as pure as the Ganges water in blue saphire. . . . A vapour appears to arise from this center, pervading the entire body and affecting its functions, nourishing the limbs and bestowing peace. This vapour is water-predominating and has a special connection with phlegm, semen and other liquids of the body that are modifications of the water element" (1997: 86–87).

In terms of structural continuity, the *mūlādhāra cakra* and the *sahasrāra cakra* are of primary importance, since the latent energy of *prāṇa śakti* manifest in the form of *kuṇḍalinī* is located at the former and is channeled upward to emerge through the latter. Here again Yogeshwaranand's description shows how the gross body is directly implicated in the subtle process of final liberation.[19]

> The ascent of *Prāṇa* is described thus. By mental force of any form the *Prāṇa* starts performing the functions in the *cakra*-s without the inner light arising. *Apāna Prāṇa,* the vital air of the lower part of the body, becomes excited by constant strokes of meditation and churns the area of nerves and tissues in *Mūlādhāra,* the basal plexus, generating a vibratory movement of *Prāṇa* from the base of the head of the spinal cord. The experience of the movement resembles the movement of ants or the flow of warm water or vapour. Sometimes this inner touch becomes very cool and the entire body is thrilled, the hair standing on end. This is called *Prānotthāna.* This practice is said to destroy the preponderance of phlegm in the areas of the bunch of nerves at the basal plexus, after which the gliding movement of *Apāna* is clearly experienced in the spinal cord from *Mūlādhāra* to the top of *Suṣumṇā,* the spinal cord. (1997: 78–79)

The sensation of *prāṇa* flowing through the *suṣumṇā* is not an end in itself, but leads, progressively, to clearer and clearer visions of each of the *cakra*s and to deeper, purer, and more subtle states of meditation.

> By suffusion of vital electricity through the wires of *Suṣumṇā* the entire inner body with all its subtleties as well as the objects of the gross body all become illuminated, *Citta* (mind-stuff) disengages from the physical body and turns inwards, linking itself to the inner world. Then the divine light passes through *Suṣumṇā,* illuminating it as it infuses the *Prāṇa*-s in the channels of the spinal cord, causing the lotuses in the area of the body plexus to swell and blossom; removing obstruction in the functioning of the knowledge and action it reveals internal processes, lights up the arteries, veins, and nerves in the skeletal cage of the body and then enters the *Sahasrāra,* the thousand petalled lotus at the crown of the head. (1997: 80)

Lest it be thought that Yogeshwaranand's use of science to explain science is unique, here is an example from Shri Surath: "The toning of the nerves is the first step. The nerves must be strong in order to hold the inrush of Divine energy. Playing with the Cakras in meditation is a scientific method for toning the nerves and as meditation progresses through this process the cells become more and more refined. Divine grace is absorbed and spiritual strength increases" (1979: 96). Not only is this described with, and in terms of, the material body, but it is of critical importance to remember that Yogeshwaranand and many others writing in the genre base their descriptions of supramental being on direct personal experience. In this context it is necessary to note that scholars such as Agehananda Bharati have argued that any attempt to somaticize the physiology of *cakra*s is nonsense, since they are symbolic representations of the relationship between human beings and the cosmos and are significant purely in terms of meditation (1965).

Whether or not it is nonsense, the somaticization of the *cakras* is made possible by the very structure of yogic logic, a logic which is not based on simple contrast—duality versus nonduality, immateriality versus materialism. Nor is it made possible by the "commonplace and easy extinction of consciousness." As Eliade points out, the somatization of the *cakras* occurs on the "plane of paradox." Eliade's comprehensive study of Yoga unambiguously shows how the body is involved in enlightenment, and how it has become possible to take the paradoxical ontology of Yoga and fashion it into a science of meta-materialism. In many ways the following may be taken as a statement which prevents descriptions such as those provided by Yogeshwaranand from being discounted as mere nonsense:

> "Taking possession of oneself" [which is what the title *svāmī* denotes] radically modifies the human being's ontological condition. "Discovery of oneself," self-reflection of the *puruṣa,* causes a "rupture of plane" on the cosmic scale; when this occurs, the modalities of the real are abolished, being (*puruṣa*) coincides with nonbeing ("man" properly speaking), knowledge is transformed into magical "mastery," in virtue of the complete absorption of the known by the knower. . . . The self-revelation of the *puruṣa* is equivalent to a taking possession of being in all its completeness. In *asamprjñāta samādhi,* the yogi is actually all Being.[20] (Eliade 1990: 94–95)

Being as being human and being all Being reflects the irony of cyborg being. Following Eliade's discussion, the "sage as metaphysical cyborg" embodies the paradox of ruptured planes of reality: "Clearly, his situation is paradoxical. For he is in life, and yet liberated; he has a body, and yet he knows himself and thereby is *puruṣa*; he lives in duration, yet at the same time shares in immortality; finally, he coincides with all Being, though he is but a fragment of it" (1990: 95).

The Gross Science of Subtleties

The narratives constructed by Yogeshwaranand, Gopi Krishna, Swami Rama, and other masters who have experienced the awakening of *kuṇḍalinī* or the enstasy of *samādhi* provide a kind of firsthand, explorers' account of *prāṇic* flow. In many ways they are a curious synthesis of self-reflexive auto-autopsy report and first-contact ethnographic discovery narrative. The authors cut into the body of flesh and bone but describe a world so different as to defy translation—which is, again, one of the many points at which science comes into the picture. In any case, these accounts mirror the standard accounts given in the classical literature, and it is often difficult to know where experience ends and textual redaction begins. Regardless, there is a voluminous literature which seeks to make modern, scientific sense of the subtle processes described by Yogeshwaranand, Rajarshi Muni, and other adepts. This modern science seeks to explain transcendence in terms of the flow of *prāṇa*, and the vast majority of the modern literature on Yoga seeks to translate the energy of *prāṇa* into the agency of healing; to harness *prāṇa* and make it function as medicine.[21]

It must be remembered here that the modern, scientific literature—which will be described and analyzed at length in subsequent chapters—is not different in kind from the literature produced by Yogeshwaranand, Swami Rama, and Rajarshi Muni. It is a matter of subtle gradation, and here Swami Sivananda's short book *The Science of Prāṇāyāma* (1997b), first published in 1935 and now in its sixteenth edition, is a perfect case in point.

Before becoming a *jīvanmukta* in the late 1920s, Swami Sivananda was a physician who published a health journal and worked as a doctor in Malaya. Although little is known about him beyond what is made available by the organization he founded—which plays down his life before 1920—it is clear that even though he was born into a family of "saints, sages, and savants," and was, therefore, exposed to classical learning in his early years, Sivananda's teachings on Yoga were thought to be based on the direct experience of enlightenment. After leaving his practice in Malaya he renounced the world. As the publicity material published on the back of most of his books points out, after practicing "intense austerities," he became "a great Yogi, saint, sage and *Jīvanmukta.*" He settled in Rishikesh in the early 1920s. He studied there for the next ten years, a decade of profound creative ingenuity in the pan-Indian Yoga renaissance. In 1932 he established a Yoga *āśram* which evolved into the Divine Life Society, a nonsectarian center for the development of spiritual knowledge that was founded in 1936, followed in 1948 by the Yoga-Vedānta Forest Academy.

Having contributed directly and significantly to the popularization of modern Yoga—and perhaps more than anyone else to its transnationalization—Sivananda, his teachings, and the work of the Divine Life Society deserve to be the subject of a separate comprehensive study (see Strauss 1997, 2000). In the context of this work, however, what is important is the unambiguous way in which Sivananda, using the language of science, physiology, and health, talks about and explains liberation in *prāṇ*ic terms, and talks about and explains *prāṇa* in terms that are very down to earth. In the introduction to his book, Sivananda points out that "*Prāṇa* is the very essence of cosmic life, that subtle principle which evolved the whole universe into its present form and which is pushing it toward its ultimate goal. To the Yogi the whole universe is his body. The matter which composes his body is the same that evolved the universe. The force that pulsates through his nerves is not different from the force which vibrates through the universe" (1997b: x). As with all others who write on the subject, Sivananda has sections in his book dealing with the classification of *prāṇa, nāḍī* structure, and the symbolism and significance of the *cakras*. As will be discussed in greater detail in later chapters, he explains the techniques for performing *prāṇāyāma* exercises as these exercises are integral to meditation, concentration, and liberation. The single significant point to make here is that Swami Sivananda, perhaps one of the most important figures in the establishment of modern institutionalized spirituality in postcolonial India, understands the relationship between mind, body, and transcendence in these terms:

> *Prāṇa,* which alternates ordinarily between *Iḍā* and *Piṇgalā*. . . . will enter the *Suṣumṇā,* the central *Nāḍī.* After such entry it is that the Yogi becomes dead to the world, being in that state called *Samādhi.* Drawing up the *Apāna* and forcing down the *Prāṇa* from the throat, the Yogi free from old age, becomes a youth of sixteen. Through the practice of *Prāṇāyāma* chronic diseases, that defy Allopathic, Homeopathic, Āyurvedic and Unnani doctors will be rooted out. (1997b: 19)

This fusion and confusion of two sciences suffuse Sivananda's writing, and it is wrong to make a distinction between his spiritual and practical teachings, just as it is wrong to interpret Yogeshwaranand's teachings as purely or even primarily metaphysical. Science enables a metonymic understanding of what might otherwise be read as an elaborate analogy. It forces the question of empirical correspondence into the domain of metaphor, producing multiple level of mimesis within and across the divide between epistemology and ontology. Thus Sivananda is able to say, "if you retain the breath for one minute, this one minute is added to your life span" (1997b: 56), and that "when you massage the liver, spleen, stomach or any other portion or organ of the body, you can speak to the cells and give them orders: 'O cells! Discharge your functions properly. I command you to do so.' They will obey your orders. They too have got subconscious intelligence" (1997b: 84). In the specific context of "yogic diet" he also provides an answer to the question about why the involuntary sound made while belching is very often transformed, voluntarily, into the intonation *"Hari Om!"* As Sivananda writes, perhaps reflecting the Āyurvedic stipulation that natural urges should not be suppressed, "Take wholesome *Sattvic* food half stomachful. Fill a quarter with pure water. Allow the remaining quarter free for the expansion of gas and for propitiating the Lord" (1997b: 33).

The work of Yogeshwaranand, Rajarshi Muni, and Swami Sivananda, among numerous other *jīvanmuktas*—including Aurobindo and Vivekananda—defines a context within which one can critically examine the writing of secular scientists who study Yoga.

Supramental Health: Rats in the Maze of Yoga and Science

Several works exemplify the objectification of Yoga by "hard science," but none more clearly than Dr. K. N. Udupa's treatise entitled *Stress and Its Management by Yoga* (1989). This book is based on clinical research conducted in the 1970s by a team of medical scientists at the University Hospital of Banaras Hindu University on over one thousand patients diagnosed with stress disorders.

Diagnosed with cardiac neurosis and subsequently finding relief through the practice of Yoga, Udupa began to study the medical literature on stress and the classical literature on Yoga. His goal was to find an explanation for what causes stress disorders and why Yoga seemed to be an effective modality of treatment. He found, however, that "none of these books could give me a scientific explanation as to how these stress disorders are actually caused and why they are increasing at such a rapid rate all over the world" (1989: vii). On the basis of his review of the literature, Udupa found that there were two schools of thought concerning the etiology of stress, one focusing on the hypothalamus and the neuroendocrine apparatus and the other on the cerebral cortex. The experiments Udupa set up were designed to measure the relative influence of these two parts of the brain on the development of various psychological and physiological symptoms associated with stress. Further, and more significantly, his team conducted experiments on humans and other mammals to evaluate how Yoga could stimulate the brain in various ways to reduce stress. Over the course of several years research attention focused on the neurohumors. In the preface to the first edition of his treatise, Udupa explains what his experiments proved.

> We are convinced that it is the cerebral cortex, specially the psychic center, which is responsible for the initiation of all these stress disorders as a result of genetic susceptibility of a person receiving excessive environmental stimulation. Thus, the cerebral cortex in response to a strong stimulus initiates the changes in the whole body through the prompt liberation of neurohumors and hormones in an excessive quantity. It is at this stage that yogic practices would greatly help the patients to get over their trouble by decreasing their sensitivity to the environmental stimulation and thereby to these neurohumoral and hormonal changes. (1989: ix)

The question of exactly how Yoga can decrease sensitivity to environmental stimulation is the central question behind Udupa's research. And it is not at all a simple question, for which the answer might be that Yoga relieves stress by providing a structured environment for relaxation.

The structure of the book itself, and Udupa's detailed discussion of the experiments, reveals the extent to which he was in search of that illusive point of transformation between subtle and gross domains. The first 130 pages provide a comprehensive overview of the physiology and pathology of stress as it is explained in terms of a biomedical paradigm. There is a discussion of the brain as a whole and each of its subcortical centers, followed by three chapters on the neurohumors and neuroendocrinal change brought on by stress and various stimuli. These chapters are followed by four more dealing with the psychology, etiology, pathophysiology, and treatment of stress disorders. In general the level of technical scientific detail is greater than what would be found in a general undergraduate biology text and more comparable to what would be found in a medical school text on the subject. Even though the neurohumors acetylcholine, catecholamine, histamine, and serotonine in particular are integral to the experiments conducted, it is not necessary to go into detail regarding the biochemistry involved. Udupa summarizes the results of his experiments as follows: "From all of this we can conclude that the main initiating factor in the development of stress disorders is the increased liberation of neurohumors by the excessively stimulated cerebral cortex. Therefore, it is now understandable that if one can learn to restrain the cerebral cortex, especially its psychic center, one can be free from the development of various stress disorders throughout one's life" (1989: 359).

Udupa's hypothesis is that Yoga reduces stress through control of the cerebral cortex and the production of neurohumors. The whole book is about Yoga, and experiments conducted on Yoga in practice, but chapters 11 through 14 are devoted "exclusively" to the practice of Yoga as such, and a discussion of Yoga anatomy and physiology. Chapter 15 is devoted to a discussion of *kuṇḍalinī*, and here Udupa provides a discussion of the *nāḍī*s and each of the *cakra*s. Overall his conclusion is that

> physiologically speaking , it seems that the main aim of the practice of *Kuṇḍalinī* Yoga is to attain at first a voluntary control over the autonomic nervous system. This is usually followed by activation of the different centers of brain by transmitting certain specific neurohumors to these areas. . . . The main principle underlying the practice of *Kuṇḍalinī* Yoga is to arrange maximum supply of oxygen to each *cakra* and other centers so that they become awakened and active. In view of this *prāṇāyāma* becomes the essential part of the practice of *Kuṇḍalinī Yoga*. (1989: 215)

In Udupa's account of Yoga physiology there is a direct and unambiguous connection between the *nāḍī*s and the sympathetic nervous system and the *cakra*s and "the six autonomic plexuses of nerves" (1989: 188). In this context Udupa defines *prāṇa* and *prāṇāyāma* as follows:

> In actual fact [*prāṇāyāma*] has a deeper meaning [than controlled intake and outtake of breath]. It actually means the control of the cellular metabolism of the entire body as a result of regulated supply of oxygenated blood to various organs and tissues leading to the optimum release of energy for performing various bodily and mental functions. In the ordinary sense *prāṇa* can be equated with breath but in a deeper sense it can also be taken as energy liberated in the body at the level of each cell. Hence breathing in and out is the visible gross meaning of *prāṇāyāma,* whereas cellular respiration leading to liberation and utilization of energy in the organs is the real meaning of the word. (1989: 215)

There are many interesting aspects to this discussion, the most significant being the link that Udupa makes between gross breath, oxygen, *prāṇa, prāṇāyāma,* and the neurochemistry of liberation, on the one hand, and, on the other, the efficient use of energy on both the cellular level of biochemistry and the structural and functional level of anatomy.

With this in mind it is possible to make sense of what Udupa is getting at in chapter 11, entitled "Studies on Physiological Aspects of Yoga." In struggling with the problem of objectivity, variable delineation, reproducibility of results, and overall standardization, Udupa wrestled with the question of whether to experiment on adepts in Yoga *sādhana,* untrained neophytes, or some group of practitioners in between these two extremes. In the end he conducted experiments using all these categories of person. But he also conducted a series of experiments that can be said to have had a profound impact on the conceptualization of Yoga as science—and science as Yoga—if only because they pose the question of what distinguishes humankind from the rest of the natural world in a radical way. In experiments with fruit flies, guinea pigs, corn, and almost anything else that reproduces, the question itself has been anticipated by Modern Science for several centuries. But not until recently—with developments in cross-species organ transplantation, genetic engineering, and cloning—has there been rapidly increasing appreciation of what the radical implications of this are for a reconceptualization of nature, and the reification by culture of nature and so-called natural categories.

Chapter 11 concerns neurohumoral changes, measured in terms of acetylcholine, cholinesterase, diamineoxidase, and catecholamine levels, before and after specific yogic procedures performed for various lengths of time per day over the course of various durations of time, ranging from days to weeks to months. The procedures include basic *āsana*s and combinations of *āsana*s as well as meditation. Summarizing the results of one study, Udupa points out that the experiment "shows a marked raise of acetylcholine in the blood after 10 days of intensive course in meditation with a slight rise of catecholamine. This indicates an increase in the capacity of these persons to do intellectual work." Another experiment on metabolic and endocrine changes shows "considerable reduction in plasma cortisol, urinary hydroxycorticoids and urinary nitrogen after a course of meditation" (1989: 156).

The purpose of detailing this here is not so much to make a point about the nature of meditation alone as an object of scientific study but simply to contextualize Udupa's more radical contribution. In order to test the validity of his experiments on human subjects, Udupa did the following:

> In order to study the effect of postural changes on various organs and tissue and also to assess the stress competence we conducted these studies on rats. In this study rats were kept on head stand posture in glass tubes with open ends. We kept these animals in the head low posture for one hour daily up to six weeks. At the end of 1, 2, 3, 4, 6 and 8 weeks, various neurohumors such as acetylcholine, adrenaline, noradrenaline were estimated in the blood and tissues. The psychological effects of this posture were also determined with the help of T-maze before and after experiment.
>
> In another experiment rats were kept in a head low posture for a period of 4 weeks and then they were exposed to various types of acute stress such as exposure to cold, electric shock, psychic shock and immobilization stress. In these studies, the stress response of these animals was compared with that of control animals. (1989: 146–47)

There is no question but that this experiment is designed to produce scientific data. The radical nature of Udupa's shift from people to laboratory rats is not in finding a malleable mammalian proxy for tests that cannot be conducted on human subjects, nor is it in factoring the messiness of culture out of what might count for instinctive human nature. The radical nature of the experiment is in its logical, philosophical conclusion—that on yogic terms humans and rats are fundamentally, rather than analogically, the same. Even though many Yoga postures are named after animals—cocks, peacocks, turtles, cows, dogs, lions—to the best of my knowledge no one has ever suggested that animals can perform Yoga. In other words, the animal basis of Yoga postures has been regarded as metaphorical and based on mythology. And yet, in many ways, Yoga *sādhana* is the embodied performance of our "animal nature," at least insofar as culture—including our cultural perception of nature—is a misperception of reality. This turns on its head the relationship between humans and animals in the context of laboratory science and allows for a realization that is integral to Yoga: that although the practice of Yoga is a construction of culture, the construction of culture is not a necessary condition for the experience of Yoga as final liberation. As in the case of Yogeshwaranand's physically manifest metaphysical *cakra*s, this, too, is a "rupture of planes" of reality. It brings into focus a paradox wherein *citta* is both intellect and beyond intellectual comprehension: "The *Citta* is present in every animal being from the lowest to the highest form, but it is only in the human form that we find it as the intellect (*Buddhi*). Vivekananda said, until the mind-stuff can take the form of intellect, it is not possible for it to return through all these steps and liberate the soul. Immediate salvation is impossible for a cow or a dog" (Majumdar 1999: 5).

In terms of a sociology of science, where science and scientific knowledge are understood as a cultural construct, headstanding rats are simply part of a much larger story in which laboratory animals are used to discover useful scientific facts, but the methods of science that go into the discovery of those facts produce a cultural account about the relationship between humans and nonhuman animals. Experimenting on nonhuman animals to test a hypothesis about neurochemistry entails a complex kind of myth making, even when one is concerned only with the neurochemistry of the animals in question, in this case rats. It is pure magic—in the sense that magic is based on the misperception of mimesis—when the difference between the animals in question is rendered either significant or insignificant depending on the level of induction being engaged in. What the headstanding rats reveal in terms of a sociology of knowledge is not that modern Yoga is pseudoscience, but that Modern Science is a kind of pseudo-Yoga insofar as it seeks endless progress and perfect knowledge—the correlates of immortality and freedom—within a framework where progress and perfect knowledge will always be illusive and therefore illusory.

But the point is not to see Yoga and science as farcically mimetic of each other, for that would entail taking neither one seriously. Headstanding rats and Supramental Beings—creatures of social reality and creatures of science fiction standing hand in hand on the threshold of a new world, to adapt and combine key phrases in the epigraphs taken from Haraway and Anantharaman—demand blasphemy.

The body of this book is concerned with the metaphysical anatomy of yogic cyborgs—Human Beings who, in some sense, have embodied or seek to embody the Universe and manifest immortality and freedom. It is informed by analytic blasphemy, where what is blasphemed is the concept of culture, the culture of science, and the culture of Yoga. I will return, in the final chapter, to broader questions of skepticism, relativism, and the irony embodied by headstanding rats.

PART 2

YOGA'S MODERN HISTORY AND PRACTICE

The method [of Yoga] comprises a number of different techniques (physiological, mental, mystical) but they all have one characteristic in common—they are antisocial, or, indeed, antihuman. . . . All of the yogic techniques invite one and the same gesture—to do exactly the opposite of what human nature forces one to do. . . . The orientation always remains the same—to react against the "normal," "secular," and finally human inclination.

Mircea Eliade, *Yoga: Immortality and Freedom* (1990: 95, 96)

Abandon *dharma* and *adharma;* abandon truth and falsehood. Having abandoned both truth and falsehood, abandon the mind by which you abandon everything.

Mahābhārata (XII.316.40)

3

SWAMI KUVALAYANANDA: SCIENCE, YOGA, AND GLOBAL MODERNITY

> It was here [Amalner] that [Swami Kuvalayananda] began to study and present Yoga along scientific lines. . . . India's age old Yoga was veiled and shrouded in mystery as also it was over-laid by numerous crusts of blind beliefs and irrelevant superstitions. In one word it was unscientific. Hence it had scant appeal to the modern mind. Shri Swamiji fully realized that its scientific presentation was indispensable to put it in its right perspective for benefit not only of India but of the world at large.
>
> S. M. Chingle (1975: 45)

Decentering the Nation: Recontextualizing Global Modernities

RECENT DEVELOPMENTS in history and the social sciences have made it clear that power can no longer be understood simply as a one-dimensional force that some people have and others do not. It is vested in culture to such an extent that it defines the framework for all social interaction. Which is not to say that all life is a struggle, but simply that there is no neutral ground on which to stand and no single perspective on truth. At the same time, as cultural reality is increasingly understood as constructed, the question of how different constructions struggle for legitimacy has become increasingly important. This is particularly so in colonial and postcolonial contexts, where the nature of power is both simplified in terms of authority and control under some circumstances and extremely complicated under others, and where the "constructedness" of culture seems to throw into question the most basic criteria of self-definition by undermining a sense of unambiguous continuity with the past.

Scholarship on colonial and postcolonial India in particular has focused on the critical problem of identity, control over identity, and the articulation of a national identity which is neither anachronistically "traditional" in an Orientalist sense nor derivatively Western—and thereby modern only by proxy—on account of colonialism and the colonial legacy. Most scholars now agree that colonial India was, and postcolonial India is, characterized by a degree of deep ambivalence concerning the whole question of modernization and development. Although there are obvious examples of those who wholeheartedly embraced various features of Western modernity and other examples of individuals and groups who have just as wholeheartedly rejected this modernity in favor of what they see as some sort of pure tradition, it is clear that numerous individuals, deeply concerned about their identity, fall somewhere in the middle and struggle to remake both the past and the future into a new, hybrid present. Some of the clearest expressions of this have been in the context of nationalism, and scholars such as Partha Chatterjee (1993), Gyan Prakash (1999), David Arnold (1993), Ashis Nandy (1995), and many others have shown that various manifestations of Indian nationalism are linked to, but not simply limited by, the whole apparatus of colonialism and the imperial legacy.

My own work over the past several years has benefited greatly from this body of scholarship on Indian nationalism and the whole question of how the terms of modernity are worked out. The question of how resistance precipitates out of hegemony and the apparent paradox of contestation through conformity is fascinating and provocative insofar as it clearly points in a direction where the problem of agency can be reconciled with depersonalized power and the construction and deconstruction of culture. Understandably much of the literature on Indian nationalism takes for granted that India, however it is defined, is the appropriate frame of reference for analysis. Indeed, one might say that it is not only understandable but a non sequitur as well—is it not only natural that India should define the framework within which Indian identity should be worked out? But is it natural that nationalism should define the limits of modern identity? Is Indian modernity bounded by nationalism, or is it, albeit located within a politically defined state, nevertheless capable of a more unbounded global vision? Is it possible for people living in India to imagine more than their community? What are their perspectives on the world as a whole?

Obviously people living in India have a didactically modern perspective on the world, but it is striking the extent to which scholarship assumes that colonialism and postcolonialism breed introspection, and that this introspection, though not passively hegemonic, is, nevertheless, viewed as comprehensive. Much of the current literature either explicitly or implicitly allows colonialism and the West to function as a mirror—if not a framework—in which visions people living in India have of themselves and the world are reflected only as nationalist, anticolonial, or postcolonial. This is even true in the case of Partha Chatterjee's seminal work which has pushed the question of nationalism about as close to the limit—as that limit is defined by colonialism and the West—as it can be pushed (1993). Many analyses of these reflected visions are extremely powerful. But a preoccupation with the nationalism/colonialism conundrum has, ironically, meant that Indian visions of what is possible in the field of *human* experience have not been recognized for what they are—alternative global modernities and not just alternative modernities for and of India.

There is a flip side to this—scholarship that has as its primary focus the question of globalization and the culture of transnationalism. Much of this scholarship is rightly concerned with the link between local cultural constructions and the transnational structure of cultural creativity. However, in showing how myths of cultural continuity are destabilized, how identity is problematized and boundaries blurred, the strength of globalization theory is also its weakness: in rightly breaking apart intellectual myths of categorical difference there is a tendency toward homogenization. At the very least, theories concerned with transnationalism are not well tuned to a consideration of how difference is maintained, even though adept scholars like Arjun Appadurai are able to build this into their analyses (1996). In other words, it is all too easy to say that Yoga has become a transnational phenomenon—much like cricket, Christianity, and democracy—but much more difficult to figure out why it takes on very different significance in different places and at different times, while still remaining the same. But the same in relation to what?

Another way of putting this is simply that in analyses of globalization it is imperative to not let "the local" stand—as a neatly binary, symmetrical balance—simply as a passive proxy for that which is not global. The implicit verticality of power in this structure needs to be critically and carefully examined so as not to restage the crimes of colonialism and reinscribe a two-dimensional understanding of power. It is also important not to let "the local" stand in and provide a "solution" to the problem of agency. It is very seductive, when trying to analyze the discursive nature of power as a transcultural phenomenon, to anchor one's analysis in the reality of a specific place, and let real people—informants—articulate answers to questions that simply cannot be localized. Obviously what people say is grist for the mill, but if theories of globalization and transnationalism are going to do anything more than simply increase the scope of study and draw attention to the complexity of transcultural constructions, then analytically "the local" must not succumb to the temptation of present-tense empiricism. It must, rather, be made to embody the shifting reality of history—past, present, and future.

Science and the Localization of Global Modernities

In his book *Another Reason*, Gyan Prakash provides an important and insightful analysis of the relationship between science and colonialism in modern India (1999). Among other things he shows how science was produced by colonialism as a means by which to both build up and modernize, and keep down and control, the population of India. As Prakash points out, taking a broad perspective on the place of science in society, Indian modernity is constituted by dislocation and disorientation as concerns the meaning and place of science in society.

> Indian modernity has always existed as an internally divided process. An aura of dislocation and disorientation has always accompanied Indian modernity's existence. I do not mean this in a negative sense; uncertainties and estrangements point to its sources of creativity and to possibilities of new arrangements and new accommodations. There is simply no way to tidy up this messy history of India and narrate it as the victory of capital over community, modernity over tradition, West over non-West. These neat oppositions exist side by side with the history of their untidy complicities and intermixtures. (1999: 234)

As I have argued elsewhere, the case of Mahatma Gandhi illustrates this point in general and more specifically shows the way in which the nationalism-colonialism-science nexus produces bodies of knowledge about the body and the place of the body in the state (Alter 2000a). Although Prakash locates the body within the discourses of modernization and science, and shows very well how the state is concerned with bodies—in the collective, and precisely problematic, sense of population—he does not go into great detail on the particular mechanics of body discipline, but concerns himself with science's objectification of the body and bodies of knowledge. As a result his analysis of Indian modernity is constrained by the Indianness of context, since that is how forms of knowledge are defined. Although the body can most certainly be linked to nationalism, it, unlike ideas and the disciplinary construction of ideas, has the advantage of not being predefined as a thing with social, let alone national, significance. For better or worse, the body can be regarded as an object of nature in the most comprehensive and putatively primordial sense of the term. It can thus signify the essential features of being, and be subject to discipline on these very broad, transnational terms, terms that are very intimate on a level that cuts across the plane of state, community, and nation by virtue of being, in essence, generically human.

Through an analysis of Swami Kuvalayananda's laboratory research on Yoga physiology, this chapter will show how research that started out as "hard-core" scientific nationalism transmuted into a universalist philosophy of science and a kind of dislocated transnational humanism rooted in the body. The work done at Kuvalayananda's laboratory manifests the kind of profound creativity Prakash speaks of, but the uncertainties, estrangements, and outright mistakes that inspired and informed this creativity are linked directly to the body on the one hand and the idea of the Universe on the other, rather than to the state or the idea of community and nation.

Although there are any number of examples of "things Indian" that have achieved a global status—Deepak Chopra comes to mind, as does New Age Āyurveda, Krishna Consciousness, and Rajneesh—they have done so as inherently Indian things. In other cases the reach of India around the globe is regarded simply as modern if not diasporically ultra-modern, as in the case of "Indian" dominance in the field of IT technology (just look at the demographics of the Silicon Valley) and disproportionate expertise in the medical field (just look at the demographics of Pittsburgh, New Jersey, and New York City), where "community" is marked—in terms of model minority status—but Culture with a capital "C" does not much matter. Unlike the export of other things Indian, Yoga can be regarded as either inherently Indian or as ultra-modern and therefore ambiguously, and "inconsistently," Indian. Consider the contrast between the government of India's essentialist representation of Rishikesh as the birthplace of Yoga, and Jane Fonda's Yoga workout for pregnant women, or almost any recent issue of the *Yoga Journal*. This contrast—magnified by virtue of the fact that Yoga of the Jane Fonda variety is taught at upscale body boutiques in Chennai, Delhi, and Bombay, among other places—can have a profoundly destabilizing effect on nationalism. Significantly, however, the instability of nationalism signals the possibility of a history of India that is not defined by the logic of colonial history, postcolonial historiography, or even the borders of the Indian state.

Kuvalayananda and his associates did not invent the kind of Yoga that has become a transnational phenomenon, but their research made it possible for this kind of Yoga to be invented. They had their sights—and their microscopes, X-ray machines, and blood pressure gauges—set on discovering new laws of universal nature. Their scientific focus on the human body enabled a translation of a branch of Indian philosophy into a form of practice that is, like Modern Science itself, putatively free of cultural baggage while clearly linked to the history of a particular part of the world. In this regard it is not so much that Yoga is postcolonial, as that it is post-Western. It is for India in its relationship to the world what science was in the global imaginary of empire. And that is both reassuring and frightening, since power is very much in flux. The unbridled capitalist ethic manifest in the pages of the *Yoga Journal* is as insidious in its implications as the nationalist rhetoric expressed in the pages of *Yog Manjari,* a magazine that promotes conservative Hindu values in the guise of embodied Universal Brotherhood (Alter 1997).

To some degree this is enabled by the way in which the universe—as well as universal space, time, and embodied experience—is conceptualized in Yoga. Fundamental to Yoga is the idea that transcendence is the experience of freedom from the binding constraints of perception, as perception, even the most cerebral, is a function of embodied, elemental being. In an important way the principle of absolute perfection, manifest as the immobilization of mind, breath, and semen, and the final piercing of consciousness,[1] produces a paradox reflected in all the magical powers known as *siddhis*. The embodied self is also the universal Self, and therefore both all pervasive in a universal, cosmic sense and manifest in the localized person and "personality" of a *jīvanmukta*.[2] As a kind of cosmicized everyman, the *jīvanmukta* is to Yoga what the scientist is to science: a person who embodies the principles of perfection, be it dispassionate objectivity or blissful transcendence.

Along these lines, it makes sense to speak of science in England, Germany, or Japan. But to speak of Japanese or German science—or even Japanese or German scientists—evokes a kind of nationalism that cuts against the very idea of science. Similarly, to speak of a *jīvanmukta* in India, England, or the United States geopolitically locates, and problematically situates and gives subjective position to, an ontologically "dislocated" universal soul. In other words, the very idea of a *jīvanmukta* is rather antithetical to the idea of bounded culture and the cultural politics of nationalism. One could, of course, say the same for a soul saved by the Holy Spirit or liberated by the grace of any particular God, but religion localizes belief under the mantel of universal truth and thereby confuses belief and transcendence, the idea of god and Truth. The beauty of Yoga is that—nominal etymology and philosophical contextualization in Sanskrit and sanskritic literature notwithstanding—is that it can be convincingly universal in universalist terms. After all, Modern Science, itself a localized product of the European Enlightenment, has succeeded in achieving this same transmutation of knowledge-apart-from-culture. Through the epic mythos of rationality and an objective, empiricist, truth-in-nature epistemology, science produces—at least in theory—a profound and powerful disinterest in value. It is this metacorrespondence between Yoga and Modern Science that inspired Kuvalayananda, and caused him, in a sense, to lose interest in nationalism, both as a political cause and as an intellectual frame of reference for experimentation. As the very idea of Yoga became more and more central to his life and work, the idea of India was absorbed into a larger vision of the world.

Although Kuvalayananda started his career as an ardent and active nationalist, over the years his perspective expanded, and much like Aurobindo, who left politics to explore spirituality, Kuvalayananda drifted away from nationalism into transnationalism—although he obviously never used the term—and used science to anchor his worldview in Yoga. Thus he made a quintessentially Indian "tradition" the basis for a global modernity rooted in the subtle body.

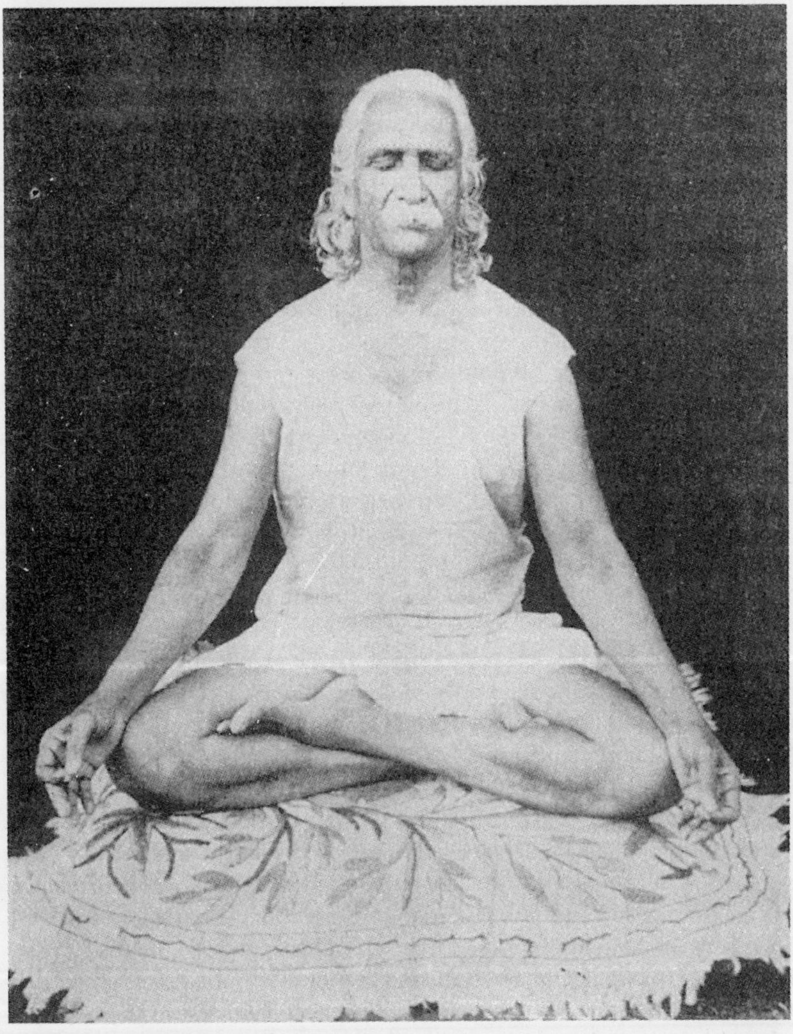

3. Swami Kuvalayananda in meditation. *Source: Swami Kuvalayananda Birth Centenary, 1984* (Lonavala: Kaivalyadhama, 1984), illus. on page 51. Reproduced with permission from Kaivalyadhama Ashram.

A crucial point in this regard, however, has to do with the degree of consciousness Kuvalayananda had about the consequences of his project. Intentionality and conscious agency are, as I have intimated above, problematic concepts to deal with precisely, because they presume coherence and rest on the assumption that actors control a particular domain of experience, be it intellectual, institutional, or ideological. Consequently, to attribute agency to local actors is to render them subject to structural forces that "transcend their consciousness," so to speak. I will return to this point in the final chapter. But as it is relevant here the attribution of agency to persons is a theoretical formulation at the base of the tragic conundrum wherein nationalism reenacts the crimes of colonialism by trying to "disarticulate" India from the West and modernity from tradition. In this regard Prakash is absolutely right to point out that an aura of dislocation and uncertainty is integral to the creativity in Indian modernity. A history of this modernity must take full account of the hybridization of community and state, science and culture, the secular and the religious (1999: 237). The analytic problem, however, is in ascribing "uncertainty" and "disorientation" to modern visionaries who embody this hybridization, without making them look naive or foolish—for they were not.

To my mind the solution is presented by the problem itself, for disorientation and uncertainty can only really be understood as creative in the public sphere, and appreciated as such from the vantage point of history. Otherwise you are relentlessly confronted by the fact—rather than by the interpretation of those facts as that interpretation produces a historical reality—that Jagadis Chandra Bose, for example, believed that plants had emotions, that Mahatma Gandhi believed that no one should have sex, and that Prime Minister Morarji Desai drank his own urine for health. You are left, in other words, with paradoxes, partitioned selves, and quirky personalities rather than with a sense of the creative possibility born of the particulate confusion manifest in human action. By dislocating creativity from agency, even the agency manifest in the multiple and multiplex words and deeds of subaltern and minor lives—which is, ultimately, where Prakash (1999: 237) and many others rest their case—one can see how "confusion" produces a coherent critique of all things that masquerade as coherent when mapped out historically in terms of what might be called—in keeping with the sense of creativity manifest in strange estrangements—disinterested and depersonalized biography.

Kaivalyadhama: Advancing beyond the "Fierce Light of Modern Science"

Upon visiting Kaivalyadhama, the institute where Swami Kuvalayananda conducted laboratory experiments on Yoga, Pandit Moti Lal Nehru, father of India's first prime minister, said: "I have been very much impressed with the work of Swami Kuvalayananda. He opened out an entirely new field of research and has shown that the different aspects of Yogic Culture Therapy could not only stand the fierce light of modern sciences but are well in advance of all that has so far been discovered in the West. His institution has already built up a reputation to the successful application of Yogic Principles and practices to modern conditions of life" (quoted in Wakharkar 1984: 8).

It was not at all unique, even in the context of the nationalist struggle, for "nationalists" like Sri Aurobindo and Vivekananda to have been concerned with the spiritual, moral, and social reform of *all* "mankind," and not just "mankind in India." Yet it is still relatively uncommon to orient analyses away from the inherently bounded idea of Indian philosophy, Indian spirituality, and Indian science and take seriously the way in which Moti Lal Nehru saw Kuvalayananda's work as being concerned with nothing less than "the modern conditions of life."

In important ways Swami Kuvalayananda's scientific work can be compared to the work of Jagadis Chandra Bose who, after making important contributions in the field of physics through the study of electrical waves, turned his attention to the analysis of plant physiology. While his work in physics was "orthodox," his study of plants was decidedly "unorthodox"—and therefore ingeniously creative. By means of scientific procedures he was trying to demonstrate that plants had emotions so as to prove that there was a rational, empirical basis to Vedāntic philosophy. Āshis Nandy has analyzed the career of Jagadis Chandra Bose from a psychological perspective, demonstrating how he struggled to reconcile the two dimensions of his personality (1995). It would be possible to find in Swami Kuvalayananda many of the same tensions between rational positivism and speculative philosophical monism. Here, however, the focus is less on the Swami's personality and more explicitly on the nature of science as he put it into practice, and how that practice—rigorously rational to the end—evolved into an implicit critique of the ontology of nature upon which science in general is founded. Following from this, the analytical goal here is to get past the personal conflicts engendered by colonial nationalism and radically deprovincialize the Swami's global vision, while keeping both its precise location and its inherently fragmentary form in sharp focus.

Swami Kuvalayananda was born Jagannath Ganesh Gune on August 30, 1883, in the town of Dabhoi in what is now Gujarat. In 1903 he won a Jagannath Shankarsheth Sanskrit Scholarship to study at Baroda University, from which he was graduated in 1910. As a young man Gune was influenced by the nationalist ideas of Lokmanya Tilak as well as by the teaching of Sri Aurobindo, who taught at the university. Most directly he was influenced by Professor Rajratan Manikrao, who was actively promoting indigenous forms of physical education for the overall improvement of youth, as well as more combative martial arts that could be deployed in the nationalist struggle. On the basis of these influences, Gune is said to have taken a lifelong vow of celibacy and set himself the following goals: "(1) Prepare the young generation for service of the country; (2) master the Indian system of physical education and integrate it with general education; and (3) bring together science and spirituality by coordinating the spiritual aspects of Yoga with modern science" (Wakharkar 1984: 3). Although these goals were congruent, and the first was an implicit feature of the second two, it is nevertheless possible to focus on each separately. Here I wish to focus on the third.

During the time when he was teaching for the Khandesh Education Society between 1916 and 1923, and at roughly the same time that he was serving as the principal of the National College at Amalner, Gune came in contact with Sriman Parmahamsa Madhavdasji Maharaj, a *sannyāsi* who, through the practice of Yoga, had acquired *siddhi*s (supernatural powers). Although Gune had been introduced to the practice of Yoga under the guidance of Rajratan Manikrao, and had undoubtedly studied Yoga philosophy, it was Madhavdasji who inspired him to conduct research on the "uncanny psychophysical effects" of various higher states of yogic consciousness. As D. G. Wakharkar, a close associate of Gune's, puts it: "the materialist in him sought a scientific explanation [for these effects] . . . and he decided to devote his life to the study of Yoga on scientific lines and its correct interpretation to the common man" (1984: 4). The problem of providing a "correct interpretation" goes hand in hand with the question of finding scientific explanations for yogic powers, for Kuvalayananda felt that mystical, secretive, and arcane interpretations of Yoga obscured the truth rather than revealed it. This was not at all to say that Gune sought to "secularize" and purely objectify Yoga or define its truth value in terms of science. Rather he wanted to reveal the basic Universal Truth manifest in Yoga by demystifying it through science. Thus, in his view, there had to be explanations for how and why yogic power could be achieved, and the idea that these powers were magical was to him anathema. What Gune wanted to do was to challenge the exclusionary teaching of so-called occultists, and recover what he regarded as pure Yoga manifest in the teaching of sages like Madhavdasji and reflected in the classical texts. In Kuvalayananda's view Madhavdasji's power proved that the classical literature revealed the truth; what he himself had to prove was that this truth was based on natural laws and universal principles. In some sense, pure, objective science was to be deployed as the handmaiden of spirituality and orthodox philosophy so as to establish what came to be the theme of his life's work: "Yoga has a complete message for humanity. It has a message for the human body. It has a message for the human mind. It has a message for the human soul. Will intelligent and capable youth come forth to carry this message to every individual, not only in India but also in every part of the world?"

The problem in trying to make science conform to spirituality was the driving force behind Gune's creativity—as it was for Bose—for he was intent on finding the objective, rational means by which to measure and test the power of extrasensory perception and transcendental consciousness—the means, that is, to link up, in a fully modern way, body, mind and soul. Although most, if not all, of Gune's experiments concern themselves with the body—at least insofar as embodied effects reflect the influence of transformed consciousness—it is important to keep in mind that a kind of profound philosophical spirituality justified the whole project.

Gune's first experiments were conducted at the State Hospital, Baroda, and were designed to measure the physiological effects of two yogic procedures, *uḍḍiyāna* and *nauli.* In *Āsanas,* the most well known of his books, he describes *uḍḍiyāna* as follows:

> [I]t is an exercise of the diaphragm and the ribs. [Assume a standing position, bent at the waist, with hands resting on thighs, just above the knees]. This position of the hands enables them to be firmly pressed against their support and thus to fix up the muscles of the neck and the shoulders. Having taken this posture the student secures the deepest possible expiration by vigorously contracting the front muscles of the abdomen. The chest also stands contracted. While the breath is held out, the muscles of the neck and shoulders are fixed up by firmly pressing the hands either against the knees or against the thighs, as the case may be. Then a vigorous mock inhalation is attempted by raising the ribs and by not allowing the air to flow into the lungs. Simultaneously the front abdominal muscles are completely relaxed. . . .
>
> In Sanskrit, *Uḍḍiyāna* means "raising up" and *Bandha* means "contracting of particular anatomical parts." This exercise is called *Uḍḍiyāna-Bandha* because of the muscular contractions described above enable the spiritual force to raise up. Anatomically this *Bandha* may be called *Uḍḍiyāna* because it raises the diaphragm. (Kuvalayananda 1993: 37–38)

In a subsequent chapter careful consideration will be given to the significance of this subtle but important conflation of the diaphragm, breath, and the spiritual force, but in the present context *uḍḍiyāna bandha* simply defines the spirito-anatomical parameters for *nauli,* which is described by Gune in great detail (1993: 88–92).[3] Basically *nauli* entails the isolated contraction of the left, central, and right abdominal recti, and then their respective relaxation, such that one "rolls" the recti first clockwise and then counterclockwise. The nature of the push is important and entails considerable practice, as does the ability to isolate the recti one from another. In any case, *nauli* is performed while the breath is being held and the diaphragm is pulled upward.

It is necessary to understand the specific features of these yogic techniques to appreciate the nature of Gune's first experiment. Using a malometer pressure gauge and an X-ray machine, and building his hypothesis on the principle of a purificatory *kriyā* procedure called *basti,* where water is drawn into the colon while performing *nauli,* Gune inserted the gauge into the rectum of an adept practitioner in order to see whether or not a vacuum was created in the large intestine. As Wakharkar notes: "[D]uring the practices of *Nauli,* the pressure inside the large intestines becomes less than the outside atmospheric pressure, thus creating a vacuum. This being a completely new finding, Swamiji associated this vacuum or negative pressure with the name of his revered Gurudeva and called [it] 'Madhavdasa Vacuum'" (1984: 5). Following on his success, Gune sent letters to Rabindranath Tagore, Jagadis Chandra Bose, and Dr. Nadgir, all of whom, he felt, would appreciate the nature of what he had discovered. And what he had discovered was, he believed, one of the precise points of convergence between gross anatomy and the subtle power manifest in yogic physiology. What made this a "completely new" discovery was not so much reflected in the data as such, as in the way in which a specific methodology of science made it possible for two different kinds of "data" to manifest themselves in the same space at the same time as a consequence of the same kind of action—a kind of empirical harmonic chord created by the simultaneous intonation of science and spirituality.

On the basis of this initial success, Gune set about trying to raise the funds to establish a research center devoted exclusively to the study of Yoga in scientific terms. In October 1924 he established the Kaivalyadhama Yoga Ashram in Lonavala, a small hill resort on the lip of the western ghats between Pune and Bombay. At this time, just as his research started to take on the form of institutionalized laboratory science, Gune retreated into his āśram/laboratory and took on the name of Swami Kuvalayananda. The "Objectives of Kaivalyadhama," which appear on all of the institute's publications, provide a perspective on his vision: "The main effort of the Kaivalyadhama is in scientifically probing the human mind and to dig deeper and deeper in the inner space, till the effort to conquer the outer and inner spaces converged and ultimately meet to solve the riddle of the cosmos."

With financial assistance primarily from the ruler of Porbandar state, Kuvalayananda established the Rana Natwarsingh Pathological Laboratory. This laboratory was divided into branches for specialized research in biochemical analysis, electrophysiology, radiology, psychology, and physiology/physical education. The laboratory was equipped with the most up-to-date equipment available, such as the Haldane gas analysis apparatus. Experiments began almost immediately following the establishment of the laboratory, and the results were published regularly in *Yoga Mimamsa,* the Ashram's journal. In addition to being designed as a journal focused on the nexus of spirituality and science, it was also designed, with sections entitled "scientific," "semi-scientific," and "popular," to cut across boundaries of readership and appeal to both specialists and the "common man." According to Wakharkar, "*Yoga Mimamsa* was received very well and highly praised not only in India but by the experts in the fields of psychology and physiology in England, France, Germany and America in the West" (1984: 5).

Careful attention will be given to the nature of the experiments conducted by Kuvalayananda between 1924 and 1966, and then to an intense period of research in the late 1970s and the 1980s, but first it is necessary to give a more comprehensive sense of the Ashram's organization. This, in conjunction with the journal's international appeal, reflects the global scope of the Swami's visionary creativity.

In addition to conducting research, one of Swami Kuvalayananda's life goals was to teach and train young people to practice Yoga in order to maintain health. Thus Kaivalyadhama was open to the public. According to the Ashram's own publications, the demand for classes in Yoga and for Yoga that could be used in the therapeutic treatment for various disease was so great that in 1936 the Iswardas Chunilal Mehta Health Center was opened in Bombay. In 1928 Kuvalayananda initiated what he called philosophico-literary work, wherein classical texts were interpreted and translated with the help of "shastric" scholars trained in Sanskrit and "doctors of literature" trained in English. In 1929 a postgraduate course was started that gave its disciples official credentials in yogic studies.

Over the years the activities of Kaivalyadhama expanded in scale and scope such that in 1944 Kuvalayananda decided to formalize the Ashram's activities by registering it as an official society under the name Shreeman Madhava Yoga Mandira Samiti (SMYMS). The Rules and Regulations of the Samiti are published in a thirty-eight-page booklet, and their extreme detail and precision provide significant insight into the way in which institutions of civil society were being imagined at this time. Of particular significance here, however, is the way in which the "objectives for which the Samiti is established," published in twenty subsections of the "Memorandum of Association," reflect the expanding scope of Kuvalayananda's vision. The work of the Samiti was to "help establish and maintain academies, laboratories, and libraries" for the "promotion of the science of Yoga"; to "establish and run colleges either independently or affiliated to recognized universities, Indian or foreign, for training recruits to join research service either under the Samiti or elsewhere to help the spread of scientific Yoga in India and abroad"; to establish indoor and outdoor clinics, publish catalogues, digests, and concordances of yogic books; to deputize Samiti members to help other institutions throughout the country develop programs in the study of scientific Yoga; and to function as a trust so as to apply for government grants, accept charitable donations, and, in turn, to give loans and award prizes and otherwise operate as a foundation (Memorandum of Association and Rules and Regulations, Kaivalyadhama n.d.: 1–3).

Under the rubric of the SMYM Samiti the activities of Kaivalyadhama were organized into three departments and a college—the departments of scientific research, philosophico-literary research, and therapeutic research and the Gordhandas Seskaria College of Yoga and Cultural Synthesis (Sathe 1975: 24). Whereas the work of the scientific department will be the focus here, this work needs to be understood in the context of the larger, more comprehensive project. Scholars working in the philosophico-literary department were assigned the task of preparing and publishing "critical editions of old Yogic Sanskrit Texts that have been lost, from quotations occurring in commentaries on other texts" (Sathe 1975: 24). In other words, this was a large-scale project designed to reconstitute the classics out of fragmentary references and make them into whole texts. Apart from making these texts available, cross-referencing various sources, and providing critical commentary, the project had the effect of making the standard canon of yogic literature more comprehensive. The publication of these texts was designed to demystify Yoga along literary lines and to constitute it as a modern, text-based philosophy, just as science was to demystify yogic physiology.

Kuvalayananda was aware of the extent to which Yoga was not just a philosophy, and not just physical culture, but rather a system of knowledge manifest in action—physical philosophy, one might say. Therefore training practitioners of Yoga who could then teach Yoga was as important as formalizing textual knowledge. With this in mind, and with a donation from Seth Makhanlal Seskaria, the Gordhandas Seskaria College of Yoga and Cultural Synthesis was founded in 1950. The college offers a graduate diploma and an undergraduate certificate, as well as month-long courses for teachers and instructors of physical education from all over the country and different countries around the world.

On the basis of the results of laboratory research, and references found in the canon, Kuvalayananda became increasingly interested in the therapeutic application of Yoga in the treatment of various diseases. With a grant from the Maharashtra State Government and a donation from Shri A. T. Gupta, the S.A.D.T. Gupta Hospital was established in 1962. With thirty-six beds, the hospital provided human subjects for studying the efficacy of *āsanas*, *kriyās*, *prāṇāyāma*, and *dhyāna* in the treatment of various chronic diseases, primarily asthma. Over the years at Kaivalyadhama there has been a shift away from treatment as such to prevention, but an ongoing concern with treatment is reflected in the establishment of a Nature Cure Center in 1994 "to complement yogic therapy." In any event, most of the purely curative work was done at Kaivalyadhama's Bombay branch where, according to a brochure published in 1999, over 100,000 people have been treated since 1936 (Kaivalyadhama n.d.).

Kuvalayananda was a tireless worker and a successful fund-raiser. Between 1924 and independence in 1947 he made his work known to nationalist leaders like Jawaharlal Nehru, Lala Lajpat Rai, Pandit Madan Mohan Malaviya, Shrinivas Shastri, Pandit Kunzroo, and Mahatma Gandhi, among others. At the same time, however, Kuvalayananda's work attracted the attention of a few researchers in the United States and Eastern Europe. Most notably, Josephine Rathbone came from Columbia University in 1928 to study Yoga as physical education, and a doctoral candidate from Yale University, K. T. Behanan, wrote his dissertation on the science of Yoga after doing research at Kaivalyadhama (see Behanan 1937). In 1957 two physicians, Dr. Wenger from the University of California and Dr. Bagchi from the University of Michigan, spent six weeks working with the scientists and are reported to have remarked: "Throughout we found an atmosphere of quiet culture and scholarship. All in all Kaivalyadhama appears to us to be unique in India and in fact in the world" (Sathe 1975: 25). In 1959 Dr. Albertson from the University of Colorado came to study at Lonavala and described Kuvalayananda—who now sported his distinctive long white "corkscrew" hair, white "walrus" mustache, and round eyeglasses—as "radiating a spirit of saintliness" (Sathe 1975: 25; see also Albertson 1969). Throughout the 1960s, when India had relatively close ties with sectors of the Soviet bloc, researchers from the Czechoslovak Academy of Sciences came to study Yoga with the Swami, as did physicians from the Medical University in Budapest. After noting his admiration for the "valuable research" done under frugal circumstances, Dr. Ctibor Dostale concluded that "it is due to the fact that these outstanding specialists sacrifice themselves for this science" (Sathe 1975: 26).

As Sathe and all of Kuvalayananda's other friends and biographers point out, the Swami was an ardent Freedom Fighter—"a nationalist at

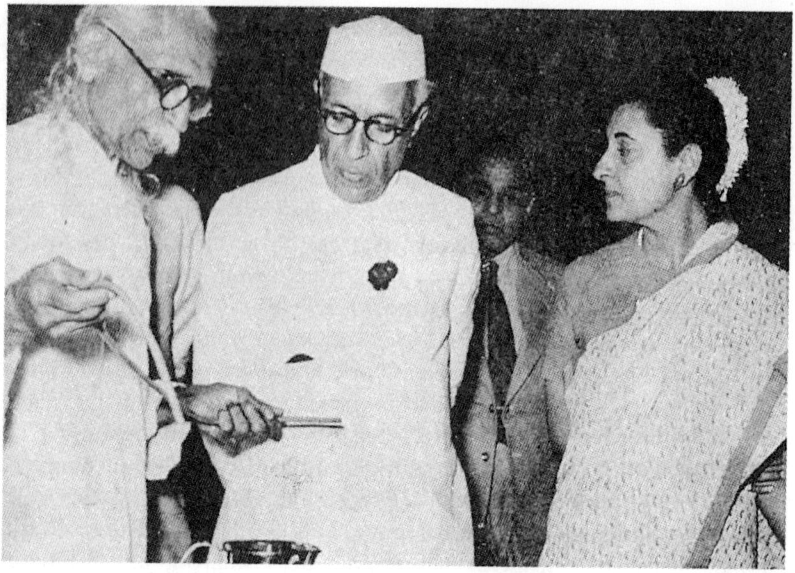

4. "Swami Kuvalayananda explaining the significance of yogic *kriyās* to Pandit Jawaharlalji and Smt. Indiraji." *Source: Swami Kuvalyanananda Birth Centenary, 1984* (Lonavala: Kaivalyadhama, 1984), illus. no. 1, between pages 8 and 9. Reproduced with permission from Kaivalyadhama Ashram.

heart and once an active member of the Indian National Congress." Although strongest in the early 1920s, some of this spirit persisted through independence. It is clearly reflected in a visit made to Kaivalyadhama by Jawaharlal Nehru and Indira Gandhi in 1958. On the occasion of this visit the prime minister applauded what the Swami was doing because "Yoga would not progress unless it was examined in light of the advances in modern science" (quoted in *Kaivalyadhama and Its Activities* 1975: 110).

Nationalism notwithstanding, after 1924 Kuvalayananda "chose to restrict himself to Yoga . . . for the betterment of human society and the world" (Sathe 1975: 29). In other words, while concurring with the prime minister, Kuvalayananda moved from nationalism to transnationalism—from composing patriotic songs, regimenting martial parades at the National College at Amalner, and advocating vigorous sports and rigorous exercise regimens for students in order to "generate a spirit of freedom and patriotism" (Chingle 1975: 109), to a more international, transcultural perspective on the relationship between "progress" and modernization. He shifted his perspective from one in which Yoga was

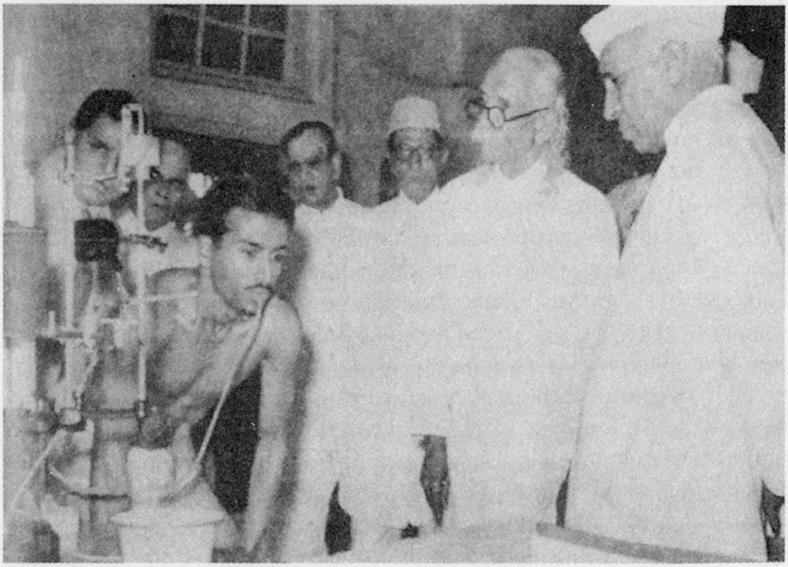

5. "An experimental set up for scientifically studying pressure changes in yogic practices being explained by Swamiji to Pt. Jawaharlalji." *Source: Kaivalyadhama Golden Jubilee Year Souvenir, 1975* (Lonavala: Kaivalyadhama, 1975), illus. no. 1, between pages 102 and 103. Reproduced with permission from Kaivalyadhama Ashram.

simply the object of a nationalist project to one in which it was the subjective means, made known through science, by which to reorient and improve human society. It was not so much a question of whether Yoga could withstand the scrutiny of science and then progress, as a question of Yoga's being able to harness "the fierce light of science" to which it was subject.

Science: Discovering the Laws of *Prakṛti*

In its total, all-pervasive, tautological, and self-referential construction of reality, hegemony by definition virtually prevents critique. Thus, as a hegemonic system, science is science, and all critiques of science are something else—philosophy, spirituality, or history, for example. Needless to say these critiques are often powerful, but here the concern is with contingencies and the disciplinary mechanics of procedural methods that produce what might be called inadvertent critiques of science, from the inside out—to mix metaphors, these are mutations within the leviathan.

This perspective opens up a space in which the construction and deconstruction of reality take place at the same time: one can be doing science and undoing science by means of a single set of experiments, even though one may be an ardent rationalist who uncritically, and unreflexively, believes in science as science. The question of how these "mutations" occur is simply a matter of the contingent convergence of historical trends—empiricism, materialism, and metaphysics—manifest in the particular interests of individuals. One can see this in the work of Einstein, as quantum physics, pioneered by Niels Bohr (1958, 1972), opened up a space for metaphysical speculation to bend reality—and for reality to bend physics—and then gave that distortion real form in the nuclear age. On a slightly different and purely theoretical register, the same can be found in Stephen Hawking's work and, perhaps, even in the tenor of Stephen Jay Gould's writings (1987, 1999, 2002), as these writings echo Teilhard de Chardin's philosophy of being.

For all their genius, however, these leading figures in the field of Modern Science have had the parochial disadvantage of seeing the World, the West, and Science as more or less coterminous. Thus metaphysical questions produced by science as it is practiced in the Academy—be it the All India Institute of Medical Sciences, New Delhi, or the Institute of Advanced Study, Princeton—do not translate into a form that changes basic assumptions about the epistemology of empirical research or the nature of nature. When "mutations" occur on the "margins" of the world rather than at its "center"—in laboratories on the fringe of science's dominion, for example—the whole structure of the hegemonic system becomes more transparent, and the relationship between margin and center comes more clearly into focus, as does the way in which ontological metaphysics forces the question of epistemology back on itself.

Swami Kuvalayananda's experiments on *uḍḍiyāna* and *nauli* were based on a hypothesis designed to challenge a conclusion reached by Dr. Bell and Dr. Meltzer of the Rockefeller Research Institute in New York after they observed the performance of the *kriyās* in question. Bell and Meltzer concluded that *uḍḍiyāna* and *nauli* produced a "sort of anti-peristaltic habit," that is, the voluntary manipulation of the large intestine's "involuntary" normal contractions. Basing his hypothesis on the principle of *prāṇa* and *praṇic* flow in yogic physiology, and understanding the relationship between *prāṇa, vāyu,* and *ākāśa*—subtle air, air, and ether—Kuvalayananda's hypothesis was that although *uḍḍiyāna* and *nauli* did involve the manipulation of gross motor functions, both voluntary and involuntary, the important effect of the *kriyās* had more to do with the relationship between *ākāśa* and *prāṇa* on a subtle register, and this could be measured in terms of the relative volume of air. Thus, in his view, the discovery of what he called the Madhavdas Vacuum not only disproved Bell and Meltzer's conclusion, but also proved that it was worth experimenting on the way in which other physiological changes could be linked to the underlying theory of yogic physiology, rather than to a theory of functional biology and structural anatomy.[4]

Given the central place of *prāṇa* in yogic physiology, it is not surprising that some of the first experiments Swami Kuvalayananda conducted at Kaivalyadhama focused on the effects of *prāṇāyāma* exercises, and the difference between simply breathing deeply and holding one's breath on the one hand, and, on the other, performing yogic exercises wherein one breathes in, locks the air in place, and then breathes out—a fairly subtle difference, but a difference of profound importance in establishing the relationship between subtle and gross features of physiology. Kuvalayananda's hypothesis was designed to challenge the notion that deep breathing simply increased the level of oxygen in the blood and the volume of carbon dioxide expired. As Dr. V. Pratap put it, in a review of the Swami's early work, "it was his view that changes in oxygen and carbon dioxide values in inspired and expired air play but a secondary role in the mechanics of *Prāṇāyāma*. According to him the main effort in *Prāṇāyāma* is not so much to manipulate the metabolic rate as to influence the respiratory feed back center" (1975: 78). As Kuvalayananda himself explained in volume 3 of *Yoga Mimamsa:* "The westerner looks to exercises in deep breathing mainly from the point of view of its oxygen value. He appreciates these exercises principally because they give him a larger quantity of oxygen to vitalize the system. With us the oxygen value of *Prāṇāyāma* is subordinate. We prize it more for its usefulness in nerve culture" (quoted in Pratap 1975: 78).

The English term "nerve culture," used here by Kuvalayananda as a scientific term, refers to the way in which *prāṇa,* as subtle air, produces psychosomatic power by flowing through the subtle body's network of *nāḍī* conduits. Later Kuvalayananda and others would conduct experiments on brain waves, pulse rates, and blood pressure to try to discover the subtle flow of *prāṇa* as it was encoded in these gross body functions, but it is significant that the first experiments focused on air, and on the crucial difference in seeing air simply as having a chemical base of relatively predictable proportions, or seeing it as an integral element with a predictable effect on the body as a whole when manipulated through the act of breathing. The difficult problem was to design an experiment that would make the invisible visible, and so Kuvalayananda measured oxygen in order to materialize *prāṇa*. This is what might be called a kind

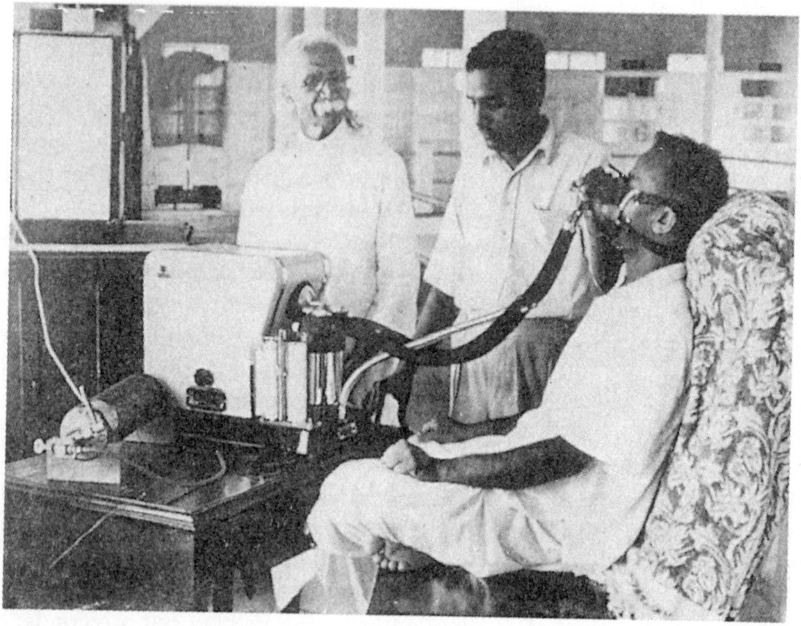

6. "Swami Kuvalayananda observing an experiment on oxygen consumption during yogic practice." *Source: Swaṃi Kuvalayananda Birth Centenary, 1984* (Lonavala: Kaivalyadhama, 1984), illus. no. 4, between pages 4 and 5. Reproduced with permission from Kaivalyadhama Ashram.

of mimetic empiricism, wherein the properties of *prakṛtic* reality—as opposed to reality as it is governed by Natural Laws—is subject to the entelechy of rational science.

To give a clear sense of this entelechy, and to appreciate the extent to which it emerged out of the procedural mechanics of specific experiments—rather than simply being theorized—it is important to trace, in some detail, the sequence of work at Kaivalyadhama.

Although Kuvalayananda classified Yoga into three categories—(1) *āsana,* (2) *prāṇāyāma,* and (3) *kriyā*s, *mudrā*s, and *bandha*s—in terms of the broader research agenda, the more comprehensive structure and function of yogic physiology was the subject of study. This is also reflected in the way in which the scientific, semi-scientific, and popular publications in *Yoga Mimamsa* intersect with one another.

Following the discovery of the Madhavdas Vacuum in 1924, Kuvalayananda conducted a series of "X-ray experiments on *uḍḍiyāna* and *nauli* in relation to the position of the colon contents" (1924b, 1925a, b, c). In 1926 he conducted more X-ray experiments, this time on *dhauti,* a *kriyā* wherein the stomach is voluntarily purged (1926c). The same year he began experiments on changes in blood pressure during the performance of *sarvāngāsana* and *matsyāsana,* showing that there was an increase in the systolic pressure when the position was maintained for five minutes, with the most significant increase in the third minute (1926a). Following this—and anticipating K. N. Udupa's research on rats—he conducted a similar study on *śirṣāsana,* the headstand pose, showing that the systolic rate changed by 4 to 10 percent whereas the dystolic change was between 14 and 22 percent (1926b). X-ray experiments continued in 1928 on the effect of *uḍḍiyāna* and *nauli* on the rib cage and the diaphragm (1928b). Having measured pressure changes in the colon, Swami Kuvalayananda became interested in other parts of the digestive system and compared the effect of *uḍḍiyāna* and *nauli* on pressure changes in the stomach (1928c). The effect of *uḍḍiyāna* was less than either one of the three *nauli* positions, and in *nauli* the isolation of the right and left recti produced the same pressure change, where as the isolation of the central recti produced the greatest change of -40 to -43 mm Hg, as compared with -25 to -29 mm Hg in *uḍḍiyāna*.

Although all of the experiments before 1928 were concerned with pressure changes explicitly, and *prāna* either directly or indirectly, in 1929 and 1930 Kuvalayananda's attention shifted to the respiratory system and the effect of *prāṇāyāma* exercises. It was at this time that he compared *uḍḍiyāna bandha* with nonyogic deep breathing and found that the yogic procedure produced a more significant change in intraesophageal pressure. To demonstrate that *prāṇāyāma* had more to do with *prāṇa* and the development of *nāḍī* conduits than with oxygen, he set up a series of experiments to measure the elimination of carbon dioxide wherein the pattern of inhalation, retention, and expiration was carefully calibrated (1930). Subsequently he began to study the effect of *prāṇāyāma* on oxygen consumption and found that even rapid, deep breathing did not increase oxygen consumption (1933). This was followed by more experiments on the composition of air, which disproved J. S. Haldane's conclusions regarding the so-called alveolar air plateau (1934).

Although some experimentation continued at Kaivalyadhama, there is a gap of twenty-two years between the publication of volume 5 of *Yoga Mimamsa* in 1934 and volume 6 in 1956, a period of time when, leading up to and following both World War II and Indian independence, the Ashram was expanding in other directions. After 1956, however, and particularly after Nehru's visit in 1958, the pace of research picked up. But it was not until the late 1960s, after Kuvalayananda's death, that scientific work again reached the level it had achieved in the decade after the Ashram was established.

The earlier studies in air composition, repeated and expanded in 1956, led Kuvalayananda and his associates to hypothesize that various yogic practices might have significant biochemical effects, and he began to experiment with how different *āsanas* decreased adrenocortical activity and thus reduced the excretion of uropepsin (Gore 1981). The performance of *dhauti,* a *kriyā* in which a cloth strip is swallowed and used to clean the stomach, was shown to increase uropepsin excretion (Gharote and Karambelkar 1975; Kuvalayananda 1926c). Other biochemical experiments focused on the effect of *vāyu-bhaksan kriyā* and *vastra dhauti* on gastric acidity (Oak and Bhole 1981a, b, 1982); changes in cholesterol levels through yogic training programs (Karambelkar et al. 1977; Moorty et al. 1978); the effect of *āsana* and *prāṇāyāma* on urea clearance and creatinine clearance values (Kesari, Vaishawanar, and Deshkar 1979); the effect of short-term yogic training on cardiovascular endurance (Ganguly and Gharote 1974; Ganguly 1981); the fibrinolytic activity of blood (Bhole 1982b); psycho-motor performance (Shahu et al. 1983) and dexterity (Shahu and Gharote 1984); and the effect of long-term Yoga training on urinary acidity (Gore 1976; Karambelkar, Bhole, and Gharote 1969) and resting neuromuscular activity (Paranjape and Bhole 1979), among many other things. After Kuvalayananda died in 1966, most of the experiments at Kaivalyadhama were conducted by M. V. Bhole, S. L. Vinekar, P. V. Karambelkar, M. L. Gharote, and M. M. Gore, many of whom served as the Ashram research directors in the 1970s and 1980s.

Although Kuvalayananda himself was interested in the therapeutic application of Yoga and published articles on the treatment of cecal constipation (1924, 1925a, b, c), appendicitis (1926c), high blood pressure (1926a), and emotions (1928b) as well as a book entitled *Yogic Therapy* (1963), it was not until after his death that clinical studies of specific diseases were conducted in ernest. For reasons that are fairly obvious given the importance of the *prāṇa*/air relationship, there was a long-term, multidimensional study of asthma (Bhole 1976; Bhagwat, Soman, and Bhole 1981) with attention given to the effect of yogic practice on the overall blood composition of asthmatics (Bhole and Karambelkar 1971), and on specific leukocyte (Bhole and Deshpande 1982) and eosinophil counts (Deshpande and Bhole 1982). Tests were conducted on breath holding (Bhole and Gharote 1977), emotional changes (Oak and Bhole 1981a), fibrinolitic activity (Bhole, 1982b), pulmonary function (Gore 1982; Gore and Bhole 1982), serum cholesterol levels (Moorty et al. 1978), and gastric responses among patients treated with *vastra dhauti* (Oak and Bhole 1981b). Although asthma was by far the most important subject of study, some research was also done on obesity (Gharote 1977), cancer (Karambelkar 1972), diabetes (Karambelkar 1976), rhinitis and sinusitis (Bhole

1970), and various emotional disorders such as anxiety (Kocher and Pratap 1971), "neurotic trends" (Pratap 1972), and hostility (Kocher 1973, 1976).

The published summary reports on each of these experiments show that, in almost all instances, the focus was on the anatomical, physiological, or biochemical variables in question and the nature of the data collected was, in all cases, empirical. For example, Bhole and Karambelkar provide the following report on their 1971 experiment on the "blood picture" of asthma patients: "One hundred and four asthmatics showed a significant increase in hemoglobin by 0.5 to 0.9 gms/cmm, and in lymphocytes by 2 to 3% per cmm while a decrease was seen in total leucocyte count by 200 to 600 per cmm at the end of 4 and 6 weeks of yogic treatment" (quoted in Bhole 1985: 108). Similarly, Kuvalayananda and Karambelkar report on a 1956 experiment testing the relationship between *bhastrikā prāṇāyāma* as defined in the *Gheraṇḍasaṁhitā* and levels of urinary acidity: "With controlled diet regimen no increase in urinary acidity was noted after *bhastrikā prāṇāyāma* for 45 minutes followed by rest for 15 minutes. One round of *bhastrikā* consisted of 40 strokes of *kapālabhāti* in 20 seconds followed by *pūrāka-kumbhaka-recaka* of 10–20–40 seconds followed by next round in the same manner" (Bhole 1985: 27).

Despite the empirical form of these experiments, and the apparent preoccupation of the researchers with gross biology, the driving force behind science at Kaivalyadhama was an ontological question about the nature of nature. Thus, in essence, urinary pH, lymphocytes, and stomach acidity are regarded as epiphenomenal in their relationship to the real object of study—the phenomenal meta-material power inherent in Yoga.

This is evidenced by two types of so-called Special Projects experiments conducted in the Ashram laboratory, one dealing with *samādhi*, the final stage of yogic realization in which the individual self is united with the universal Self, and the other with nostril dominance—a deceptively innocuous-sounding phenomenon.

In the late 1960s there were a number of studies conducted in India and the United States on the ability of adept yogis to perform seemingly miraculous feats, such as changing temperature in different parts of the body, manipulating various "involuntary" nerve and brain functions, stopping the pulse, and being able to survive without air. The belief was that when a person achieved a state of *samādhi* his or her body manifested a condition of death, but that an adept yogi could bring his or her own body "back to life" at will. Breathing, and the ability to survive without breathing air, came to be regarded as a kind of litmus test to measure the "degree" of *samādhi,* most likely because one who has achieved the highest state of Yoga can survive on *prāṇa* alone.

It is of great importance to point out that the term used in these experiments was *samādhi,* and the reference point for designing the research, postulating hypotheses, and measuring and interpreting data was, both discursively and meta-discursively, the state of enstasy which characterizes the final goal of Yoga. *Samādhi,* as we have already seen in the context of the previous chapter and as we will see again in the chapters that follow, is an embodied state that is saturated with mystical and magical significance. As David White puts it, in *samādhi* breath, semen, and mind are all stabilized, "but more important, when through breath control (*prāṇāyāma*) the base of the medial channel is opened, that same breath causes the reversal of mundane polarities. Rather than descending, semen, energy, and mind are now forced upwards into the cranial vault, effecting total yogic integration (*samādhi*), a reversal of the flow of time, immortality and transcendence over the entire created universe" (1996: 45). In describing what is involved in *sālambana samādhi,* or *samādhi* with support—which may be regarded here as the mystical analog for the empirical experiments conducted at Kaivalyadhama—Eliade, referencing both Vyāsa's and Vācaspatimiśra's commentary on the *Yoga Sūtra* (I, 44, 45) provides the following comment: "When thought 'identifies' itself with the *tanmātras* without experiencing the 'feelings' that, because of their energetic nature, these *tanmātras* produce, . . . the yogin obtains the state of *nirvicāra.* Thought then becomes one with these infinitesimal nucleuses of energy which constitute the true foundation of the physical universe. It is a real descent into the very essence of the physical world, and not only into qualified and individual phenomenon" (1990: 83).

In 1967 Bhole, Karambelkar, and Vinekar observed as four practitioners—who had, at least on the level of discursive knowledge "descended into the very essence of the physical universe"—were buried underground and six others placed in air-tight boxes under the ground. The researchers recorded their observations in *Yoga Mimamsa,* concluding that the subjects buried under ground entered into "states akin to suspended animation through specific physical techniques for a predetermined period of time" (Bhole 1985: 127; Bhole, Karambelkar, and Vinekar 1967). Subsequently an experiment was conducted measuring and comparing the oxygen consumption of yogic subjects—but not adept yogis—and a control population sealed in air-tight boxes, each 6 feet long by 3 feet 6 inches wide, for between twelve and fourteen hours. The summary of the experiment is as follows: "Reduction in oxygen consumption in subjects practicing Yoga was found to be less than control subjects. . . . Increase in respiration, blood pressure and heart rate was observed when carbon-dioxide reached beyond 5% level. Galvanic skin resistance decreased initially, but it increased in the end and electrocardiography showed a strain on the heart" (Bhole 1985: 128).

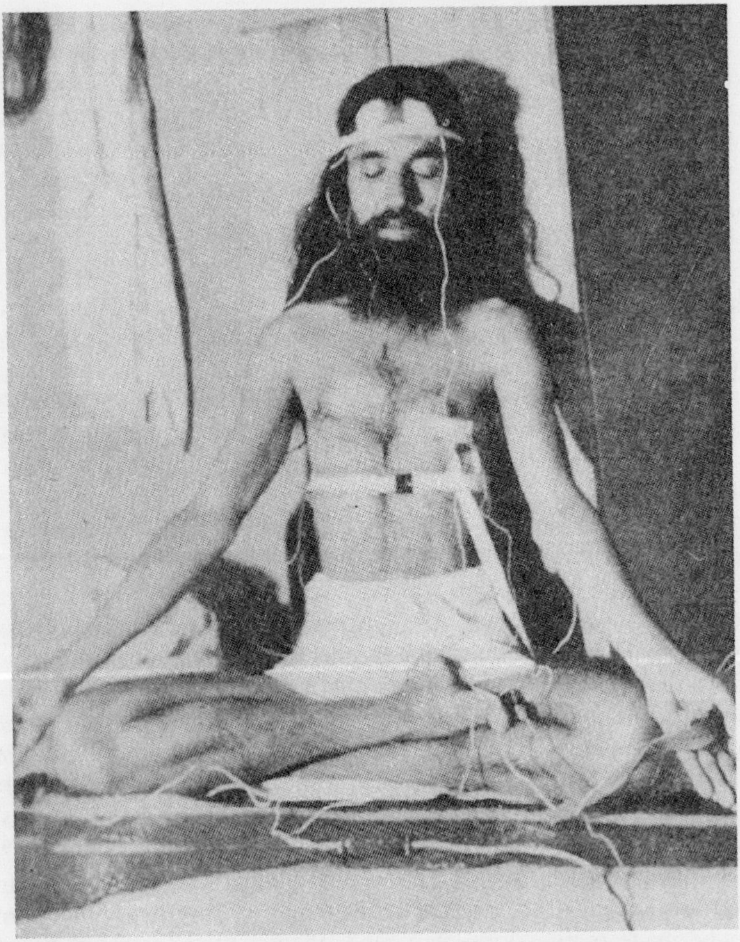

7. "Subject VNR sitting in Yogic condition with necessary attachments." *Source:* "Difference in Magnitude of Response in Yogic and Non-Yogic Conditions," *Yog Mimamsa* 12, no. 2 (1969): 9–18, fig. 1. Reproduced with permission from Kaivalyadhama Ashram.

The following year Karambelkar, Vinekar, and Bhole conducted another experiment on "one professional [yogic practitioner] and three control subjects" sealed in air-tight boxes for between twelve and eighteen hours. The researchers published their results in the *Indian Journal of Medical Research* (1968: 1282–88) and drew the following summary conclusions:

> Staying in an air tight pit was seen to reduce oxygen consumption by 2 to 34% below the basal requirement in one professional and three control subjects. The reduction is believed to be related with the gradually raising levels of carbon dioxide in the pit air over a period of time. The carbon dioxide level in the pit had reached 7.2 to 7.73% when the subjects preferred to terminate their stay at the end of twelve to eighteen hours. Practice of *prāṇāyāma* definitely helped to withstand higher concentrations of carbon dioxide in the pit air. (Bhole 1985: 128)

These experiments were designed to prove that "supernatural" yogic powers—*siddhi*s—were not magical. At the same time, the experiments took for granted that *samādhi* was real, and that yogic power could be understood and analyzed in rational, logical terms. What Karambelkar, Vinekar, and Bhole were doing, in some sense, was expanding the range of human experience by explaining its outer limits through a synthesis of Yoga and science.

If the synthesis of Yoga and science took shape in the relationship between air and *prāṇa,* and the influence of *prāṇa* on the "nerves," the structure of the relationship was realized in nostril dominance. The hypothesis here was as simple as it was important. In yogic physiology the three primary *nāḍī* conduits run parallel to the spinal column, with the vertical *suṣumṇā nāḍī* being intersected at the *cakra* centers by the *iḍā* and *piṅgalā* conduits. According to the *Gheraṇḍasaṁhitā,* the *iḍā* and *piṅgalā* terminate in the left and right nostril, respectively.[5] *Prāṇāyāma,* which is at base a procedure for the purification of all the *nāḍī*s, entails various techniques for alternately closing and opening the nostrils to breath in through one and then out through the other, for example. On a fairly obvious level, then, the gross physiology of the nose mirrors the subtle physiology of the *nāḍī*s and, furthermore, the nostrils function—or can be made to function—as a kind of interstitial threshold between subtle and gross domains.

In 1966 S. L. Vinekar devised a technique for measuring changes in the electrical amplitude of the nasal mucus membrane as these changes in amplitude corresponded to various kinds of sensory stimulation. His thesis, published in the journal *Neurology,* was that electro-nasography provided a new approach to neurophysiological research (1966: 75–79). Vinekar's experiment was followed up by three other studies. In 1968 Bhole and Karambelkar tested 96 subjects to provide a statistical profile on nostril dominance and found that 47.8 percent had a dominant right nostril, 37.7 percent a dominant left nostril, and 14.5 percent had balanced nostril dominance (1968: 1–12). Subsequently Pratap, testing a thesis put forward in the classical literature on patterns of change in nasal dominance, compared the breathing patterns of 89 patients and 10

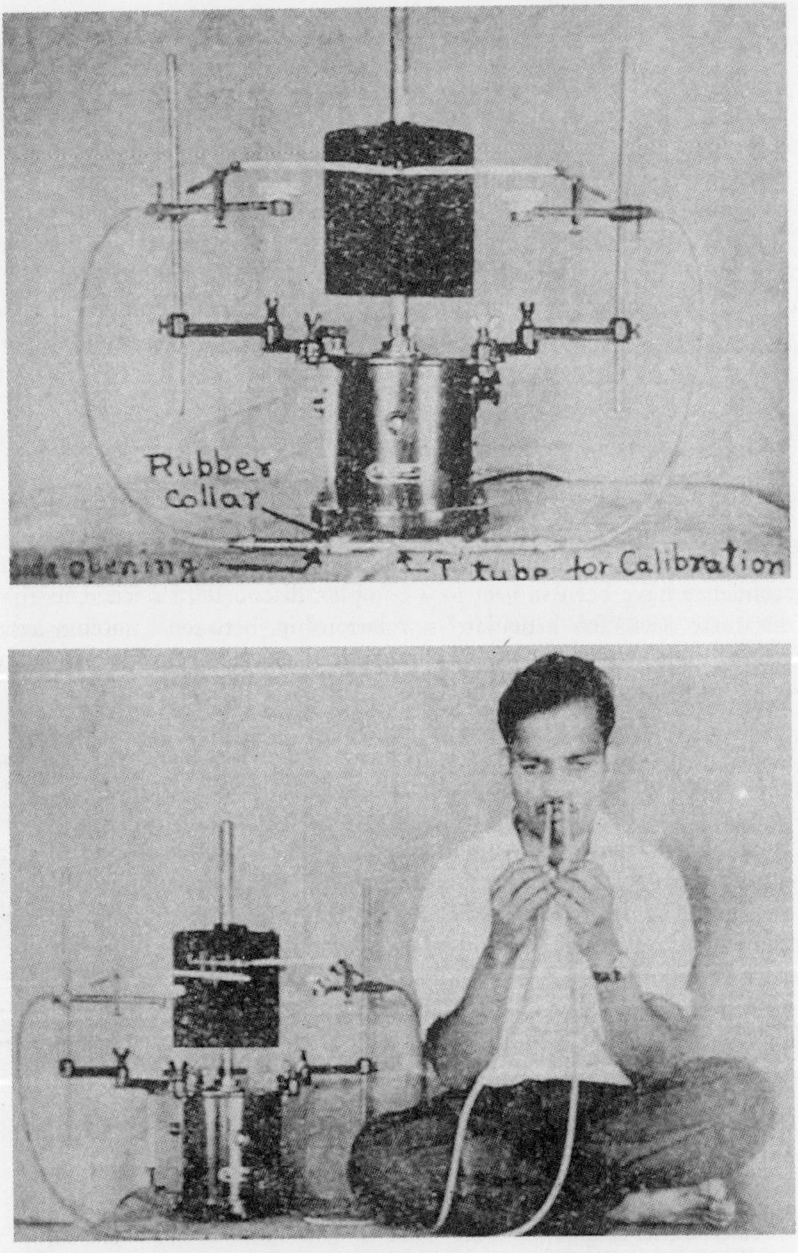

8. "Experimental set up for recording the force of breathing through each nostril." *Source:* M. V. Bhole and P. V. Karambelkar, "Significance of Nostrils in Breathing," *Yog Mimamsa* 10, no. 4 (1968): 1–12, fig. 1. Reproduced with permission from Kaivalyadhama Ashram.

normal, control subjects to study the rate at which sick and healthy individuals experienced a shift in dominance from left to right nostril (1972: 1–18). Finally, in 1982 Moorty, Ganguly, and Bhole, testing a hypothesis that the effect of nasal breathing on the *nāḍīs* would affect neuromuscular patterns, undertook a study of the relationship between nostril dominance and grip strength in healthy and sick individuals. Their conclusions, published in *SNIPES,* India's primier journal for sports research and physical education, are as follows: "Static grip strength of both the hands was more when the right nostril was open for breathing in thirty physical educationists while thirty four asthma patients showed just the reverse trend. In thirty nine Yoga practitioners the grip strength was stronger on the same side as the nostril [in dominance]" (1982: 77–80 in Bhole 1985: 129).

Alternative Ontology: *Citta, Prakṛti,* and the Laws of Nature

It was pointed out in the previous chapter that the metaphysics of transcendence have been subject to a complex discourse of science, as that discourse seeks to articulate a relationship between consciousness, cosmic transcendence, mind, and body. Key aspects of this discourse are reflected in the research at Lonavala.

As it is defined in the *Yoga Sūtra* Yoga is "the cessation of the modification of *citta* as an outcome of *prāṇa*'s movement through the *suṣumṇā nāḍī,* being preceded by the purification of the *nāḍīs.*[6] *Citta* is consciousness, and in yogic psycho-physiology consciousness distracts from true awareness. In these terms, the final goal of Yoga is understood to be "a cessation of modifications of consciousness," which is synonymous with the state of *samādhi* described above. In a state of *samādhi,* when all consciousness has ceased, Truth is realized when observer and observed become one and there is a dissolution of subject and object. As R. H. Singh, professor in the Department of Kayachikitsa and director of the Center for Yoga at Banaras Hindu University puts it in his book *The Foundations of Contemporary Yoga,*

> When the *Citta* becomes one with the object and its own form of existence and when there is realization of nothing other than the object of meditation, then such a meditation is called the state of *Samādhi. . . . Samādhi* is achieved after the disappearance of self awareness while progressing in meditation. One's self awareness starts disappearing, higher consciousness starts emerging and the Yogi starts realizing the ultimate truth situated beyond the object of meditation. Here the meditator and the object of meditation become united as one. (1991: 43)

Consciousness is understood as having emerged out of *prakṛti* (primordial matter) and is, therefore, constituted by the three *guṇa*s, *sattva, rajas* and *tamas*. Apart from the fact that *citta* is agitated by subliminal desires and tendencies (*vāsanā saṃskāra*s), as well as by direct sensory stimulation that gives raise to emotional responses, and is "polluted" by the five *kaśaya*s of false knowledge, egoism, attachment, hate, and fear of death, it is on the fundamental *prakṛtic* level that *citta* is understood to manifest impurity and imperfection by its very nature. The gradual purification of the mind through meditation is thought to produce all of the numerous supernatural powers associated with yogic practice. But the final state of union is a kind of dematerialization of nature through what might be called "de-creation," since it entails a realization of the universal truth that "predates" the creation of all apparent truths, including the laws of nature that apply to time, space, and matter. Thus when *samādhi* is described as a state of bliss, it is the bliss of *mokṣa* or final liberation from bondage to the material world, as that bondage is manifest in the cycle of births. It is the bliss of absolute nothingness reflected in the synonymous term *kaivalya,* from which Swami Kuvalayananda derived the name of his Ashram laboratory.

Needless to say, scholars of Hindu philosophy, spirituality, and metaphysics have analyzed and reanalyzed Yoga philosophy in great detail. Without rehearsing all that might be relevant, the simple point to be made here is that Yoga is based on an ontology that subverts the laws of nature, and this necessarily undermines the epistemology of science, at least in the final instant of self-realization. Thus in the degree to which *prāṇa* manifests the agency of a prospective realization of universal truth, its manipulation by means of Yoga-subject-to-science will manifest a denouement wherein science is made subject to Yoga. This is an instance where the problematic effect of the relationship between observer and observed in the epistemology of science is resolved in terms of an ontology in which they are both, in fact, fundamentally the same.

For this reason, I think, the experiments conducted at Kaivalyadhama had the paradoxical effect of "proving nothing," thereby establishing transcendental laws rather than the universal laws of nature. Consider again Kuvalayananda's prime objective: "The main effort of the Kaivalyadhama is in scientifically probing the human mind and to dig deeper and deeper in the inner space, till the effort to conquer the outer and inner spaces converge and ultimately meet to solve the riddle of the cosmos."[7] The ontological paradox manifest in the relationship between *prakṛti* and nature creates a kind of Mobius strip wherein science and Yoga are both subject and object of each other. However, the embodied riddle of the cosmos undoes science and makes Yoga a powerful alternative for understanding the convergence of inner and outer space. The more Yoga is subject to science, and the closer one gets to discovering the nature of *prāṇa,* the more powerful Yoga becomes as a means by which to discover truth.

It is of critical importance to keep in mind that Kuvalayananda saw no paradox. Nor did Bhole, Karambalkar, Vinekar, or any of the other directors of research at Kaivalyadhama. The consequence of what they did is, in fact, more profound than was their stated goal of subjecting Yoga to scientific scrutiny. To put this another way, Kuvalayananda could have simply founded an *āśram,* as did Aurobindo in Pondicherry, or established a mission, as have the disciples of Ramakrishna. Thereby he could have "revived" and "reformed" a branch of Hindu philosophy on its own terms, at least putatively. Alternatively he could have done what researchers at the All India Institute of Medical Sciences did, and study Yoga purely and simply in physiological terms. Anticipating the work of K. N. Udupa, the director of Medical Sciences at Banaras Hindu University, he might have incorporated Yoga completely into the disciplinary system of science within the framework of academic research and development. But what he decided to do was to localize and harness the power of Western science in order to translate the physiological philosophy of Indian Yoga into a "complete message for humanity." He took the "culture" out of Yoga, so to speak. But in making it speak the language of science in order to get the message across to all humanity, what he ended up doing was making it clear that science is not a universal language of truth. *Prāṇa* is *prāṇa* and oxygen is oxygen, but in trying to "make the twain meet" in the human body he made it impossible for science to play colonialism to Yoga's nationalism. Yoga's position within the discourse of nationalism made it possible to imagine—in terms of the body and embodied practice—a global community.

Global Health, Universal Happiness, and the Limits of Science

An exploration of scope, scale, and vast diversity manifest in the transnational global community of people who practice Yoga—to adapt Sarah Strauss's apt phrase (1997, 2000)—is well beyond the scope of this book. The simple but important point to be made here is that the research at Kaivalyadhama enabled Yoga to be understood, practiced, and embodied as a profoundly important but generically human activity. Let me put it this way: it would be completely inconceivable and impossible for Yoga to be taught as a form of physical fitness training in the Jewish Community Center in Pittsburgh—just to cite one of several hundred thousand possible examples of localized practice—if Yoga were only conceptualized in terms of metaphysical transcendence or embodied perfection. And yet if Yoga were simply reduced down to a set of physical postures and deep breathing exercises—by explaining their function in terms of gross anatomy alone—what would account for the fact that people all over the world find Yoga to be of particular interest and value when they have access to all kinds of other forms of healthy recreation? Kuvalayananda's research helped to make it possible for Yoga to contain within itself, and within itself in relation to embodied practice, the dynamic ellipse of physical science and metaphysical experience.

This Mobius ellipse was first set in motion during the heyday of the Yoga Renaissance in the 1920s, and then was reproduced and reinforced time and again throughout the period when others like Shri Yogendra pioneered the self-help manual (1928, 1930, 1936) and Swami Sivananda combined Haṭha Yoga with Vedānta to produce an embodied society of Divine Life, with its own subsequent transnational scope and significance. Thus Kuvalayananda's contribution was to "modernize" Yoga not just in practice, but on the level of the body, and this configuration of modernity enabled what seems to be Yoga's phenomenal ability to grow, expand, and transmutate. If Yoga and Yoga physiology were simply subject to science as science authorized by the West, the reductive process of experimentation would have quickly produced conclusive results—one way or the other—thus circumscribing and limiting the range of Yoga's effectiveness. If Yoga were not subject to science and was promoted simply as an articulation of exotic Indian culture, its spread throughout the world would be in terms of what might be called New Age postcolonial Orientalism, of which there are, most certainly, many varieties. But each of these—New Age Orientalism and hard-core Western science—suffers under the burden of nationalism and the culture of colonialism in one one form or another.

At the risk of being reductive in a different way, and also of universalizing on the basis of a single case, the following, taken as a random sample from the search engine of my University website (www.pitt.edu/` mcenter/Salute.html) is, nevertheless, precisely exemplary of what must be hundreds of thousands if not millions of cases in which Yoga is being practiced virtually without reference to science or Indian culture as such. It is, thereby, being practiced as a mutated somewhat disarticulated "message for all humanity:" On April 19, 2002, at the University of Pittsburgh at Johnstown, in a program at the Living Learning Center called "Salute to Working Women," there was a "Breathe Your Stress Away" workshop. It was described as follows: "The final portion of our program will teach us the benefits of deep breathing and achieve deep relaxation and concentration. We'll also find out how we can use deep breathing to conserve and increase energy, reduce muscle tension, lower blood pressure and heart rate, and create more positive attitude. So, turn off your pager, put your cellphone away, sit back and . . . breathe your stress away."

In the thousands upon thousands of similar examples that could be given, there is an implicit connection made between such things as stress and the principle of suffering that is central to Yoga philosophy. It follows from this that the practice of Yoga enables one to embody the bliss of transcendence as a "solution" to the banal problems of everyday life.

In order to work toward a conclusion, it is worth considering how it is that the principle of bliss provides a global vision of universal health happiness that is—to use a new "Mobiotic" term—spiritific.

In a volume commemorating the golden jubilee of Kaivalyadhama, Dr. K. S. Joshi, professor of yoga studies at Sagar University, points out that

> Science cannot tell what is right and what is good. Thus with all its excellence in moulding the nature outside us, science so far has met with a failure in moulding our inner nature. . . .
>
> Science has given us the cars, aeroplanes and nuclear weapons. But the inner control which must go with the use of them cannot be the product of science. . . . [I]nner control, restraint, understanding, and tolerance, which are all the more necessary in a scientifically advanced society, are not attainable through science. There is no science of inner richness and beauty.
>
> We are in need of some kind of discipline which will be scientific, yet not crippled by the limitations of the scientific method. . . .
>
> Can Yoga do this? It is a super science which can overcome the shortcomings of the particular sciences while at the same time preserving the marvels of their method of investigation. (1975: 204)

Joshi, writing with a clear sense of Kuvalayananda's legacy, is not simply articulating the commonplace rhetoric of New Age pop philosophy. Nor is he simply a pseudoscientist. By raising the issue of inner richness and beauty, as well as happiness, he is evoking the yogic literature on *sukha, ānanda,* and *ānanda samādhi* (see Eliade 1990: 81, 121; Whicher 1998: 238–39, 242–43), as well as the primary and now paradigmatic reference in the *Yoga Sūtra: saṃtoṣādanuttamaḥ sukhalābhaḥ,* or superlative happiness from contentment (Taimni's translation [1961: 247–48]).

Although there is no need to go into the specific difference between *ānanda samādhi,* which is conditional, and the "formless enstasy" of *nirvikalpa-samādhi* (see Feuerstein 1990: 23), it is clear that Joshi is pointing out how it is that dispassionate, value-free science is subsumed by a kind of happiness and bliss that places ultimate value beyond the distinction between pleasure and pain, right and wrong, good and evil. What Joshi seems to be suggesting is that a fundamental problem in the logic of yogic philosophy as concerns the experience of pure bliss as different from pure enstasy—and the extent to which bliss is conscious, supraconscious, or located in the "cloud of *dharma*" (see Feuerstein 2001: 253)—can be used to problematize the epistemology of science, but not reject it as such.

After defining inner richness and beauty as the constituent elements of an alternative modernity made possible through yogic science, Joshi makes it clear that he knows what science as science really is, by explaining the epistemological principles of observation, induction, logical reasoning, verification, and the construction of theoretical models. He then asks, rhetorically, if, in terms of the "peculiarity" of science as such, it is possible to imagine a "science of happiness." Yoga, Joshi points out, is "a science of happiness *par excellence*" but only when—to adapt Moti Lal Nehru's phrase to show how, after fifty years of research, the ends have changed the meaning of the means—it has absorbed, and not just withstood, the harsh light of science.

> The findings of ancient sages regarding the working of the human mind, its impurities, the techniques of making the mind pure and enlightened, and the state of *jīvanmukti,* if subject to rigorous scientific scrutiny, can definitely show us a way out of the ills the human society is today suffering from. . . .
>
> Yoga practices are found, for instance, to influence our endocrine glands and the nervous system so as to bring about emotional integrity and psychological balance. . . . Yoga influences our attitudes and brings about a change in the core of our personality. It teaches us to be good human beings, free from conflict and war, within as well as outside. Yoga, verily, is destined to be the pinnacle of the age of science. (1975: 204)

Here, it seems, the bliss of transcendental consciousness—*cittavṛttinirodha*—is materialized in the endocrine glands to produce better human beings. It is the embodiment of bliss that matters. And so the nerves and endocrine glands must be understood by means of science and improved through the technology of Yoga so as to fuse knowledge and power in the gross function of subtle anatomy.

Quite apart from what might be said about the quality of research at Kaivalyadhama, since the question of quality applies to all laboratory projects, there can be no question but that it is scientific in the narrow, empiricist, reductive, and fully modern sense of the term. While the experiments are unique, they can be conducted by anyone, anywhere, and are no more restricted to Lonavala than quantum physics is to Princeton. However, the fact that research was done in an *āśram* laboratory, and not just any laboratory, by a swami scientist and not just any scientist, and that it systematically "confused" *prāṇa* and oxygen, nerves and *nāḍīs*, organs and *cakras*, has meant that the knowledge produced by this research requires a new vocabulary—spiritific, "glocal," and "physiosophical."

The programmatic features of this research, as its creative confusion reveals the parameters of a distinctive ontology, has more to do with an alternative global modernity than with the manifest tension between colonialism and nationalism, East and West, as these tensions are localized in India. The global reach of science makes this possible, but the cosmic scope of Yoga's ontology prevents Yoga from being subsumed by the epistemology to which it is subject. Moreover, science moots the question of self-reflexive nationalism. Obviously Kuvalayananda's research was something "India" could be proud of, as Nehru's visit in 1958 made clear. But as Joshi's comments indicate, the whole business was concerned with a redefinition of humanity and the problem of being human, rather than with any question of being Indian or some derivative thereof.

Yoga was not simply modernized by Kuvalayananda; Yoga was analyzed in such a way that it has come to harmonize with the modernity manifest in science to create an alternative. And to a large extent it is this harmonic hybridity that has enabled Yoga to colonize the West, so to speak. And not just in the phenomenal scope of its appeal and scale of worldwide practice, but by providing scientific answers to questions that science does not ask. In this case the "aura of dislocation and disorientation" that constitutes, as Gyan Prakash puts it, the creativity in Indian modernity, means that one can simply drop the non-Western, residually nationalist qualifier "Indian" and be left with a kind of modernity that is neither singular nor intrinsically Western.

Lest there be any confusion, let me state in conclusion that the point here is not to trump a European science of concrete universals with an Indian science of embodied cosmic abstraction. If one may speak, even somewhat cynically and ironically, of India's oblique colonization of the Western mind through the medium of Yoga, the process of colonization involves transmutation and ambiguous translation. Echoing the perspective of Talal Asad, Gayatri Chakravorty Spivak, Homi Bhabha, and others, Dipesh Chakrabarty has pointed out in the introduction to his collection of essays entitled *Provincializing Europe,* "that what translation produces out of seeming 'incommensurabilities' is neither an absence of relationship between dominant and dominating forms of knowledge nor equivalents that successfully mediate between differences, but precisely the partly opaque relationship we call 'difference'" (2000: 17). To write about difference is to produce a translucent analysis. Just as Chakrabarty points out that the provincialization of Europe must, of necessity, work from within European thought, the provincialization of science—or its radical localization—must, as Paul Rabinow (1996a) and

Donna Haraway point out (1991), be done without rejecting science in terms of either its epistemology, the knowledge produced by that epistemology, or the technological products of applied scientific knowledge. Although the yogic subjects of Kuvalayananda's experiments may well be quite different from the cyborgs that figure in Haraway's analysis, or the genetically-mapped-out actors in what Rabinow calls the politics of biosociality, the yogic subject produces "difference" in terms of the incommensurability of the two kinds of materiality he or she embodies.

On the one hand Kuvalayananda's scientific study of Yoga produces what Rabinow, following Foucault and Gilles Deleuze, refers to as postdisciplinary rationality manifest in the figure of the postmodern "afterman" in whom the finitude of empiricity gives way to a "play of forces and forms"—*prāṇa*, oxygen, self, Self, *cakra*s, and neurobiology. What Rabinow has to say about the human genome project and the meaning-structure of DNA applies just as well to the scientifically produced physiology of Yoga: "In this new constellation, beings have neither a perfected form nor an essential opacity" (1996a: 92). The translucent imperfection of the adept's analyzed body allows for a critique of universal law and the facticity of nature upon which those laws are established. Along these lines Haraway points out how situated knowledge—in this case Yoga as an alternative science of life—may be understood in terms of "the apparatus of bodily production" (1991: 200). Although this apparatus, manifest in the intersection of Yoga and science, is imperfect and translucent, it is also, very clearly, linked to the actual "production and reproduction" of bodies as organic things. Despite its ethereal, translucent form, the Madhavdas Vacuum is embodied. Most significantly, however, it is not the organic form as such that constitutes the base of knowledge. Rather it is "bodies as objects of knowledge [that] are material-semiotic generative nodes. . . . independent of intentions and authors" (1991: 200). Materiality signifies reality; it is not itself really real.

This distinction between intentional authorship and embodied knowledge as it relates to the production of meaning brings me back to where I began, with the apparently oxymoronic notion of depersonalized, dislocated biography, confusion as against coherent cultural meaning, and the principle of estranged agency. It brings us back to Gyan Prakash's notion of the impossible-to-clean-up, messy history of modern India. There is no point in trying to argue that Kuvalayananda succeeded in proving that Yoga is really real, that *cakra*s are factual rather than artifactual. However, it is clear that Kuvalayananda thought he was using science to prove that Yoga was not mystical or magical. Therefore there is no point in trying to argue that he himself, as an intentional author, articulated an alternative nationalist Indian science. And although I have not been able to go into it here, there is no evidence that anyone else has either. On account of this, however, what has happened is that the incommensurable difference between Yoga and science as materially based ways of knowing and as empirically grounded perspectives on the nature of universal truth has produced a structure of meaning that is creatively inconclusive in the sense that hundreds if not thousands of studies have been done over the course of the past three-quarters of a century and will continue to be done indefinitely. This global parochialization of truth—to adapt and extend the sense of Chakrabarty's thesis concerning the provincialization of Europe—is in keeping with Nietzsche's call, quoted as an epigraph to part 3, for a medical critique of physiology such that philosophers may take over the work of science and work toward a solution of the problem of value.

4

BIRTH OF THE ANTI-CLINIC: NATUROPATHIC YOGA IN A POST-GANDHIAN, POSTCOLONIAL STATE

> I believe the great fantasy is the idea of a social body constituted of the universality of wills. Now the phenomenon of the social body is the effect not of consensus but of the materiality of power operating on the very bodies of individuals.
>
> Michel Foucault, *Power/Knowledge* (1980: 53)

European Nature Cure in the Early Nineteenth Century

AS A SYSTEM of medicine, Nature Cure was "invented" in central Europe during the nineteenth century. Granted, there were important eighteenth-century antecedents to this invention, and to understand Nature Cure as a modern phenomenon it is necessary to look into the medieval history of water cures, sacred springs, and the practice of spirito-therapeutic bathing, as well as into the heterodox practices involving hydrotherapy that were current between 1850 and 1900 (Bradley 2002; Gruber 1992; Hampel 1998; Rolls 1988). Nevertheless, the "system" of Nature Cure, defined in terms of nineteenth-century theory, is based on the exclusive use of natural elements to treat illness by facilitating the body's ability to heal itself. Under the direction of experienced practitioners, and often with the aid of elaborate technological devices—saunas, pressure showers, hot and cold compresses, enema douches, and tubs of various sizes, shapes, and configurations—the body is exposed to air, earth, sunlight, and water so as to purge toxins and restore natural balance and integrity. Vegetarianism and the consumption of raw, unprocessed foods prevent morbid toxification and are, therefore, integral to Nature Cure.

Nature Cure in general and hydrotherapy in particular became popular in Europe near the end of the nineteenth century (Whorton 2002), at least in part as a response to the increasingly specialized, invasive, and iatrogenically dangerous forms of allopathic practice that were current at the time (Bynum and Porter 1987; Cooter 1988).[1] For some of the same reasons—as well as because they served to de-link medicine, health, and colonial governmentality—they became very popular in India during the early part of the twentieth century. This popularity is due in part to Louis Kuhne's work on hydrotherapy (1893), which, through translation, became the foundation of both theory and practice in South Asia (Alter 2000a: 56) . Without a doubt, however, it was Mahatma Gandhi's advocacy for Nature Cure (Alter 2000a; A. Misra 2001)—based on a close reading of Kuhne, Adolph Just, and numerous English advocates of vegetarianism—which gave this system of medicine a degree of prominence, permanence, and official respectability in modern India.

Significantly, as I have pointed out elsewhere (Alter 2000a: 55–82), Nature Cure and Yoga are completely integrated, at least from the vantage point of practitioners of Nature Cure and the government of India, if not, by any means, all practitioners of Yoga. This integration is based on a number of incipient congruities on the level of both theory and practice. On a practical level, Nature Cure's concern with detoxification and purgation is similar to the idea of internal and external purification in Yoga, such that enemas and *basti*—in which a tube is inserted into the rectum and water sucked up into the bowel and then expelled—can be understood simply as minor variations on a theme. Theoretically, Yoga's connection with *pañcabhūta* physiology is thought to link it directly to the elemental structure of Nature Cure. Similarly, as the subtle form of air, *prāṇa* and *prāṇāyāma* can be easily understood, through direct translation, as vital breath and dynamic breathing exercises within the framework of Nature Cure therapy. Perhaps most significantly, the etheric element *ākāśa* in Yoga can be conceptualized as an extremely rarified fifth element, thus making Yoga a kind of penultimate natural therapy, perfectly congruent with earth, water, air, and solar modalities of treatment, wherein the body provides the "technology" for self-manipulation.

Although accurate comparative figures are not available, there is no question but that Nature Cure in India, as a distinct "system of medicine"—rather than as a generalized amalgam of New Age practices—is, relatively speaking, very popular. Perhaps more so than in other countries, it enjoys a significant degree of official recognition.[2] It is supported by the government of India, there are state-certified Nature Cure hospitals in different parts of the country, and medical degrees and diplomas are granted from a network of teaching and research hospitals. There are also numerous Nature Cure doctors in private practice (Central Council for Research in Yoga and Naturopathy 1996).[3]

In this chapter my goal is both to provide a perspective on Yoga as alternative medicine, as it has been integrated into Nature Cure in the context of private practice, and to provide a perspective on the institutionalization of alternative medicine in a context where institutionalization and medicine are pushed—by the force of "alterity" in what is counted as alternative—to their logical limits.

If Nature Cure Is the Answer, What Was the Question?

Despite Gandhi's vision of public health in India as a low-cost, easily available, self-treatment method of Nature Cure, as an institutionalized system of medicine Nature Cure is more popular among the urban middle class than among the rural masses. In terms of the Gandhian vision, expressed most directly in *Key to Health* (1948), this is painfully ironic, since one of the primary ideas behind Nature Cure is to avoid expensive drugs and promote a simple, healthy way of life based on a vegetarian diet and various therapies using only the natural elements air, earth, water, sunlight, and ether. In calling for a "return to nature" Gandhi imagined that it was rustic, earthy peasants—true sons and daughters of the soil—who would be most likely to accept and adopt the principles of Nature Cure (see Gandhi 1921, 1949, 1954).

However, for most peasants, as well as for the urbanized working poor and impoverished "slum dwellers," Nature Cure is as alien, if not more alien, than Āyurveda, allopathic biomedicine, Homeopathy, or any of the other permutations of healing that are available in the marketplace of medicine. In fact, one might even say that there is an element of bitter irony in advocating a form of treatment such as hydrotherapy in places where drinking water is in short supply and contaminated, and in promoting breathing exercises to treat asthma in congested inner-city neighborhoods where air pollution threatens to retard the neurological development of young children and causes chronic respiratory ailments in a large percentage of the population. It may even be regarded as not simply ironic, but just plain ridiculous, to treat those who "live closest to nature" with a few hundred grams of raw fruit, nuts, and vegetables when their access to things of greater value is structurally constrained. One could say that it is not simply ridiculous but downright unconscionable, cruel, and unself-consciously cynical—in a way that only modernity makes possible—to prescribe fasts for the treatment of tuberculosis, typhoid, cholera, and dysentery of one kind or another, when those who suffer from these ailments have very limited access to even the most basic of basic resources.

Taking a conservative, critical perspective, one could say that Nature Cure turns the tragedy of modernity into a postmodern farce, and that its institutionalization as an alternative system of health care is pure commercial exploitation, wherein people pay money to starve themselves, cover themselves with mud, submit to daily enemas, and "learn" how to breathe, among a host of other things. Alternatively, taking a partisan stand, one could argue that Nature Cure is the answer to all of the world's health problems, since it makes use of only readily available, inexpensive elements and is based on the principle of prevention. In these terms it is simple, economical, effective, efficient, and environmentally sound.

My argument is that by forcing these two perspectives together it is possible to show how the "farcical simplicity" of institutionalized Nature Cure/Yoga can pose a serious challenge to medicine's modernity by destabilizing the structure of biopower upon which postcolonial governmentality is based. This destabilization is significantly inadvertent, in the sense that it is not the direct consequence of Nature Cure/Yoga's radical position as an alternative to other forms of medicine. As Nature Cure/Yoga is institutionalized as an alternative to medicine—as an alternative both to the class injustices of capitalist medicine and to the epistemic violence of allopathic medical practice—its ontology subverts the structure of biopower that authorizes the apparatus of institutionalization within the framework of the state. In this sense, its consequences are more radical than its stated goals.

If someone is unable to afford drugs to treat cholera, for example, at least this is the familiar injustice of capitalism played out in the local environment of clinics and pharmacies. And if the state, with aid from the World Health Organization, promotes sanitation and immunization campaigns for the collective benefit of the population at large, one is dealing with a form of institutionalized benevolence for the public good. As Foucault has pointed out, however, care and coercion get confused as the state's interests come to define what is good, who constitutes "the public," and how the population as a whole is subdivided into meaningful/useful categories. This is particularly so with the socialization of medicine, where the state, through a ministry of welfare, or a department of human services, takes on the role of caregiver and provides free or heavily subsidized health care. But even in states where medicine is not socialized, there is keen interest in maintaining the health and welfare of the population as a whole in order to prevent epidemic diseases and, at least in principle, to improve the living conditions of the people who collectively constitute society at large. The problem—or at least one of them—is that the state produces, in order to authorize itself, a false sense of concern for individuals, and for the equality and shared interest of individuals as a social collective, by imposing benevolence. To adapt Foucault's terminology: when immunization, sanitary guidelines, and nutritional standards are mandated by law, the wolf of police sovereignty is in the sheep's clothing of pastoral governmentality.

What Foucault and others have not fully explored, however, is the problematic relationship between the ontology of various forms of medicine and the nature of power as it is infused in biogoty. The reason for this is that in Foucault's genealogy of health care in the eighteenth century—as in all of his other studies—the body is prioritized as a locus of power and is subject to all manner of disciplinary mechanisms, but is, itself, regarded as more or less powerless: it is acted upon, so as to effect various results, but does not itself act. It is also regarded as intrinsically whole, even when only parts of it are subject to various disciplinary strategies. Needless to say, Foucault's analysis of health care and the disciplines of biology and medicine within science hinges on the historical significance of Descartes and of the paradigmatic distinction Descartes made between mind and body. However, while recognizing the historicity of this shift in thinking, Foucault then seems to treat the body as if it were in fact distinct from the mind, rather than socially constructed as such in the context of the Renaissance. This is particularly true with regard to the key relationship between body and power. What Foucault has to say about ideology clearly betrays his "uncritical" prioritization of the body: "As regards Marxism, I'm not one of those who tries to elicit the effects of power on the level of ideology. Indeed I wonder whether, before one poses the question of ideology, it wouldn't be more materialist to study first the body and the effects of power on it. Because what troubles me with these analyses which prioritize ideology is that there is always presupposed a human subject on the lines of the model provided by classical philosophy, endowed with a consciousness which power is then thought to seize on" (1980: 58). From this it would seem that Foucault posits the body as an analytical alternative to the "human subject endowed with consciousness" so as to dislocate power, reveal its complexity, and make it more intelligible. Although this was a brilliant move, one could reflect Foucault's somewhat cynical anti-Marxist skepticism back on itself by saying that what is troubling about studies that prioritize the body is not only that they presuppose that the body is *not* endowed with consciousness, but that power, acting upon the body, creates multiple human subjectivities, only one of which is modeled on classical philosophy, and that too by means of a different exercise of power.

David Arnold has rightly criticized Foucault for not factoring colonialism into the conception of the clinic and its subsequent birth in Europe, since in many ways the colonies provided contexts in which the body and public health presented specific problems of control and management (1993). And yet, in using Foucault to make sense of colonial biopower, Arnold and others have taken for granted that medicine—be it biomedicine, Āyurveda, or some combination thereof—can only work to produce disciplined, docile bodies. To be sure, the nature of docility is different, and there are examples of various local contestations and forms of subaltern resistance to the corporeal technologies of the colonial regime, but in all of this there is a nagging sense that resistance is reactive rather than proactive and, furthermore, that, in being enmeshed in the microphysics of power in local contexts it has a limited reach and does not fully engage with the nature of power as such. In his discussion of science and modernity in colonial and postcolonial India Gyan Prakash deals with issues of medicine and health, but although he clearly articulates how the struggle over public health in India manifests a struggle to define and institutionalize an alternative modernity, he, like Arnold, seems to accept the basic Foucauldian formula concerning the relationship between bodies and biopower, health and governmentality (1999).

To fully engage with the nature of power one must, I think, not think in terms of resistance or even in terms of alternatives, much less in terms of colonial institutions—although obviously all of this has its place.[4] Each in its own way, several recent studies have succeeded in breaking out of the nationalist-leftist-subaltern conception of historiography-in-the-shadow-of-colonialism, and point research in a new direction. Waltraud Ernst challenges any conception of a medical system as seamlessly integrated unto itself or as set apart from, and thereby politically configured only in relation to, other institutions and practices (2002). Contributors to a volume edited by Biswamoy Pati and Mark Harrison (2001) focus directly on the details of specific cases, an approach that always has a way of revealing larger truths (see also Ernst and Harris 1999; Meade and Walker 1991). Deepak Kumar (2001) works against the hegemony of colonial and postcolonial historiography, broadly defined, by extending and connecting questions of power and politics across the span of premodern and modern India, an approach that also has the virtue of radically historicizing the link between medicine and culture.

Working harmonically against these and other developments in the history of medicine in India, the argument made here—which is historical in a theoretical sense if not in a temporal sense—is that to understand power apart from its specific effects, analyses should be concerned with the unconscious meta-consequences of inconsistent unconformity. Just as Foucault deconstructs and dislocates a priori assumptions about the nature of the human-subject-endowed-with-consciousness to fully engage with the nature of power/knowledge in the world—rather than just in Europe, or Europe-in-Asia-in-Europe—it is necessary to conceive of the body as having multiple materialities. It is necessary to hold that "consciousness" is the product of at least one of these materialities. There may also be a kind of consensus based on this consciousness that reproduces a social body that stands in such a close relationship to the individual body that it makes it difficult for power to work its way in between the two.

As I understand it, the unstated—and thereby seemingly commonsensical—assumption in *The Birth of the Clinic* (1973) is that as a figuration of modernity—as a discipline—medicine conquers disease, corrects problems and restores health. Most significantly, a person is healed through outside intervention, whereby a disease is cured through the introduction of medicine into the body, or the body as a whole is restored to balance through the application of humoral therapy. A whole apparatus of knowledge informs practice of this kind. Healing in this mode extends directly out from the body of individual patients into the social body of various groups through the practice of public health. Medicine confronts pathology both on the singular level of individual organisms and on the meta-collective level of society at large. Thus in a sense, medicine stands in opposition to the nature of the body, even though it is understood as integral to the restoration of health, both public and private. Played out on a large scale, and complicated by various forms of institutionalization, this destabilization of the relationship between agency, body, and self is the underlying paradox manifest in biopower, one manifestation of which is the "useful" confusion of coercion and care. Another—and one that can be regarded as paradigmatic in Gandhi's struggle with the social implications of health and healing—is the way in which modern medicine heals through destruction and violence.

But what if it were possible to discover a system of health care, institutionalized in a clinic, which did not conform to the structure of the paradox upon which biopower is based? One place to look would be in the development and establishment of some of the first hospitals in Baghdad during the ninth and tenth century C.E., or in the building of similar institutions under the influence of Buddhist practice in South Asia (see Zysk 1991). Another, which has the simple advantage of being unambiguously engaged with modernity as such, rather than complicated by a legacy of so-called traditional practice and ancient history, is Naturopathy, as Naturopathy in India, as a modern pluralistic system of medicine (Ernst 2002), has incorporated the science of Yoga.[5]

Promoted by the central government—albeit with moderate and somewhat self-conscious enthusiasm—as a radical alternative to allopathic medicine; promoted by various nongovernmental organizations (NGOs) and private sector physicians; promoted, specifically, as a solution to the problem of public health associated with poverty in India; and promoted as a curative system that places control of health back into the hands of common people, Nature Cure/Yoga complicates the relationship between health and wealth, care and coercion, personalized self-help and professionalized institutionalization. It also subverts the logic in which health is the opposite of disease, and the corresponding rationale that diseases must be destroyed in order for health to be restored. In destabilizing the relationship between body and person, and in shifting the dynamics of agency, self-control, and the control of health, Nature Cure/Yoga also confounds the very concept of population upon which governmentality is based. Therefore, despite the ironies and "cruelties" it might be seen to manifest on the level of personal experience, and despite the farce that modernity, having first defined the very concept of nature, has subsequently made of that concept's applied logic, there is something in the nature of Nature Cure/Yoga as a system of medicine that enables it to function outside the powerful nexus of capitalism, state public health policy, and nationalism, while still being intimately, and uncritically, linked to this nexus.

The question, then, is how does a perspective on health, the body, and population taken from the vantage point of institutionalized Nature Cure/Yoga help to clarify the nature of the sociohistorical problems underlying public health? If Nature Cure/Yoga is a radical solution, can one "read backward" through this solution to a better understanding of the nature and scope of the problem that is common to all forms of medicine, as medicine is situated at a particularly critical intersection between the interests of the state, the interests of various social groups, and the concerns of people who get sick? What does Nature Cure/Yoga tell us about the nature of power if it is a system of health care that acts like medicine, but attacks the ontological basis of both medicine *and* the bodies of people who get sick?

The Bapu Nature Cure Hospital and Yogashram

Established in 1984, the Bapu Nature Cure Hospital and Yogashram (BNCHY) is, in many ways, a unique institution. This is not because it is a Nature Cure hospital. There are hundreds, if not thousands, of these throughout urban India. It is not because it combines Yoga therapy with Nature Cure, since these two forms of alternative medicine have been almost completely integrated in practice (Alter 2000a). Nor is it unique in paying homage to Gandhi, since Gandhi's advocacy for Nature Cure is, to a large extent, responsible for the authority granted this system of medicine in contemporary India. The BNCHY is unique because it is neither privately owned nor government run but managed by a charitable trust that functions as a nonprofit voluntary organization designed to "promote and propagate naturopathy as a way of life."

What makes the BNCHY most unique, however, is the way in which it appeals to the middle and upper middle classes, through media, high-profile government authorization, and an aggressive fund-raising strategy, in order to subsidize a project of health care and health reform designed for the poorest of the poor. Administrators of the Nature Cure and Yoga Trust, in particular Dr. R. M. Nair, have been very successful in garnering support for their enterprise from various sectors of the government, and in raising funds through tax-exempt donations solicited from corporations and wealthy patrons. Whereas most, if not all Nature Cure/Yoga institutions in India reflect an ideology of socioeconomic reform derived from the teaching and practice of Gandhi, the BNCHY is one of the few institutions that has tried to put into practice a kind of post-Gandhian constructive program that combines social, personal, and health reform.

Located on 1.5 acres of land in the trans-Jamuna colony of Patparganj, in the densely populated working-class neighborhood close to the Mother Dairy factory, the BNCHY has twenty inpatient beds for specialized care and facilities for the daily treatment of fifty outpatients. It has separate male and female wards and provides "scientific body massage, Japanese massage, enema, mud pack, sauna bath, steam bath, whirlpool bath, chromotherapy, osteopathy, acupuncture, electrotherapy, magnetotherapy, dietetics, acupressure, [and] yogic *kriyās* like *kunjal, sūtra neti* and *jal neti*" (BNCHY n.d.a: 2). Along with standard Nature Cure therapy, the hospital includes a gymnasium with "a multigym, rowing machine, treadmill (jogger), vibrobelt, twister, exercycle, [and] automatic roller (fat churner)," a physiotherapy unit with facilities like "diathermy, ultrasound therapy, and paraffin wax therapy" (BNCHY n.d.a: 2), and a drug de-addiction-cum-rehabilitation center. The BNCHY is recognized by the Ministry of Welfare's Central Government Health Services program, through which government employees can be reimbursed for the treatment they receive. In 1993–94 it provided services to 120 inpatients and 480 outpatients and by 1995–96 this had increased to 173 and 982, respectively. Since it began the hospital has treated 125,000 outpatients and approximately 7,500 inpatients.

According to one of its 1998 promotional publications, the BNCHY provides free and affordable "treatment facilities for the poor and needy. Presently 25% of the facilities are kept open for the deprived sections of society." In addition to this, since the early 1990s the BNCHY has been running an aggressive promotional campaign with free weekly lectures on Yoga and Nature Cure, the primary objective of which is to "reach the poor and needy from the slums and resettlement colonies." For example, a series of ten camps was organized in ten East Delhi "slums" to teach preventative Nature Cure/Yoga techniques; regular summer camps are organized "for the benefit of the poor and needy"; a "mega program for the benefit of slum dwellers" was organized on the 125th anniversary of Gandhi's birth; and copies of the monthly magazine published by the hospital are "circulated free of cost to voluntary organizations and other benevolent groups who are serving the poor and needy." From the perspective of conceptualizing the relationship between Nature Cure/Yoga and poverty, the BNCHY has organized several seminars to which leading medical practitioners were invited. By the mid-1990s drug de-addiction was an integral feature of the hospital's work, providing detoxification and rehabilitation therapy to 230 people between 1995 and 1996, almost all of whom were slum dwellers from nearby trans-Jamuna colonies.

Although it is modestly appointed and, in keeping with the ideal of Nature Cure, relatively inexpensive—inpatients were charged Rs 300 (US$8.00) and outpatient treatment was approximately Rs 80 (US$2.00) in 1997—it is clear from the glossy brochures published by the hospital, as well as from the overall design and bilingual content of the monthly magazine, that the BNCHY is meant to attract English-educated, middle-class patients. This is reflected in one brochure which contains a color photograph of the hospital that strategically includes lots of greenery and excludes other buildings in what is, in fact, a very dusty, congested working-class neighborhood surrounded by small-scale industry and commercial enterprises. The photograph is shot at an angle, from the ground up, to enhance the perspective on the garden. A conscious effort is made to make it look as though the hospital is situated in a lush environment that has been aesthetically landscaped. Inside the brochure are color photographs of young men in Western-style gym clothes working out in the modern gym under the supervision of a trainer. On one page, two fashionably dressed young women sit at a desk in consultation with Dr. Nair. On another the president of India, with other government officials, is shown touring the hospital and receiving copies of the magazine. In listing the hospital's achievements, the brochure makes note of a long list of "glitterati and VIPs" who have presided over various functions, including then Prime Minister P. V. Narasimha Rao, Rajiv Gandhi, former presidents of India Gyani Zial Singh, S. D. Sharma, and R. Venkataraman, and numerous union and state cabinet members. Above a picture of Dr. Nair at the Beijing Airport, and below pictures of a young Chinese boy in shorts and a singlet performing Yoga *āsana*s, the brochure also points out that "the doctors of the hospital have attended many national and international seminars and conferences."

The international, upper-middle-class "glitterati" orientation of the BNCHY becomes even clearer when considering plans the Nature Cure and Yoga Trust has for future expansion and development, plans that are "titanic in size and would require financial, technical and administrative assistance from governmental, international and corporate bodies."

> The trust has embarked upon a program which would require an investment of Rs. 1.45 crores [one crore = ten million] for expansion of present hospital buildings, construction of new wards to accommodate 100 indoor patients, a multipurpose spacious hall, offices, doctor's dutyrooms, hostel for trainees, doctor's residence, laundry, guest house, reading room etc.

> The trust has a plan to establish an "International Institute for Research and Development in Naturopathy and Yoga" in the Gandhi Nidi Complex to develop and coordinate scientific research in the fields of Naturopathy and Yoga. The estimated cost for the research institute is Rs. 8.25 crores.
>
> The dearth of qualified Naturopathic Physicians and absence of a college imparting Degree in Naturopathy and Yogic sciences in the north India has forced the Trust to contemplate the establishment of a degree college of Naturopathy and Yogic Sciences at Gandhi Nidi, Patparganj, which would be affiliated to any one of the Universities located nearby. The proposed college would provide education and training to aspiring Naturopaths and confer on them the Degree of Bachelor in Naturopathy and Yogic Sciences. (BNCHY n.d.b: unnumbered back page)

The architectural model for the new institute-cum-hospital makes it look ultra modern in design and palatial in scale, with gardens, manicured lawns, and ample parking for private vehicles.

Significantly, the BNCHY is closely affiliated with the Resort Nature Cure Institute (RNCI) at the Resort Country Club in Gurgaon, a suburb of New Delhi in Haryana that has undergone rapid development since 1985. Dr. Nair, who is both director of the RNCI and general secretary of the BNCHY, took over the facilities of a failing golf course and transformed the main clubhouse into a "3 star holiday resort" where individuals and groups can come to receive treatment. Although primarily providing hydrotherapy, solar therapy, and mud baths, "the club has opened a Āyurvedic Health Club where experts from Kerala in āyurveda and herbal oil therapy treat patients with body massage. Herbal massages [are] effective in treating rheumatic ailments and allied manifestations such as arthritis, paralysis, spondylitis, muscular dystrophy, gout, sciatic, slip-disc and asthma. Patients are given comprehensive lessons and training in Yoga and meditation to help cope with the stresses of modern life at the Stress Management Center" (Varadpande 1997).

Of particular interest with regard to the dynamics of poverty and wealth in the relationship between the BNCHY, the RNCI, and the proposed development of the Naturopathy Institute at Gandhi Nidhi, is the way in which donors of various amounts of money are offered package-deal incentives. For a donation of Rs 50,000 one gets a free 30-day treatment for rejuvenating and cleansing the body at BNCHY, plus 1 day's free stay at the Gurgaon resort every year. For Rs 100,000 the package is for a 60-day treatment and 2 days' free stay, and so on, accordingly, for donations of increasing amounts. The top-line donation of Rs 750,000 comes with 365 days of free treatment, 21 days at the resort, a 10-day package of holistic treatment at a "5 star" facility in Manesar, free advertising in twenty-four issues of the magazine *Naturopathy*, and two blocks of the new institute building named in your honor.

It seems, at least to some degree, that funds from wealthy patrons are being used to support the development of an institute designed, at least in large part, to serve the needs of the poorest of the poor. Of course, a cynic could see it the other way around: a rhetoric of service to the poor is being used to provide moral justification for what is in reality an elitist, capitalist venture. However, it is clear from the trust's publications that "50% of the new facilities [are] to be kept open for the poor and needy of the slums [and that] 50% of the seats in the [proposed] diploma and certificate courses [will be] reserved for the economically deprived scheduled castes, scheduled tribes and slum dwellers."

There is no reason at all why an institute such as this should not serve the poor. Discussions with Dr. Nair and a tour of the facilities make it clear that the BNCHY is guided by Gandhian ideals. It functions more like an *āśram* than a health resort. As a number of Dr. Nair's associates pointed out, it cost a great deal to enable the Mahatma to live a simple life. The important point, however, is that the BNCHY has instantiated a system of health care which at once makes a farce of class disparities by literally "treating everyone the same way." Yet it also reinscribes class difference—with a kind of reverse, "three-star" vengeance—through extreme, albeit extremely well intentioned, classist paternalism. What is interesting about the BNCHY is that it is distinctly "capitalist" in form, but radically "Gandhian" in terms of the social ideals to which it aspires. What is important about this Nature Cure/Yoga hospital is that the simple solution it proposes for the problem of inequality—take from the rich and give to the poor—redefines the very nature of a more basic human problem concerning equality and health on the one hand and, on the other, both the enumeration of the population and its corollary, the administration of public health. Nature Cure/Yoga tends to blur class boundaries by producing a system of self-discipline that is inherently egalitarian. But it also blurs class distinctions by redefining "economy" in terms of embodied health.

One may well be able to purchase relatively inexpensive drugs for hypertension in a small-town pharmacy, but on the level of institutionalization there is a fairly direct correlation in biomedicine between the cost and complexity of treatment on the one hand and the seriousness of the medical problem on the other. Despite its more humoral, herbal basis Āyurvedic medicine reflects a similar correlation in terms of the relative scarcity of those herbs and minerals needed to treat the most serious cases of humoral imbalance. As with mercury and gold in Siddha medicine, the elixir *soma*, to be sure, is quite dear, and just as hard to come by for most people as a kidney transplant or expensive drugs for the treatment of AIDS. Consequently the institutionalization of Āyurveda, Siddha (alchemical medicine), and biomedicine tends to reproduce extreme social inequality, particularly in a free market. There is no mystery in the fact that one can receive the world's best medical treatment in Delhi, Bombay, and Calcutta, but only if one has enough money. And one should never lose sight of the fact, particularly in the context of Yoga and miraculous *siddhi* powers, that money is inherently magical.

With institutionalized Nature Cure, one can certainly have more or less lavish facilities, and the technology used to administer steam baths and hydrotherapy can be quite elaborate. However, in keeping with Gandhi's ideal—and what is more significant, working through the logic of the Mahatma's physical philosophy of social reform—what Dr. Nair is trying to do at the BNCHY is not simply "take from the rich and give to the poor." He has tried to establish a scientific research institute that embodies the balanced, universal principles of nature upon which Nature Cure and Yoga are thought to be based. The idea is to strip away the toxic accretions of civilization, both in the body and in the clinic, that are produced by wealth on the one hand and poverty on the other—the nonbinary relationship between the two being of critical importance—and put everyone back in touch with nature on an equal footing. If the BNCHY were simply a benevolent organization meant to serve the poor, Dr. Nair could run the RNCI in Gurgaon as an upscale, high-class, spa-like resort with better food and more "high-tech" forms of treatment, and maintain the Patparganj hospital as a hospital only for "slum dwellers." But even though "the gymnasium is more frequented by middle class people [and] the physiotherapy unit . . . by the poor and needy," the services provided by the BNCHY are explicitly meant to blur class distinction. There is something in the very nature of Nature Cure/Yoga that subverts hierarchy and makes this possible, at the same time that it makes hierarchy perversely visible. In essence this "something" is the curative, therapeutic, and inherently public, but categorically antimedical and ontologically embodied, nature of Nature Cure/Yoga.

Curiously, as well, Nature Cure as a system of medicine defies categorization as either traditional or modern, Eastern or Western. Although its origins can be traced back to eighteenth-century Central Europe, it was very popular in both India and the United States during the early twentieth century (Gevitz 1988; Whorton 2002; Wrobel 1987). With some permutations, it is currently seeing a revival as an alternative, holistic "New Age" therapy. Similarly, Nature Cure renders the standard contrast between science and nonscience somewhat problematic, since it claims to be an alternative science of health based on the laws of nature. In practice, then, Nature Cure cannot easily be denounced and discarded as anachronistic, as many forms of "traditional" medicine can be by their detractors. This makes it rather well suited to question the assumptions of modernity in general and modern medicine in particular, even when to do so is not the conscious objective of its practitioners.

Bodies and Persons: Revolutionizing the Science of Life

Most significantly, however, Nature Cure/Yoga is not just antimedical and is not just a different kind of science. Nature Cure/Yoga defines the nature of curing in such a way that the body as a natural organism, functioning in harmony with the world at large, can heal itself. As the history of European medicine makes clear, the idea that the body fights off diseases and infections and repairs itself is not unique. But in biomedicine as well as in all other systems of medicine there is a distinct tendency to try and "outdo" the body, so to speak, and heal it, rather than let it heal itself.

Historically speaking, the principle of letting the body heal itself is an extremely radical proposition—and an extremely modern one—since almost all modalities of treatment other than Nature Cure/Yoga entail the intervention of some kind of outside force that has been explicitly modified and engineered by culture to make it better than nature.[6] Furthermore, in Nature Cure/Yoga emphasis is given to the prevention of disease through healthy living. Healthy living becomes a comprehensive way of life that often entails radical changes in diet, exercise, and other regimens of everyday life.[7] As Dr. Nair points out in an article entitled "Living the Nature Cure Way," echoing almost every Nature Cure doctor from the early-nineteenth-century "Silesian peasant" Vincent Pressnitz up to Gandhi himself, by way of Adolf Just (1903) and Louis Kuhne (1893): "Nature cure, apart from being a way of life, is a distinct system of healing based upon its own philosophy of health and disease. It does not limit itself to curing aches and pains. It is a complete revolution in the art and science of living, as it is a realization and application of all that is good in natural science, philosophy and religion" (1997: 11). To a large extent the basic rules for healthy living—eating a moderate, unspiced, vegetarian diet, getting daily exercise in the fresh air, and not consuming any intoxicants—are also the primary modalities of treatment. It is not just the whole body that must be restored to health. In some sense the body restores a person—who is much more than a body, and this is where Yoga comes into the equation most dramatically—to a condition of life lived in tune with nature. The importance of this cannot be emphasized too much, and its significance is all too easy to miss from a perspective where medicine, even under the mantle of public health, concerns itself with the body as a self-contained system. When a person does get sick—which is, in Nature Cure, only symptomatic of a much larger problem of environment—the specific symptoms are understood as the body's natural reaction to disease, and treatment often entails using the disease to restore health through fasting and enemas that purge the system of toxins. This is usually followed by a series of different kinds of baths using either sunlight, air, earth, or water, as well as by changes in diet. The body's natural "defense mechanism" is thought to be the best, most powerful medicine, including, in many instances, the symptoms of illness as such. The simple idea is to heal *through* disease, rather than to destroy the disease to restore a person to a default condition of "health" defined as the absence of disease.

Before we turn to a consideration of the relationship between bodies and persons, and the way in which this relationship complicates the "self"—as the self is located at the nexus of health, relative wealth, and the problem of population manifest in public health—some examples, drawn indiscriminately from various issues of *Naturopathy,* the monthly magazine of the BNCHY, will illustrate how Nature Cure/Yoga is put into practice.

After pointing out that drugs can be used to treat "kidney congestion," but that patients recover in spite of the drugs and not because of them, and often suffer chronic problems as a result of drug treatment, Dr. R. M. Nair writes: "The proper treatment for congestion of the kidneys is *fasting*. The patient should be fasted on water and orange juice for as long as the acute symptoms last, and [a] warm water enema should be used nightly during that time. Then the *all-fruit diet* can be adopted for a further few days, and finally the *full weekly dietary* can be begun when convalescence is well advanced. This full weekly dietary should be adhered to rigorously thereafter if future kidney trouble is to be effectively prevented and sound health restored" (1992a: sec. 4, p. 20).

Although "simple" in theory, Nature Cure treatment can be very complicated. For example, Dr. Rukmani Nair published the following case history of Mrs. Urmila Devi, a fifty-seven-year-old "Hindu housewife" suffering from rheumatoid arthritis. Mrs. Urmila Devi was overweight, had great difficulty walking, and had been taking painkillers for a year. The case history starts with a list of the results of various tests on the "vital data" of blood pressure, pulse rate, and respiration, and an appraisal of sleep patterns, appetite, and digestion. Results are then given on "systemic examination," showing that the cardiovascular, respiratory, renal, and nervous systems were functioning normally at the time, but that the patient's feet were swollen and that she had difficulty walking. On the basis of this Mrs. Devi was put through an intensive, extremely precise month-and-a-half-long course of fomentations, mud packs, compresses, hip baths, spinal baths, hot foot and arm baths, steam baths, infrared lamp treatment, and massage, along with fasting, enemas, and daily dietary prescriptions. To give some sense of the precision of the treatment as a whole, consider what is said about just three modalities—mud pack, hip bath and Yoga *āsana*.

> Mud pack or direct mud was applied to the lower abdomen daily for 10–15 minutes. Mud pack was given to the eyes when the patient had no complaint of common cold or cough. Special facial mud pack was applied on the face on alternate days to remove the blackish pigmentation on the face. Mud was directly applied on inflamed joints for 20–30 minutes. Sometimes mud pack or mud was kept on the head if there was complaint of heat on the head or tension. . . .
>
> In the first two weeks [the] patient could not tolerate hip bath. Hip bath was given for 10 to 15 minutes everyday from the third week onwards. During the previous two weeks the patient was given [a hip bath] only thrice for ten minutes. The scheduled time for the hip bath was from 3:30–3:45 in the afternoon. (1994: 10–12)

For one hour every day, except when suffering from fever, the patient was prescribed the following *āsana*s: *uttānapadāsana, pavanamuktāsana, tāḍāsana, katicakrāsana, trikoṇāsana, sukhāsana*. As her condition improved she advanced to *gomukhāsana, ardhasalabāsana, bhujaṅgāsana,* and *dhanurāsana*.

The precision of treatment is the same for all of the other baths and massages, while careful and extremely detailed attention was also given to diet. For the first eleven days the patient was given 200 ml of *nim* juice at 6 A.M., followed by a glass of lime juice and honey at 6:30. At 9:30 she was given a glass of vegetable soup without salt or spices. At noon she ate three to five chapatis, 200 gms of vegetable porridge, 200 gms of steamed or boiled vegetables, a cup of soup, and between 50 and 100 gms of raw vegetables. At 2 P.M. she was given a glass of lemon juice with honey, followed at 5 P.M. with a glass of seasonal fruit juice. For dinner, at 7 P.M., she had three or four chapatis, 200 gms of boiled vegetables, and 50 gms of salad. Every day she drank between six and eight glasses of water. On four of the first eleven days she ate only raw vegetables in order to increase her appetite. From the tenth through the fourteenth of May the patient underwent "fast therapy," drinking a glass of lemon juice and honey at 6 and 10 A.M., and 2 and 5 P.M. After breaking the fast on the fifteenth, she began a five-day diet of raw fruit and vegetables, with the main two meals, at 11 A.M. and 7 P.M., consisting of between 500 and 700 gms of vegetables, roots, sprouts, and fruits. At the end of this regimen she went back on the cooked diet for another ten days, and then underwent another five-day fast. After this she went back on the raw diet for a week before shifting again to the cooked diet, all the time drinking six to eight glasses of water. She was advised to continue this diet along with the

Yoga exercises after being discharged. The case study concludes by pointing out that Mrs. Urmila Devi "was able to walk without pain and support, could sit on the floor without any difficulty, had an improved appetite, showed no signs of depression, had a radiant complexion, no foot oedema, and required no medication" (1994: 13). She was, in other words, cured and rejuvenated. She had also changed her way of life.

An article on asthma starts by noting that the incidence of the disease is increasing at an alarming rate. Citing a report published in the news magazine *India Today,* the authors point out that between 1979 and 1994 there was a 15 percent increase among children, and that in Delhi 75 percent of all asthma patients are young children. The physiopathology of asthma is defined in the following terms.

> The trouble starts when the immune system becomes sensitized to allergens, usually through heavy exposure in early life and gets it treated as a threat. The allergens, on entering the body, the immune system's B Lymphocytes release antibody molecules called immunoglobulin E (IgE) which surges through the blood stream that attach themselves to mast cells and respond by pouring out histamine and other inflammatory chemicals. When localized in the nose the victim suffers no more than itching and running nose. The real trouble starts when the reaction extends down into the lungs, the results become lethal.

The increase in incidence is attributed to a deterioration in the quality of air, and to allergic reactions, dust mites, mold and pollens. This is followed by a discussion of treatment.

> Naturopathic treatment of asthma is more patient friendly and encouraging [than treatment with drugs]. Here the principle lies on total elimination of the ailment rather than giving symptomatic relief to the patients. Through diet and Yoga a change in the body physiology and immune mechanism could be modulated. This will develop the capability to encounter allergens.
>
> Yoga is not primarily a method of asthma treatment but is associated with the curative and prophylactic values. *Śavāsana* [corpse posture] with *Padmāsana* [lotus posture], *Makarāsana* [crocodile posture] and *Matsyāsana* [fish posture] are helpful.
>
> *Neti Kriyā* (nose cleaning) with salt and milk is advocated to the patients with chronic cold and sinusitis. When done with salt the mucous membranes develop the resistance (immunity) to variation in environmental temperature whereas *neti kriyā* with milk is to build up resistance against proteins. In patients with wet cough *Dhauti*s like *Jaldhauti* (cleaning with water), *Vamanadhauti* (cleaning with stick) and *Vastradhauti* (cleaning with cloth) are recommended to remove excessive mucous from the stomach. *Kunjal* and hydrotherapy improves the recovery process significantly.

> Diaphragmatic breathing or so called *Kapālabhāti Kriyā* effectively removes sputum from the lungs. Further research and investigations are still needed to completely unlock the mystery behind the disease. Areas of interest will be on Yoga and genetic identification to control asthma, the disease of modern and civilized culture. (Nair and Nair 1997: 11–13)

Much has been written in the popular press about the radical potential of holistic health to combat the reductive fragmentation and attendant depersonalization manifest in biomedicine. One of the basic principles in holistic health is to make medicine more humane and less alienating, the idea being that the natural state of being whole is to be a health-conscious person. There is a tendency, however, to conflate such things as wholeness, happiness, health, and well-being, and to assume that it is individuals unto themselves who are, or should be, in a position to restore wholeness and achieve health and happiness. One may think of this as personal responsibility with a vengeance. Much of the Nature Cure literature follows this tendency. Patients such as Mrs. Urmila Devi, or those who wish to prevent themselves from getting sick, are instructed on what to eat or what kind of yogic exercise to do. Underlying this is a basic assumption that one can and will choose to do and eat different things, and that these choices will affect one's health in certain ways, both positively and negatively.

One could argue that in all of these examples of holistic, natural health care there is the familiar problem of medicalization, in which patients like Mrs. Urmila Devi are enmeshed in a certain configuration of power. Their bodies are disciplined and made the object of a panoptic, scientific gaze. Manifesting patient docility, they participate in the production of knowledge by subjecting themselves to various therapies, and live within the fields of force defined by that knowledge. One could argue, in other words, that even though Nature Cure is a different kind of medicine it still conforms to the overarching principle of biopower by disciplining bodies. Mrs. Urmila Devi's treatment is, in many ways, as radical, as invasive, and as directly linked to a discourse of power as any regimen of chemotherapy.

A problem presents itself, however, in the fact that in Nature Cure the body is assigned a curious kind of agency that is localized in persons but is not a feature of the self. Or at least the body's agency is not a feature of the self associated exclusively with that "human subject . . . endowed with a consciousness" that so vexed Foucault in his analysis of power (1980: 58). Although the disconnection of body and agency was probably an issue in nineteenth-century central Europe, where the agency of nature was thought to be more powerful, more benevolent, and closer to the truth than anything contrived by "modern man," it was certainly true in early-twentieth-century India. Throughout the twentieth century and into the beginning of the twenty-first this significance has increased. It has served to draw Yoga and Nature Cure together to produce a kind of proactive health care that is medical in practice but that does not simply or easily "medicalize" the patient, on the level of either the person or the body.

Nature Cure is based on a theory of prevention and cure in which choice is epiphenominal to a more basic, impersonal form of phenomenal agency manifest in the natural elements. As a product of civilization the self cannot be entrusted with the health of the natural body. Strictly speaking, therefore, the standard Nature Cure injunction to "cure yourself" is inaccurate. It should be "let your body cure itself," and let your health heal the culture and society to which your body is subject.[8] This entails more passive sacrifice and submission than conscious self-control, or at least it involves a kind of self-control keyed to natural laws rather than to cultural codes of health consciousness. In being natural and in submitting to the laws of nature when sick, the body, as an aggregate of nature, disciplines persons. It does not, itself, become the object of a disciplinary project manifest in the logic of medicine defined as a cultural system. Whereas biomedicine fragments the body and thereby does epistemic violence to the person as a whole, to the extent that selfhood is an embodied experience, Nature Cure/Yoga disaggregates bodies and persons in terms of a natural ontology that does not see that disaggregation as problematic or violent. Nature, in this scheme, is more humane than humankind, and its holism is not confined to the biology of persons or the self-consciousness of individual selves. This is a kind of "positive" mind/body duality that does not carry with it the negative implications of Cartesian logic, and—at least in principle—it inhibits a whole apparatus of power derived from that logic.

How does this work? In a brief statement entitled "Fundamental Principles of Nature Cure," reproduced in *Naturopathy,* an American naturopath named Harry Benjamin clearly locates the agency of health in the body. In his and many other such statements a sense of the person is almost completely absent.

> The second principle of Nature Cure is that the body is always striving for the ultimate good of the individual, no matter how ill-treated it may be. . . .
>
> The third principle of Nature Cure is that the body contains within itself the power to bring about a return to that condition of normal well-being known as health, providing the right methods are employed to enable it to do so. That is to say that the power to cure disease lies not in the hands of the doctor or specialist, but within the body itself. Within this will be

found the source of the healing power which Nature is ever ready to bestow on all who are willing to accept her laws and live in accordance with them. (1992: 2–3)

The Embodied Laws of *Prakṛti:* Self, Nature, and the Nature of the Self

While it was the German inventors of Nature Cure who first devised a whole system of medicine built around the idea that the body could heal itself, this system of medicine found ready acceptance in India, where ideas of animate and animating nature, in the guise of *prakṛti,* were well developed.[9] Although it is usually translated as nature, *prakṛti* has a broader and more complex denotation than its English gloss. Most significantly it is active and dynamic unto itself, albeit in the inherently compromised mode of an illusion. Although the point has been made in other contexts, it is worth reviewing the important features of *prakṛti* with specific reference to the fact that it is more of an "unstable" process than a stable thing as such. Referring to *prakṛti* as "creatrix," Georg Feuerstein writes:

> Nature in all its aspects is utterly insentient. Whereas the Self is perfectly and eternally immobile, the pure witness (*sākṣin*), Nature is inherently in motion. Its dynamics is due to the interplay of its three types of "primary constituents" (*guṇa*), namely *sattva, rajas* and *tamas.* In combination, they weave the entire pattern of cosmic existence, from high to low. The *guṇas* underlie all material and psychic realities. The mind and the ego are counted among the material phenomenon. (1990: 263–64)

A concept of *śakti* is used in one very common theorization of the relationship among *prakṛti,* the self of lived experience, and the transcendental cosmic Self, to explain the "dynamic force" whereby a singular Reality continually creates and re-creates the multiplicity of forms in a world of multidimensional experience. In manifesting, by its very nature, the meta-material agency of *śakti,* an embodied person can submit to the *prakṛtic* "laws of nature," so to speak, and yet maintain a kind of self-control that is consciously embodied, but not simply the product—or by-product—of personal consciousness. Where *prakṛti* is concerned, an idea—the thought "I think, therefore I am," for example—is an elemental material thing of the same organic substance as water, earth, sunlight, air, and ether.

What may well have made Nature Cure so popular in India around the turn of the last century was its direct, unmediated appeal to "nature," understood as a modern concept denoting the purity of many things—the past, precultural and primordial purity, integrated holism—and the way in which this appeal synchronized with the concept of *prakṛti* manifest, most clearly, in *Sāṃkhya* philosophy. This synchronization transformed *prakṛti*/nature into a construct directly relevant to contemporary Indian concerns, cut against the grain of colonial modernization, and allowed for the development of a modern discourse that was critical of the particular kind of modernity manifest in British India.

While resonating within the social body of hospitalized patients such as Mrs. Urmila Devi—who seems to have had no particular qualms about the nature of her treatment—the harmonics of *prakṛti*/nature undermines the ontogenic dichotomy of self and substance, mind and body, that is integral to clinical practice. A disciplinary regimen that understands the self to be a manifestation of the body's essential nature renders Foucault's perspective on power highly problematic. In effect it short-circuits the reproduction of power's "capillary form of existence, the point where [it] reaches into the very grain of individuals, touches their bodies and inserts itself into their actions and attitudes, their discourses, learning processes and everyday lives [as] a synaptic regime of power, a regime of its exercise *within* the social body, rather than *from above it*" (Foucault 1980: 39). Although "the clinic" medicalizes nature—to be sure, as anyone who has undergone hydrotherapy knows—*prakṛti* "naturalizes" medicine in a way that draws attention to numerous fault lines that cross-cut a postcolonial world that is sutured together with a Cartesian logic of pure and practical reason.

Although it subverts the "capillary form" of power's existence and thereby destabilizes the structure and function of biopower, it would be wrong to conclude that Nature Cure/Yoga is liberating. Quite the contrary. Nature Cure/Yoga produces a regime of power "from within" whereby the body is made to get back in touch with nature. Once it cures itself in this way, it articulates the laws to which it has conformed. In a sense what happens through the institutionalization of Nature Cure/Yoga is that the kind of power "from above" that reflects an absolute need to control in toto takes the form of a regime that exercises power from within. Nature defines an absolute rule of law, and Nature Cure/Yoga manifests the mechanics of a kind of despotic self-control, wherein one is liberated from the rule of Western science and cured by adopting a way of life structured by a new science of life. Consider what Dr. J. M. Jussawalla, one of the pioneers of Nature Cure in India, has to say in his article in *Naturopathy* entitled "Vis Medicatrix Naturae":

> The healing forces of or powers of nature within the body are a gift from the Creator to all his creatures for the purpose of preservation of health and life

> and protection from destruction by evil forces. Man being the product of nature, is definitely governed by natural laws; his life, his health and his very being are influenced by it in one form or another. . . .
>
> The present generation is so overpowered by the word "Science" that it will not open its mind to the simple and rational truths of the natural healing forces embodied in the body. . . .
>
> Health is the normal, natural state of the human being, and it is maintained quite without conscious control by the wonderful, normalizing, building, healing "intelligence" which is sometimes called "Nature" or "Vital Force. . . ."
>
> Violation of Nature's laws may be due to ignorance, lack of self-control, self-indulgence, indifference, resulting in a lowered vitality, abnormal composition of blood and lymph, accumulation of the waste matter and poisons in the system.
>
> Obedience to law is [by] far the best healer and real health will be the reward for all who heed Nature's warning and obey its laws. (1992: 5–7).

Nature Cure/Yoga as a way of life is, most certainly, holistically healthy. But precisely by virtue of being that, it is strictly and rigidly circumscribed. It defines itself with the authority of supreme law, and deploys the rule of law into "the very grain of individuals" and "inserts itself into their actions and attitudes." Governmentality takes on new significance as a kind of post-eighteenth-century notion of sovereign power—Jussawalla's prose resonates well with the sermons of John Wesley and the moralism of late-nineteenth-century health reformers—is built into the body. This mutation in significance is made possible because of the way in which the body is assigned a curious kind of agency that is localized in persons but is not a feature of the self as a thing apart.

Although the case of Mrs. Urmila Devi clearly illustrates this, it is worth examining some other examples of what happens when life and nature come together to constitute a kind of power that works from above, below, and within the social body all at once. Consider the case of Mr. Swarajya Prakash, who for two years suffered from arthritis and sciatica. He went to BNCHY, where he was treated for a fortnight with "Yoga, enema, massage, infrared, vibrator, steam/sauna bath, sun bath, wax bath, and sometimes diathermy." As he recounts:

> I was also put on juice fast for 5 days, fruit fast for another five days and then I started taking only two meals containing two *capātīs* in the morning with almost very little salt and oil in vegetables.
>
> In two weeks I lost about 6 kgs and now I am more than 95% cured. I get only little trouble in the morning for about an hour and then after doing exercises I am feeling very well. I am doing all these regularly in my home. (1996: 62)

Discharged from the hospital, he embodies a new life and gives birth to a new kind of clinic in his home and his body where Yoga exercise imperatively reinforces nature's rule of law—imperatively, since to choose otherwise would be to break the laws of nature and revolt against the body.

Another example of how the body disciplines its person when it is imbued with the power of "nature-called-upon-to-do-her-duty" may be taken from an innocuous-sounding article entitled "Care of the Hair":

> A thorough scalp massage exercises the papillae, relaxes the hair-follicles, stimulates the circulation and thus ensures the health and beauty of the hair. Put the fingers through the hair until they grip the scalp. Use the pads of the fingers and be sure that the scalp moves.
>
> Describe firm pressing circles, beginning at the center of the forehead and continuing backward along the hair line to the nape of the neck. Now repeat these movements with the palms of the hand, and, for good measure, give the hair some sharp tugs. For the hair was meant to protect from pressure and shock and, as Nature thrives when it is called upon to do her duty, so such treatment will convert straggling, lank, lusterless hair into a radiant halo for the face and thus add to the beauty and charm of one's personality. (Jussawalla 1991: 7)

The pure force of embodied nature as having a kind of meta-human agency that stands in a complex relationship to the person who occupies that body is most clearly reflected in the way in which Yoga is combined with Nature Cure. Although I have discussed this merger elsewhere with specific reference to the elements in general and the importance of ether in particular (Alter 2000a), the critical issue here concerns nature, the dynamics of embodied nature, and self-consciousness. Simply put, in yogic theory embodied *puruṣa* consciousness is controlled by the force of *prakṛtic* nature until the circumscribed *jīvātman*ic self becomes disembodied and merges with *paramātman*ic universal consciousness. Until the final goal of Yoga is achieved, however, *puruṣa* consciousness is experienced through the mind, which is a product of devolved *prakṛti*. As Dr. Naresh K. Brahmachari, director of the Central Council for Research on Naturopathy and Yoga, puts it in an article published in the first volume of *Naturopathy:* "To have the experience of nature, every *puruṣa* is assisted by mind. . . . The mind, galvanized into life, knowledge and action because of its proximity with the self, is the sole cause of misery and affliction, bondage and liberation." Dr. Brahmachari then explains how the mind, when it is dominated by *rajas guṇa*—one of the three constituent properties of *prakṛti*—"is marked with . . . mental diseases like lust, anger, avarice, arrogance, spite, egoism, envy and jealousy." When dominated by *tamas guṇa,* "it is tainted with ignorance, lassitude, dullness, sleep, inadvertence and stupidity." He then points out that "when the mind is filled up with Sattvic traits like humility, faith, devotion, righteous conduct, truth, contentment, knowledge and detachment through the practice of Yoga all the afflictions, miseries, diseases and psychosomatic dysfunctions start gradually attenuating and the individual develops the competence to experience enlightenment, detachment, utter contentment, sound psychological attitude toward life situations and perfect mental health" (1991: 10).

Several important points emerge from this. First, the mind is part of the body, as the body's anatomical structure and metabolic function is keyed to the balance of *guṇa* manifest in *prakṛti*. Second, the self experiences nature through the mind. Third, and perhaps most significant, a *sattvic* state of mind ultimately only establishes a contingently healthy state of being. Although embodied self-consciousness can lead to "liberation," it also produces—by its very relationship to nature—"misery, affliction and bondage." Ultimately, then, Yoga is oriented toward the transcendence of even the most pure, "uncontaminated" *sattvic* state of embodied self-consciousness. "When the yogi . . . transcends the *sattvaguṇa* . . . by the practice of utter detachment, the self abides in itself and the mind, having performed its function[,] merges into its material cause[,] the nature" (Brahmachari 1991: 11). The final goal of Yoga is understood, not as a disaggregation of mind and body, but as the disassociation of self-as-the-Self from nature, and it is this final possibility that illustrates the power of nature over the self in the state of being human *prior* to final liberation. This translates into the discipline of persons by means of the subtle metabolic balance of embodied *sattva, rajas,* and *tamas* and the five *mahābhūta* elements from which these three constituent *guṇa* are derived.

In the following example, taken from an article entitled "The Science of Yogic Postures (Yog Mudrās) and Their Benefits," the body is clearly animated with a kind of suprahuman—but not supernatural—power, and it is the mindful person who gets disciplined by the way in which the body-so-animated is thought to work.

> We all know that our body is composed of five elements—the earth, the water, the fire, the air, and the ether (*ākāśa*). All these are governed by bioelectricity of human system. The imbalance of these elements causes disease. The five elements of our body are represented by the five fingers of our hands—the thumb representing the fire (sun); the index finger the air; the middle finger the ether; the ring finger, the earth; and the little finger, the water. Joining of these fingers with each other makes the life current flow and bring changes in the body system removing imbalance. The science of touching fingers in a particular fashion is called the science of Yogic postures or *Mudrā Vijñān*. (Chanana 1995: 59)

The author goes on to provide a comprehensive list of *mudrās*, showing how the body activates itself in different ways. *Prāṇa mudrā,* for example, where the tips of the thumb, little, and ring fingers touch, "switches on the flow of life force in the body mechanism and is very beneficial to both healthy and diseased persons. It enhances the natural resistance of the body" (1995: 60). Although it is easy to think that what is involved here is simply a person doing *mudrās*, the power of the *mudrā* is completely dependent on an understanding in which the *mudrā* recreates the body through a person's actions.

Returning to Dr. Brahmachari's analysis of the relationship between self and nature, one further point about individuals and individualized care is noteworthy. Although personalized therapies are not unique to Nature Cure/Yoga, other forms of medicine instantiate them on an epistemic level. Adjustments are made for blood pressure, allergies, pain tolerance, cholesterol levels, genetic patterns, and so forth, but "difference" on the level of biology is trumped by species-specific uniformity. It is this uniformity, constructed through a discourse of science, upon which medicine depends. To think differently is to confound the basis of clinical practice, among many other things. In this regard Dr. Brahmachari points out that in the context of Yoga it is *prakṛti* rather than biology that is universal and standardized, and every body contains the elemental structure of nature. However, both embodied consciousness and the mind, which together link consciousness as such to the material world, are understood to be unique in every organism. If this were not the case and everyone and everything had the same consciousness, Dr. Brahmachari goes on to reason—drawing on the concept of *saṁsāra,* "the constant flux of events in which no permanence and security can be found" (Feuerstein 1990: 308), but looking for order nevertheless—that "there would be no orderly arrangement of birth and death, pleasure and pain, release and bondage" in the world (1991: 10).

To a significant extent, therefore, each person's inherent difference is a necessary precondition for the continuity of life as a process, a social process that is built on the irreducible difference of each person, but which makes sense only in terms of the abstracted structure of "base pair" patterns reflected in each mind on the one hand and transcendental consciousness on the other.[10] Consequently there is a fundamental tension in the practice of Nature Cure/Yoga between the standardization of treatment reflected, for example, in categorical statements about what *prāṇa mudrā* is good for, and how "everyone" should massage his or her hair, and the kind of radically personalized treatment regimen prescribed for Mrs. Urmila Devi and most other patients.

This is a critical point to which I will now turn in order to consider the way in which Nature Cure/Yoga problematizes the "problem of population" and complicates the way in which postcolonial governmentality functions to address that problem. It is a point that can be defined by turning to reconsider the epigraph from Foucault on body/power at the beginning of the chapter.

What Nature Cure/Yoga seems to make possible is a conflation of body and will to produce a kind of social body defined by the materiality of consciousness manifest in individual bodies. Given the materiality of consciousness, the link between the individual body and the social body is relatively unmediated, thus both restricting and expanding the way in which power operates to produce consensus.

Naturopathy and the Language of the Anti-Clinic

> I am happy to learn that the Bapu Nature Cure Hospital and Yogashram, Patparganj, Delhi decided to bring out a monthly magazine with the title *Naturopathy* from July 1991. Naturopathy is increasingly gaining popularity since the treatment based on this system is completely free from any adverse effect. This is a drugless system.
>
> M. L. Fotedar, Minister of Health and Family Welfare, Government of India, New Delhi (1991: 3)

A question is suggested by the way in which bodies cure people—how does this translate into public health, or, more properly, what happens to the problem of population when public health is translated into the language of Nature Cure/Yoga? Just as the body takes on disciplinary agency in Nature Cure/Yoga practice, and thereby preempts the exercise of power upon it, the argument in this section will be that language—in the form of words that are written down and disseminated to the public—comes to take on the kind of clinical significance that in other forms of medicine is strategically localized in experts, hospitals, and research centers. Through the publication of knowledge about Nature Cure/Yoga, and its consumption by individuals who seek to heal themselves—but who find that they will be healed by nature—the materiality of the individual body and the printed word go hand in hand, as the signifier of knowledge and the signified of power converge in public consciousness.

Since 1991 the BNCHY has published a bilingual Hindi/English monthly journal entitled *Naturopathy* under the editorship of Dr. R. M. Nair. The articles in the journal almost all deal with a specific feature of Yoga and Nature Cure treatment: how to treat bronchial asthma with steam baths, enemas, and arm and leg baths, along with fasting and yogic *kriyās* (Anonymous 1991: 15–28); how to recognize and use pure honey

(Hiralal 1991: 29–31); the virtues of mangos (Niraj 1995: 2–6); different techniques for mud treatment (George 1995: 29–30); exercises and diet for natural childbirth (Jeyaram 1993: 32–34); the treatment of systemic lupus erythematosus (P. Reddy and Vimaladevi 1993: 35–37); pain relief (Bhatt 1992: 4–6); emphysema (Charu 1994: 30–34); the health value of dietary fiber (Singh, Nair, and Nair 1997: 14–17); and many, many other topics. There have been special volumes on the treatment of liver and kidney disease (Nair 1992c), diseases of the heart and lungs (Nair 1992b), and Yoga, spinal baths, pimples, and the bad effects of tea (Nair 1993), for example. Early volumes contained subsections on diet, health care, and therapeutics as well as one for "messages" from various government officials—such as the epigraph above—letters from readers, opinions, editorials, and research reports. In recent years there have been fewer subsections and an increasing trend toward reprinting extracts from the nineteenth- and early-twentieth-century publications of leading German, American, and Indian naturopaths such as Kuhne, Kniepp, Kellogg, Jussawalla, and, of course, Gandhi himself.

What is most significant about the magazine is the way in which it consolidates a wide range of information of different kinds in order to produce knowledge that is authoritative on the level of the social body and yet extremely useful to individuals who suffer from migraines, back aches, bladder infections, diabetes, typhoid fever, cancer, and so on.

Much of the writing in the magazine is distinctively bilingual in the sense that the articles in English—such as those quoted above—do not conform to "standard" English, and the articles in Hindi contain numerous English words. Many of the articles draw on the sciences of biology, physiology, and anatomy as well as on biomedical diagnostic procedures to explain the nature of disease, while using the science of Nature Cure to explain treatment. For example, Dr. Ram Kirin writes:

> Hypertension in one of the direct outcome of modern ways of living during the past fifty years. Improper and wrong life style and getting into the trap of various social stigmas, wrong habits of living are the direct precursors of high blood pressure. . . .
>
> Blood pressure is a state of health is the resultant of a number of forces, the important of which are the contraction of the heart and the peripheral resistance provided by the arterioles, large arteries and also capillary bed, Hypertension can be grouped into two major classes. . . .
>
> So long as the underlying causes are not removed there is no radical cure, Hygienic living is the answer. As Nature Cure begins with a fast of 4–7 days on excessive fresh fruit diets a depending upon the individual patient condition. (1997: 3–4)

Unless it is to be dismissed out of hand, this must not be seen as an example of partly assimilated Western medicine being imperfectly localized in the misspellings, odd capitalizations, strange punctuation, bad grammar, and poor syntax of some cheap magazine published under the auspices of a not-quite-modern, postcolonial, alternative clinic in the back allies of some underdeveloped Third World city. *Naturopathy* is, after all, approved as a "scientific journal" by the Indian government's Council of Scientific and Industrial Research. It should be read as an example of how struggles over the terms of public health, and struggles over the kinds of knowledge that should be relevant for the practice of modern medicine, are reflected, with deadly seriousness, not just in the substance of what gets said but in the very grammar of the languages that have to be used to debate clinical issues. As it seeps into the public sphere—and it is in the seepage factor that power lies—this hybrid language, speaking of bodies whose agency transcends that of persons, articulates a kind of modern vernacular, anti-clinical knowledge.

It is common for Nature Cure/Yoga institutes, societies, hospitals, and centers, along with their purely yogic counterparts, to publish journals in which the articles define and promote these forms of therapy, primarily as "self-help" prevention and treatment. Although it is common for many different kinds of groups to publish journals, it is particularly significant in the case of Nature Cure/Yoga, where practitioners advocate their cause with missionary zeal. Perhaps most significant is the way in which these publications function as a kind of proxy alternative structure for the institutionalization of public health programs, and present themselves as clear alternatives to institutionalized health care. To the extent this works, it works, simply, because a key idea in Nature Cure/Yoga is that one can, and in fact should, learn to let one's body cure oneself and develop a lifestyle that works through the nature of illness to experience the nature of health.

As is often stated in the literature, one should become one's own doctor. If this were to happen on a large scale, the whole infrastructure of remedial health care would become obsolete. One by one, the public would take back health from hospitals, departments of sanitation, and health departments, as well as from other government and nongovernment, national and international, bodies. Think of it: "health for all in the year 2000"—as the WHO would have wanted it—turned into "all for health in the domain of nature." This could happen if the scale of consciousness, about health as well as about immortality—including the future of time—were configured in terms of a different structure of power. This is the radical, populist potential at the heart of Nature Cure/Yoga. It is a potential that becomes more and more radical with increasing subscription rates, growing readership, and the possibility—the hope, as Gandhi put it—that collective knowledge of nature and nature's laws will eventually translate into health for all. The dissemination of knowledge about Nature Cure/Yoga stands in sharp contrast to the production and dissemination of highly specialized, technical knowledge within communities of biomedical and Āyurvedic physicians. What is even more significant is the way in which the dissemination of knowledge about Nature Cure/Yoga stands in sharp contrast to the dissemination of medical knowledge to the public at large. Experts who control the ways and means of health control knowledge by virtue of the fact that they control the technology of medicine. Control of technology is a particular kind of control when that technology is understood as ultracultural rather than natural.

There is, however, a contradiction in the growth and development of Nature Cure/Yoga as institutionalized medicine. Although many groups preach complete self-reliance in their publications, there is a growing tendency, reflected in the BNCHY, to build hospitals and train specialized naturopathic physicians who can treat others. To some extent the very nature of Nature Cure/Yoga should undermine the logic of institutionalization. But since, in fact, it does not, the production and dissemination of knowledge function as a kind of nagging critique of bureaucratization and state-mandated forms of consensus derived from policy. Rather than resulting in a crisis, this critique produces what may be characterized as a vital, creative tension within the practice of Nature Cure/Yoga. Thus, along with the growth of Nature Cure/Yoga as a modern system of alternative medicine—and it would not be possible otherwise—has come what I am calling, with apologies to Foucault, the birth of the anti-clinic.

Biopower as Addiction to Health in the Anti-Clinic

The anti-clinic does not take shape as a tangible entity, except in the shadows of institutions like the BNCHY. It comes into being as a kind of power/knowledge wherein individualized care of the individual is all important. Here I am explicitly using the highly problematic notion of "individual" to mean not only that state of being human which is inherently linked to various ideologies, such as nationalism and capitalism—and thereby charged with great cultural and political significance—but also to mean a kind of reified, materialized personhood that is neither intrinsically social nor inherently defined by "itself."

In sharp contrast to all other kinds of medicine, in the anti-clinic care *of* the individual is care *by* the individual as well. And this produces a different kind of biopower, both with regard to the way in which the self is thought to be embodied, and also in terms of how the problem of population is defined. Along with a "self-governing body," the radical, "short-circuit" nature of individualized individual care produces a sustained critique of governmentality by promoting a kind of publicized private surveillance of subtle body functions, rather than a discipline of the body through gross fragmentation and the externally authorized regulation of its movements.

Individualized surveillance is focused on the same subject as is surveillance at large—the health of the public—thereby making for a kind of pastoral power wherein, to extend and mix Foucault's metaphor, the parishioners break ranks and let their bodies become themselves. It is not so much the self-help nature of Nature Cure/Yoga that matters here, as the scale on which that self-help is imagined as a project for the public good. What matters is the way in which knowledge materializes the anticlinic's powerful potential to aggregate and disaggregate population, in terms of more and more or fewer and fewer individuals added together. The goal is to solve the "problem of population," as that problem is defined in terms of the more complex, predetermined mathematics of class, ethnicity, race, and language or even specific health problems—those with or at risk for diabetes, those with or at risk for asthma, those with or at risk for tuberculosis. This enables Nature Cure/Yoga to work *not* as an alternative form of medicine, but as an antimedical modality of public health treatment that instantiates itself, precariously to be sure, both within and against institutions of the state, within and against clinics like the BNCHY in Patparganj, and within and against upscale "three-star" health resorts in Gurgaon. It turns a radically inclusive, undifferentiating form of public health into the most extreme form of private practice.

As many advocates point out, Nature Cure/Yoga may well be the only way to realize "health for all in the new millennium." But this absurdly utopian—and dangerously totalizing—goal of the WHO will not be achieved because Nature Cure/Yoga is simple, economical, effective, efficient, and environmentally sound; not because it is "drugless" and free from "adverse effects." If it is achieved, it will be in terms of a radically disarticulated "dictatorship of the masses" in which each person abides by the law of nature that he or she embodies. In this regime—which might be called anatomo-anarchism—difference only comes to matter on the level of individual physiology, making it possible to treat everyone differently in exactly the same way. The price of health for all, be it the year 2000 or 3000, will be, I think, a state—probably without borders, and certainly with no laws or economy—where, to adapt Dr. Brahmachari's yogic view, everyone and everything has the same consciousness and where there will be no orderly arrangement of birth and death, pleasure and pain, release and bondage. It would have to be a state of nature.

To conclude, let me invoke an image that was invoked at a conference I attended. An organization very much like the BNCHY has developed a program using Yoga along with dietary and lifestyle changes for effective drug de-addiction in a number of cities throughout India. The organization models itself on the work of Mother Teresa rather than on Gandhi's program of social and moral reform, and is based on the Iyengar method of Yoga practice. Using *āsana, prāṇāyāma,* and various meditation techniques, and both dietary and lifestyle changes, the organization takes in those who have reached rock bottom—heroin addicts and alcoholics—and provides them with a radical and revolutionary approach to health that is also an approach to life. The image that was invoked during the conference—ruefully, by a researcher who wanted to see more dramatic results—was of several dozen *bīṛī* (hand-rolled, inexpensive cheroots)-smoking ex-addicts from the slums of Bombay practicing *prāṇāyāma.*

There are many different ways to make sense or understand the implications of this image. The one I wish to focus on is the radical way in which it represents holistic health as both personal and highly impersonal. Addiction is the problem and Yoga provides a solution, as the problem and the solution are forced to intersect in the body of the addict/ex-addict. Clearly the organization sees Yoga, along with dietary and lifestyle change, as a "cure" for addiction and a solution to self-destructive behavior. But as I talked with the young physician who made the presentation, we also laughed about the way in which the addicts get addicted to Yoga, and how this "addiction" transforms their lives. In many ways the metaphor of addiction provides the best characterization of biopower in the anti-clinic of public health reform. It is, in any case, a way to conceptualize health that is not easily reduced down to metaphors—and the medical instantiation of these metaphors in practice—of fragmentation, medical warfare, the destruction of disease, and the kind of reactive and almost clandestine stealth that is required to walk through the minefields of modern risk.

Addiction to health is a useful concept, since the idea of addiction displaces agency and confuses not only the question of responsibility but the relationship between mind and body that factors directly into the question of individual responsibility and medical care. To the best of my knowledge, Gandhi did not think of a lifestyle structured around the practice of Nature Cure as a kind of addiction to health. And yet his obsession with questions concerning the embodied virtue of diet reform, the social value of celibacy, the political efficacy of fasting, and the public health value of the friction sitz bath clearly conveys a profound desire to be "in tune with nature." This desire extended beyond the simple realm of self-conscious "rational choice." In terms of this obsession with health, Gandhi sought to put into practice a program of socio-moral reform that was not only radically egalitarian, but egalitarian in the radical and somewhat utopian sense that what was required was institutionalized poverty. Here again a term that is usually used reactively, derivatively, and pejoratively can be used to purposefully confuse the relationship between ideas about progress and ideas about a possible future that is different from progress as such.

In his *āśrams* Gandhi institutionalized the practice of Nature Cure as a way of life. As is well known, he institutionalized poverty and sought to make a lifestyle of self-conscious simplicity and poverty the moral standard for public life and public service. He admonished those who were wealthy, as well as those who were simply "comfortable," to empower themselves through selfless service. One must keep this in mind when trying to understand the complex and confusing mix of poverty and wealth in the institutionalized structure of the BNCHY. Granted, the three-star Nature Cure "spa" facility in Gurgaon is no Gandhian *āśram*, but what Dr. Nair is trying to do there is, in many ways, significantly different from what is going on in the unself-consciously modern, elitist Yoga resorts located in the mountains above Rishikesh in North India. (Bhanutej et al. 2002: 22–27) or in the so-called Bhajan Belt of the Catskills in New York (Healy 2002: D1, 7)

Until a "Gandhian" state of nature is realized, and everyone eats only a modicum of steamed vegetables, everyone realizes the virtue of fasting, everyone accepts the premise that ultimately disease is good for the restoration of natural health, and until everyone adopts Nature Cure/Yoga as a "way of life," the tension between the laws of nature, public health policy, and the economics of private health care will continue to produce a kind of ironic, farcical, cruel dissonance in which significant differences like hunger and gluttony, basic needs and taste, both matter and don't matter—where *bīṛī*-smoking, drug-addicted trans-Jamuna slum dwellers must aspire to breathe the fresh air that their not-quite-in-Gurgaon, less-than-one-star bodies demand. But in this post-Gandhian, modern regime—in the publication, and subsequent mass consumption of Nature Cure/Yoga's anti-clinical ontogeny—there is at least the possibility of something that engages with the power/knowledge nexus of medicine's violence, the state's welfare governmentality, and health care's commodification.

In many ways the BNCHY mirrors the emergence of new state-of-the-art, pay-for-service, profit-oriented elite hospitals in urban India, all of which are funded by donations and investments from so-called Non-Resident Indians, most notably the wealthy Hinduja family group. These hospitals are appointed with the newest medical technology, are staffed by highly trained health care professionals, and provide some of the best biomedical care available anywhere in the world. In explicitly linking the quality of care and medical service to the five-star world of global tourism and luxury living, hospitals in the Apollo Group are often referred to as Super-Deluxe (www.apollohospitals.com/). Catering to the elite and the rapidly growing upper middle class—charging Rs 885/day for a general ward bed and Rs 5,600 for a deluxe room (www.apollo hospdelhi.com/)—these hospitals simply reflect the broader trend in modern India toward privatization and away from socialized medicine. They reflect the phenomenal rate at which, in the past twenty-five years, the gap between rich and poor has not just widened, but widened as a direct consequence of the abandonment of a Gandhian ideal that was institutionalized as socialist policy by Nehru, albeit with many radical modifications based on the two men's very different conceptions of modernity. This gap reflects, in every way, a far more profound perversity and cruel lack of concern in the social body than anything that could be imagined in institutionalized Nature Cure/Yoga, including the regimen prescribed for Mrs. Urmila Devi and the practice of *prāṇāyāma* by habitual *bīṛī* smokers.

There are, of course, many complex issues involved in the modernization of medicine and changes in government policy toward health care in contemporary India (Jeffery 1988). But viewed simply with reference to the body—and the disciplinary mechanisms whereby medicine creates and tries to solve the problem of population—it seems clear that the relationship between money and disease in the configuration of biomedicine is mirrored by a relationship between nature and health in Nature Cure/Yoga. Clearly the BNCHY is not a radical solution to the perceived failure of biomedicine, just as super-deluxe hospitals are not a solution to the perceived failure of socialized medicine. But in deflecting the "materiality of power," Nature Cure/Yoga transforms the key relationship in clinical medicine between individual bodies and the social body, producing a kind of mutated biopower. This biopower, as a kind of healthy-addiction regime, is reflected in the fact that medicine is not medical, everyone is a doctor and doctors only treat themselves, self-help magazine articles function like medicine, therapy is lifestyle and lifestyle is therapy, and bodies are "liberated" by their conformity to natural laws and by their submission to the will of nature.

To nervously echo India's minister of health and family welfare, quoted at the beginning of this section, there are enormous problems produced when the deinstitutionalization of medicine is institutionalized and made more or less "popular." However, the cruel irony of treating malnutrition with a regimen of fasts, or asthma with *prāṇāyām*ically breathed inner-city air, for example, will probably produce less social violence than will the well-known but obscured and elided problems manifest in the birth of all clinics, but most certainly the super-deluxe, ultramodern bastards of postcolonial India.

5

DR. KARANDIKAR, DR. PAL, AND THE RSS: PURIFICATION, SUBTLE GYMNASTICS, AND MAN MAKING

> *Bhūta-śuddhi* ("purification of the elements") . . . is often used synonymously with *kuṇḍalinī yoga,* which attempts the gradual transformation of the body into a quasi-divine body (*divya-deha*) endowed with supernal faculties. As the "serpent power" (*kuṇḍalinī śakti*) ascends from the base center to the crown of the head, it is thought to successively "dissolve" the five elements—earth, water, fire, air and ether. This is interpreted as a process of gradual purification.
>
> Georg Feuerstein, *Encyclopedic Dictionary of Yoga* (1990: 59)

> Our concept of *Dharma* is based on the universality of spirit. . . . It is a principle of universal harmony—harmony between and individual and society, harmony between human society and outward nature or *Prakṛti,* harmony between individual soul and universal soul. . . . The mission of the RSS is to unite and rejuvenate our nation on the sound foundation of *Dharma.* This mission can be achieved by a strong and united Hindu society. . . . Rejuvenation of the Hindu nation is in the interest of the whole humanity.
>
> Mission Statement of the Rashtriya Swayamsevak Sangh (www.rss.org/mission/htm)

The Body and Hindu Nationalism

SINCE THE MID-1980s Hindu nationalism has emerged as a pervasive and dramatically influential cultural force in contemporary India. Many people are deeply concerned with the numerous political, moral, and juridicial implications of this development. Given the rise to prominence and public attention of the Rashtriya Swayamsevak Sangh (RSS) through its direct links to the ruling Bharatiya Janata Party (B. Chakrabarty 2001; Jaffrelot 1993; Sathyamurty 1997), and its involvement in the destruction of the Babri Masjid mosque in Ayodhya—and more recently the riots in Gujarat—there have been a number of studies focused on the ideology and political structure of the organization, both unto itself (Andersen and Damle 1987; T. Basu et al. 1993; Hansen 1999: 71–133) and within the broader context of colonial and postcolonial nationalism (Brass 1996; Corbridge 1999; Hansen 1999; Jaffrelot 1996; Ludden 1996; Malik and Singh 1995; McKean 1996; Nandy 1997; Pandey 1990, 1993; Pennington 2001; P. van der Veer 1994; Varshney 1993).

There is obviously much to be said for trying to understand the RSS as a militant Hindu organization in and on its own terms in order to understand nationalism and communalism in modern India. But there is also great value in looking at the way in which the RSS has influenced cultural practices beyond the framework of its specific and self-consciously masculinist and militaristic agenda. This is particularly so since the body is integral to RSS ideology, but that concern with the body—its health, energy, and vitality—spills over, so to speak, into other areas of experience, carrying with it elements and aspects of its nationalistic regimentation.

Through an examination of the institutionalized practice of two doctors—Dr. Karandikar of Pune and Dr. Pal of New Delhi—this chapter is concerned with the "spillover" of RSS ideology into the arena of health and healing. Each in its own way, the cases under consideration provide a perspective on the RSS that is not limited to or by accounts of the organization as such, or even by what might be called formalized "nationalism." I take this to be important because nationalism, like Yoga, is most powerful when it is, in some sense, least recognizable, and because nationalism, like Yoga, is often least recognizable when it is embodied. Beyond the important and primary perspective that Dr. Karandikar's and Dr. Pal's work provides on the problem and process of embodiment, an analysis of their work, set against a more comprehensive analysis of the nationalist North Indian Yoga society Bharatiya Yog Sansthan (Alter 1997), also illustrates the extent of influence the RSS has had in modern India, and the ambiguous forms of knowledge and practice it produces in society at large. Therefore I begin with a discussion of how the body is implicated in RSS ideology and practice, and conclude—reflexively, it is hoped, after a deep consideration of parallel themes—with a discussion of Yoga's ambiguous position within the disciplinary program of the "mother organization."

The RSS: Life Force, Health, and the Hindu Nation

Since it was established by Dr. Keshav Baliram Hedgewar in the early 1920s, the Rashtriya Swayamsevak Sangh has been involved in a project of social and nationalist reform based on what it regards to be the development of Hindu cultural ideals. The RSS is often referred to as a Hindu nationalist organization that is anti-Muslim, anti-Western, and against the idea of secularism. It is often accused of participating in, if not also directly organizing, communal riots. There are a number of scholarly works and journalistic reports that have criticized the Sangh for various manifestations of fundamentalism (T. Basu et al. 1993; Goyal 1979). As might be expected, the response of the RSS is to deny any involvement in violence—except that which is defensive—and to eschew labels associated with fundamentalism in favor of those that invoke the idea of selfless service (Deshmukh 1979; Malkani 1980).

Whatever else it is—an organization for moral and cultural reform, an organization to establish national unity, an organization designed to root out power politics and corruption in government, or a "fascist" organization calling for the reconversion of Muslims and Christians to Hinduism—the RSS claims to be an organization primarily concerned with "man making," a phrase borrowed from Swami Vivekananda.[1] This "man making" is linked to what is called "organic" self-discipline and a kind of selfless self-improvement that is referred to as "character molding." As H. V. Seshadri, general secretary of the organization, put it in a 1992 publication:

> Hindu thought and practice has accorded the pride of place to the "man" and not power. Here, all out emphasis was laid on strengthening the moral, cultural and spiritual *saṃskāras* (character) of every individual in society—right from the humblest to the highest. The ruler himself was not excluded from the strict training of the character-molding. It was this tradition of the blossoming of the highest human virtues that had made the Hindu Nation the cultural and spiritual mother of the entire humanity for millennia. (1992: 10)

Man making is directly linked to an unconditional love for the Hindu Nation on the one hand, and disciplined participation as a *swayamsevak*—volunteer—in the activities of the Sangh, on the other. These activities are conceived of as being in the service of society. The idea is to develop each man's moral character and then, through the work of that man, to establish a kind of moral and ethical standard that brings society up to a level that reflects the ideals of the Hindu Nation. The explicitly gendered dimensions of this and related projects have been critically analyzed by a number of scholars (Banerjee 1999; T. Basu et al. 1993; Hancock 1995; Hansen 1996; Pierson and Chaudhuri 1998).

The cornerstone of RSS organization is the smallest unit of association known as the *śākhā*. Each *śākhā* is linked to a higher-level association such that the central leadership is efficiently connected to each *śākhā* through a series of clearly delineated and extremely well organized administrative links. On a day-to-day basis the training of *swayamsevaks* takes place in the *śākhā*, and, as I have indicated elsewhere (Alter 1994), this training directly engages the body. It involves singing patriotic songs, playing team games and sports, listening to lectures, performing volunteer public service, and taking part in mass paramilitary drill exercises. Song texts and tunes, rules for games and sports, and detailed drill instructions are standardized in various RSS publications (Anonymous n.d.a, b, 1992a, b). On account of this militaristic, chauvinistic training, it is often said by critics that *śākhā*s are implicated in communal riots. In fact, historically speaking it was in direct response to communal riots that Dr. Hedgewar organized the first *śākhā*s, drawing inspiration from Sister Nivedita's admonition: Hindus should "congregate and pray together for 15 minutes, every day, and Hindu society will become an invincible society." As Basu et al. note, "this was developed in course of time into a single format of ritual-cum-physical training, to be performed at identical times by RSS branches (*śākhā*s) all over the country. The notion of a spiritual energy generated by universal, time-bound prayer and ritual draws inspiration from a concept of an invisible congregation" (1993: 16).[2]

Although it is possible to debate the question of what is and is not construed as violence, and what, if anything, legitimatizes the use of violence and force, there is no question but that in the rhetoric of the RSS a great deal of emphasis is placed on the development of physical strength, athletic prowess, and martial arts. This comes across most clearly in essays published just before and after independence in the organ of the RSS, aptly called *Organizer:*

> What a sin weakness is! Any time you are punished for this sin. A weak person can have no place in the world today. This world where survival of the fittest is the law of nature does not tolerate weak people. The world is full of gold and silver, beauty and charm, joy and pleasure, but all for the strong, nothing for the weak.
>
> The weak commands no respect, no dignity, no esteem. He is always at the mercy of the strong. He cannot go against his will. He cannot maintain and enjoy even his most basic civic rights. He is always in danger of being crushed. (Anonymous 1947: 11)

In advocating "compulsory military training for self-preservation," Rup Chand Kapila writes: "The men who have undergone military training leave the ranks with bodies steeled to resist disease and minds capable of prolonged concentrated effort. Hence they will be able to do better work and for longer time. A few years military training greatly improves a man's physique" (1947: 9).

The issue of muscular Hinduism as it is linked to the RSS is an important one that I have dealt with directly elsewhere (1994; see also n.d.a.).

But the issue of strength and fitness fits—albeit problematically—into a broader discourse of health and vital energy. In part, but only in part, this discourse is linked to the RSS's advocacy of celibacy.[3] As an anonymous contributor to the *Organizer,* addressing himself "to youth," puts it, "self-control is the most important factor in the growth and maintenance of health."[4] Echoing Gandhi's words, if not his political views, the author then goes into a long, polemic discourse on the nature of a good, wholesome diet, as diet is linked to celibacy. He concludes with the following point: "*Brahmacharya* [celibacy] not only bestows upon us health and long life but develops our many latent faculties. . . . It transforms our sex energy into mental and spiritual energy. And, as our spiritual energy grows our capacity to understand and master the mysteries of nature grows wider and wider" (Anonymous 1947: 4).

These perspectives on health and physical fitness, as they are an integral part of *śākhā* training, are expressed in more general terms by the general secretary of the organization. In describing the relationship between the RSS and the nation's "life force," H. S. Seshadri writes:

> The RSS seeks to play the role of the Life-Force—*Prāṇa-śakti*—in the body of the society.
>
> Let us explain: Living bodies live and grow so long as the Life-Force is vibrant. Every single organ and limb—every living cell—carries out its respective function only when that force pulsates in it. When that throb becomes feeble, the eye sees not, the ears hear not, the hands move not, the brain thinks not. More potent the Life-Force, more dynamic the functions of the organs. (1992: 13)[5]

Seshadri's collection of essays entitled *The Way* is infused with the metaphor of society as an organism, and organic unity is clearly his perspective on national unity—everyone engaged in a common purpose bringing the nation to life. He calls on people to cultivate "physical health through *yogāsana* and . . . athletics" and to establish "general health education and home remedies" at the grass-roots level. Once this concern for health and physical fitness gains momentum it will "turn into a mighty national movement" (1992: 33).

Seshadri's cryptic and smooth conflation of Yoga and athletics notwithstanding, Yoga is integrated into the *śākhā* drill regimen in a very problematic way. Its integration produces ambiguity. Several training manuals simply describe seventeen "*āsana*s" without much commentary (Anonymous 1994a, b). Interestingly, a few of these *āsana*s are "adapted" and many are identical to calisthenic stretching exercises and isometric physical training (Anonymous 1992b: 21–39). For example, the first seated posture, *ardhanāvāsana,* is depicted as an extended-leg, unsupported sit-up such that the stomach muscles are forcibly contracted in

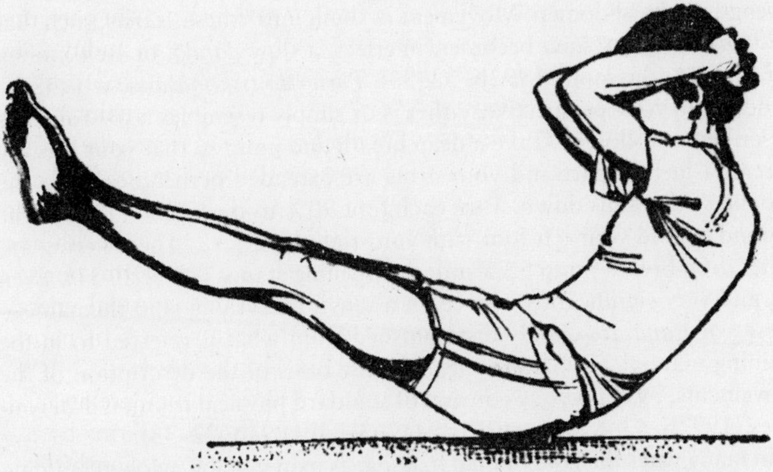

9. *Ardhanāvāsana. Source: Śarīrik Śikṣa: Dvitīya Varṣ* (Nagpur: Madhav Prakashan, 1992), p. 24. Reproduced with permission from Madhav Prakashan.

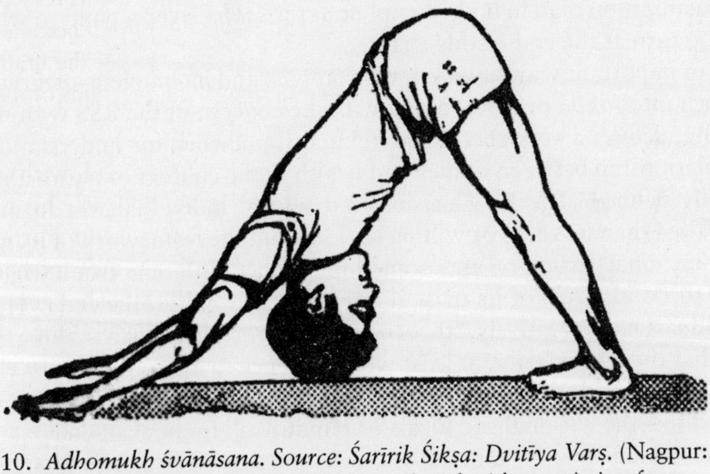

10. *Adhomukh śvānāsana. Source: Śarīrik Śikṣa: Dvitīya Varṣ.* (Nagpur: Madhav Prakashan, 1992), p. 33. Reproduced with permission from Madhav Prakashan.

what is often called a "crunch" (Anonymous 1992b: 24).[6] The effect is to strengthen the abdomen. Movement is "built into" these *āsanas*, such that *adhomukha śvānāsana* becomes, in effect, a slow *daṇḍa*, or jack-knifing push-up (Anonymous 1992b: 32–33). *Parivṛtta trikoṇāsana*, which, depending on your perspective, either is or simply resembles a toe-touch, is described as follows: "Take a deep breath and jump so that your legs are spread a meter apart and your arms are extended perpendicular to the ground with palms down. Turn each foot 90% to the left. . . . [Touch the ground behind your left foot with your right hand]. . . . Then, taking another deep breath jump back into the opening stance" (1992b: 21). Even so, and very significantly—since, in a sense, everything is in the name—these *yogāsana* are clearly distinguished from what is referred to in the training manual as *vyāyām yoga*. On the basis of the description of the movements, *vyāyām yoga* consists of standard physical training drill routines (1992b: 62–67; see also 1994a: 63–64; 1994b: 22–33).

In many ways the goal of man making, as man making involves building up *prāṇa śakti* on the level of individual cells, individual people, and the indivisible nation, makes it very difficult for the RSS to accommodate Yoga as Yoga. The difficulty is compounded since, on one level, the RSS seeks to define itself within the rubric of classical civilization and classical, sanskritic learning. This difficulty is reflected less in the discourse of the organization than in body discipline at the *śākhā* level, a point to which I will return at the end of this chapter.

In an important way, however, the complex and incomplete integration of Yoga into *śākhā* practice, along with the concern of the RSS with man making, defines a very specific contextual framework for understanding the relationship between bodies and health in the context of nationalism, broadly defined. The RSS has inspired several individuals to do more with Yoga than it is able or willing to do within the framework of its own organizational structure and something rather different from what it seeks to do in terms of its masculinist, muscular cultural agenda. These individuals have creatively "theorized" the principle of man making in a way that the RSS has not, at least with reference to Yoga. Moreover, they have put it into practice as a kind of therapy that is inspired by—but not limited to—the nationalistic ideals of Hindutva (Hindu character).

Whereas an overtly nationalistic organization such as the Bharatiya Yog Sansthan manifests the kind of organizational structure of the RSS applied to the development of Yoga as an alternative form of public health (Alter 1997), Dr. Karandikar's work is an example of how the vital life force is theorized on both a cellular and an organizational level. Dr. Pal's case illustrates the ambiguous connection between the vital life force, physical training, and Hinduism. Dr. Karandikar's affiliation with the RSS is relatively unmarked, but clearly stated. He is a sympathizer and has been an active member. Dr. Pal's affiliation is clearly marked and openly discussed, but his attitude toward the RSS is ambivalent and complicated. As he put it in an interview, the principles of Yoga are incompatible with RSS ideology, because Yoga is not limited to Hinduism. Thus his case provides a perspective on one man's moral commitment to health, well-being, and Hinduism, as well as an "insider's" disaffection with the cultural politics associated with that commitment.

Sunderraj Yoga Darshan: Yoga, Cosmic Biochemistry, and the Fitness of Cells

Sunderraj Yoga Darshan is a private enterprise located on the grounds of, and directly affiliated with, the Kabir-Baug Matha Sanstha Trust founded in 1952. The Sanstha is directly modeled on—if not directly affiliated with—the RSS. Though named in honor of B.K.S. Iyengar, Sunderraj Yoga Darshan was established by Dr. S. V. Karandikar to commemorate the birth centenary of Dr. Hedgewar, the founding chief of the RSS. The regional chief of the RSS inaugurated the completion of the Smriti Bhavan building in 1995, and the Sanstha's activities are clearly "nationalist" in keeping with the cultural priorities of the RSS. According to the published list of achievements on the Sanstha's web page, "many high dignitaries in different fields such as Prof. Rajendra Singh of RSS, Mr. Nanaji Deshmukh of Deendayal Sanshodhan Sanstha, Late Shri P. L. Deshpande the well known writer in Marathi . . ." have participated in and benefited from the Yoga technique developed by Dr. Karandikar (www.kabirbaug.com/Achievement.htm). The stated purpose of the Sanstha "is to improve the Nation through social enlightenment by means of cultural enrichment. The plan for cultivating a better society rests in the creation of a range of programs and activities staffed by a cadre of devoted and strong volunteers. Accordingly the trust has initiated various projects and programs based on these objectives: a hostel for students from rural areas, a nursery and play center for children, as well as programs for moral and cultural education" (Karandikar 1997: 24, counted; pages unnumbered).

It was under the auspices of the Sanstha that Dr. Karandikar—who recently took the name Acharya Yoganand—founded an organization called the Manav Sanshodhan Vikas ani Sanshodhan Manch in 1986. In turn this society "for the purification and development of human kind" provided the platform for establishing his prop-based Yoga clinic, now known as Sun-Jeevan Yoga Darshan. Dr. Karandikar's concern with "purification" is an extension of RSS ideology, in which social, moral, and embodied purification is also a primary concern. His concern with purification—and the therapeutic use of purified elements—is reflected in his theory of etheric space, cosmic biochemistry, and the physical fitness manifest in cells. As the website of the organization pointed out in 2003: "Sun-Jeevan Yoga, propounded by Acharya Yoganand is a fusion of traditional yoga philosophy, modern objective medical thinking and ultramodern energy thought process in subatomic particle physics" (www.kabirbaug.com). The volunteers who work in his clinic are, in a profound sense, concerned not just with health and welfare but with the development of humankind through "subatomic particle physics" and yogic genetic engineering.

I recorded the following note in my field diary on June 3, 1998:

> *The yoga clinic/gymnasium known as Sunderraj Yoga Darshan in Pune is something to behold! If I had to imagine a facility that fit my image of a modern yoga clinic this would be it! It is obviously the brainchild of Dr. Shrikant V. Karandikar, a trained physician and disciple of B.K.S. Iyengar. The clinic itself is a modern, three-story facility built on top of and encompassing the* samādhi *of a saint on the grounds of Kabir Baug Matha, an eighteenth-century temple complex. Dr Karandikar could not say which saint was buried in the "*samādhi *tomb" but he had fond memories of playing around the grounds when he was a child in the 1930s.*
>
> *The clinic is set up much like a modern gymnasium and appears to be heavily influenced by the Iyengar school of equipment-assisted yoga. Each floor is fully equipped with various apparati—ropes, free weights, folding chairs, wooden blocks, bolster pillows, straps and weighted pulleys—to assist practitioners in achieving and maintaining a pose. The most noticeable equipment is double-strand rope "swings" from which patients appear to hang themselves or suspend various appendages. There are also beautifully crafted curved benches which patients bend backward on to support themselves while performing* āsanas. *On the walls, in addition to the ropes and pulleys, there are numerous anatomical diagrams of the body showing organ and nervous systems, muscle physiology, and skeletal structure.*
>
> *The ground and first floor of the clinic were fully occupied and operational as Dr. Karandikar took me on a tour of the facility. He pointed out a man, assisted by one of numerous volunteers, dressed in shorts and a blue "yoga darshan" tee-shirt, who was pulling his leg up backwards after attaching it to a harness connected to a self-controlled pulley. The contraption looked like a modified version of the pulleys used in hospitals to suspend and immobilize broken arms and legs. Beside the man was a woman with a rope that was attached to the wall tied around each shoulder. She was pulling against the rope to pull her shoulder blades back and expand her chest. On the same floor a twelve-year-old boy with cerebral palsy was being helped by an older man to fit his feet into rope loops in preparation for an assisted pos-*

ture of some kind. Most of the people in the building were, however, sitting on pillows with the soles of their feet pushed together and pulled up as close to their groins as possible. In this position they were all lying back with arched backs on bolster pillows with their eyes closed.

After the tour of the facilities, Dr. Karandikar took me up to his office on the top floor, part of which was equipped with the standard medical equipment of any biomedical doctor's examination room. From the window he pointed out a large, 300-bed dormitory cum hostel facility nearing completion that would accommodate students to be trained in yoga therapy.[7]

The whole complex gave me the impression of a very smoothly run, well-funded operation. Dr. Karandikar has been on several trips overseas, including Russia, Canada, and most recently the United States. His wife has also traveled and taught abroad, and she was earlier introduced to me by him as a colleague.

One of the most interesting things Dr. Karandikar said was that he had recently begun to focus most of his attention on ākāśa *as he felt that "space" was the most important but least understood of the five elements. As he explained, Āyurvedic theory provides a good understanding of the relationship between earth, air, fire, and water but it does not explain the origin of these elements very well. Nor does it deal adequately with the properties of space. In Dr. Karandikar's view space or* ākāśa *is the special purview of yoga.*[8]

He went on to explain that each āsana *is "the genetic form of a particular species," by which I think he meant that an* āsana, *such as the peacock pose, does not simply reflect the shape of the bird, but is more intimately linked to its "genetic form."*[9] *Following on this he said that "each cell of the human body" intuitively knows every possible* āsana *posture, but that every individual must learn how to perform the posture.*

*Overall I was very impressed by Dr. Karandikar's articulate and comprehensive discussion of his theory of yoga. He used the language of physics to talk about space—*ākāśa*—in the body, pointing out that a lack of space or "the experience of nearness" manifest in physical contact created the element fire. As he explained, space is most apparent in the digestive tract, and fire in the density of tissue and bone. Air escapes from the body through the mouth and water and earth through the anus and urethra. The diaphragm is important insofar as it regulates the flow of air.*[10]

Dr. Karandikar has a very interesting and innovative perspective on yoga therapy. For example, if a person is suffering from a disease such as diabetes, one approach is to try and treat the symptoms. Since the disease is genetic, a second approach is to try and cure the disease by preventing the genes from being inherited by the next generation. What makes Dr. Karandikar's perspective unique is that he believes that yoga therapy can be used to treat those who carry the genetic traits for the disease so as to produce immunity in the next generation. That is to say, the beneficial effects of yoga are inherited.

> *This is based on a distinctive theory of causation which derives, in part, from the dynamics of* tridoṣa *theory in Āyurveda. Illness, according to Dr. Karandikar, is caused by "anatomical distortion," which in turn leads to physiological dysfunction which ultimately leads to pathological change. When anatomical distortion is genetically based, there is an internalized circle of causation.*[11] *The circle is normally thought to be closed, except for the fact that yoga, as a mechanism for the manipulation of intellectual and spiritual power, makes it possible to influence genetic make-up. According to this theory, genes are subject to yogic power even though they "determine" everything else. In effect this is a kind of "natural" biogenetic engineering. According to Dr. Karandikar, all forms of medicine, including Āyurveda, homeopathy, nature cure and biomedicine are limited to pathology and the mechanical manipulation of change on this level. Yoga, which is more subtle, goes deeper and is designed to "open up space" and thus resolve the problem of anatomical distortion, be it on the level of genes or on a more macro-biological level.*
>
> *Perhaps as an indication of the latter, Dr. Karandikar pointed out that he was currently involved in producing a video demonstrating how people could manipulate their scapulas. He said that all animals have scapulas, but bipedal humans, unlike dogs and other four-legged creatures, don't move theirs. Building on the idea of the scapula's movement opening up space, he hypothesized that it could have some health benefits.*

While there are numerous clinics where Yoga is used for treatment, and numerous examples of Yoga's being tested to prove efficacy, there are relatively few examples of a theory proposed to explain why Yoga is more effective—or effective in a different way—than other modalities, and even fewer examples of treatment regimens based on such a theory. Thus almost all research done on Yoga evaluates outcome, and is not designed to explain the physiological process that causes that outcome. Indeed there is often a tacit assumption, based on biomedical diagnostic procedures, that asthma is "caused" by respiratory function and allergic pathology even when the cure is based on a manipulation of *prāṇa*. In this there is a degree of incompatibility between two different theories of the body, one used to explain the agency of cure and the other the pathology of disease. What is clearly apparent in Dr. Karandikar's work is an effort to reconcile this difference. This is somewhat ironic, since Dr. Karandikar's method, which is based on B.K.S. Iyengar's technique, is extremely "mechanical" in the sense that the body is manipulated into yogic postures by technological means. Yoga is, in some sense, done *to the body*—if not also to various parts of the body—rather than *by a person,* although I am sure this is not how either Dr. Karandikar or Iyengar would see it.

There is no sense in which Karandikar's program is simplistic. In fact, it is an exemplary case of the ingenious synthesis of ideas that characterizes modern Yoga as a medium through which people in India are reimagining the relationship between health, modernity, and the body. Nevertheless, based on interview material, observation, and an analysis of Dr. Karandikar's published and privately circulated papers, the following is a simple analysis of the relationship between a theory of physiology, a theory of cure, and the way in which technology-assisted Yoga—Yoga engineering, it might be called, since things so basic to life as genes are now subject to this transitive verb—makes perfect sense in terms of Dr. Karandikar's theory of health and human welfare.

Dr. Karandikar earned his M.B.B.S. degree from Pune University in 1962, after which he served first in the Medical Corps of the Indian Army and subsequently in private practice as a family physician in Pune. After suffering from heart disease he began to study Yoga with B.K.S. Iyengar and was cured. He traveled with Iyengar to many parts of the world and participated in numerous Yoga workshops. Responding to a request from his *guru,* he established the Sunderraj Yoga Darshan in late 1989, and this soon after became Sun-Jeevan Yoga, a clinic for therapeutic, restorative Yoga. As of late 2000 the clinic had treated over twelve thousand patients and conducted basic research on hypertension, asthma, problems of the spine, diabetes, neurological problems, and kidney disease (www.kabirbaug.com). Although this approach is very much in keeping with the basic principles of Iyengar Yoga, which is characterized by him as "physically sound, physiologically rewarding and psychologically [the] most suitable to present day vibrant atmosphere," Dr. Karandikar points out that in his own experience, "[Iyengar's technique is] rather difficult to follow for those who [are] suffering from different physical and psychological ailments due to their physical constraints" (n.d.b: 1). He continues: "Therefore it was necessary to modify this teaching method so that it can be practiced by those who are diseased. It was also essential to improve the technique as Iyengar method is more stressful on joints and may harm those who are unaware of this. . . . [In the Iyengar method] not much attention is given to functional anatomy and physiology of a human body" (n.d.b: 1).

Dr. Karandikar's method is based on functional anatomy and physiology. What he means by this, however, is somewhat different from what others have meant in invoking the same terms. According to him the gross human body comprises the elements earth, fire, and water. Gross medicine addresses itself to the body through the medium of these elements in the sense that surgery is by nature an earth-based modality, since it deals with gross anatomy, and psychiatry is based on air, since words—

the gross medium of healing in this case—are conveyed through sounds made by displacing this element.[12] Following a distinct precedent found in Āyurvedic literature—though not using Āyurvedic terminology or categories—Dr. Karandikar holds that disease is caused by an imbalance of elements. Creatively breaking with precedent, he holds that the root cause of imbalance is distortion in *ākāśa,* which constitutes the elemental plane upon which the body exists as a mass.[13] Drawing on Patañjali's *Yoga Sūtra,* he points out that *citta* is a kind of energy flow that links the human body mass to ether, and this enables people to adapt to their environment.[14] Etheric distortion disrupts this flow and causes disease.

> Therefore to know the cause of the disease it is essential to understand the disruption in the flow of energy which is guided through pathways of learning through proof, inference, imagination, memory and sleep. All of these pathways have limitations of understanding [based on the purely sensory nature] of the five organs of perception and action. Therefore the real cause of disease cannot be recognized by modern medical philosophy which is entirely based on knowledge of the organs of perception and action. (n.d.b: 2)[15]

It follows from this that Yoga, which is not limited by the five organs of perception, provides a means by which to recognize ethereal distortion, restore balance, and adjust energy flow to cure disease. As Robert Walker, who interviewed Karandikar for the *Yoga Journal,* explains, "as we grow older, our body shrinks, and the spaces between the body tissues and joints decrease. . . . This distortion leads to physiological dysfunction and pathological changes. Yoga restores the space and length, enabling nature to rearrange and repair the diseased parts of the body the natural way" (1998: 105). Contrary to what one might expect, the focus on joints does not at all mean that Dr. Karandikar's practice is particularly concerned with arthritis.

On the basis of his training and practice as a biomedical physician, Dr. Karandikar has refined his theory of disease causation in terms of the effects of Yoga on cell metabolism: "This body mass consists of billions of cells and each cell has a well defined form. [Each] cell has a self-energizing force called 'bio-cosmic energy' or '*prāṇaśakti*'. [The] energy of a particular cell lasts from the birth of the cell until its death. This stored biocosmic energy controls the existence, survival, growth, function, reproduction and ultimately the death of the cell" (n.d.a: 1).[16] Significantly, this micro-biocosmic activity is "carried out through [the] different biochemical processes" of anabolism and catabolism. This critical point of transfer between cosmic and chemical planes controls patterns of growth and decay. Overall the human body is in a constant state of decay caused by "gravitational force . . . as well as other celestial forces that act on [it] from ten different directions (*dasadik*)" (n.d.a: 1). In short, "it can be said that there are a number of forces that destroy the human body. Only biocosmic energy in each cell resists these destructive forces and makes it grow and function" (n.d.a: 1–2). According to Dr. Karandikar, Yoga provides the means by which to promote the body's natural resistance, since "*āsana*s [have a] direct effect on the metabolism of the diseased cell."

> Every chemical reaction in a cell requires energy which is obtained from glucose, water and oxygen. Since different chemical reactions in the cellular metabolism are disturbed in a disease, physiological function of the individual cell slows down. The cell cannot store enough energy which is required for its function, and [this] ultimately leads to premature death of individual cells.
>
> Practice of *āsana*s can avert this disaster. In each physical posture different organs are placed in different anatomical architecture for considerable lengths of time. [This] results in [a] disturbance in the physiological activity of each individual cell. In short, each cell is subjected to starvation without tormentation. This process teaches every cell to function normally even in abnormal circumstances created intentionally in an *āsana*. (n.d.a: 6–7)

The principle of "starvation without tormentation" is something like a combination of diet, disciplinary regimentation, and physical fitness training on a cellular level. The ultimate goal of Yoga is to enhance the volume of *prāṇ*ic energy, regulate its flow, and thereby enable each cell to work against the forces of degeneration and decay. A cellular "workout" is achieved by means of the stretching that is integral to Yoga *āsana*s as reflected in the way in which each muscle spindle can be stretched to a maximum point of relaxation without damaging the tissue fibers. This has the effect of working against the force of gravity and the body's natural response of muscle contraction and the stretch reflex. As one learns to perform each *āsana*, the performance becomes more and more "natural" until it is learned by the body on a cellular level.

There are many facets to this process, but one involves holding each posture long enough so as to "bring about physiological changes in the functioning of different involuntary systems" (n.d.a: 5). Over time and through disciplined Yoga training, these physiological changes produce control over the autonomous nervous system.

> Each cell in the involuntary vegetative system in the body is taught to survive and function under the condition congenial to the system. . . . Perfection in each *yogāsana* brings . . . chemical equilibrium in every cell which results in conservation of energy. . . . Chemical equilibrium in an individual cell attained by practicing the sound physiological technique of the Iyengar

> method results in storage of energy [that is] made available for anabolic [metabolism]. Perfection in the technique [of] performing any *āsana* modifies the functioning of an individual cell. . . . New proteins, [and] nucleic acids are absorbed in a cell to improve its functioning. (n.d.a: 8)

I think it is possible—if not necessary—to make sense of this logic with reference to RSS ideas about disciplinary man making, on the one hand, and an Āyurvedic theory of metabolism that is invoked when Yoga is incorporated into the world of biochemistry and cellular pathology, on the other.

With reference to RSS ideology, it is fascinating to see the complex mimesis of the organic body as a diseased entity and society as a diseased organism: both can be cured through disciplinary reform and regimented training on the most basic, elemental level. In Karandikar's formulation the cells are subject to a *śākhā*-like drill routine, so that they will manifest *prāṇa śakti* and thereby provide service to the body as a whole.

It is not surprising that Dr. Karandikar frames his functional theory of cellular health in terms of biochemistry, since he is a biomedical physician. It is noteworthy, nevertheless, that in the context of his nationalist sentiments he does not make reference to a concept of functional metabolism known as *dhātu* transubstantiation in the Āyurvedic corpus, since *dhātu* transubstantiation is homologous to the process whereby the body "cooks" itself into shape and becomes *ātivāhika-deha* or "superconductive."[17] As a biomedical physician convinced of Yoga's natural organic efficacy, the overtly medical structure of Āyurvedic knowledge, though quintessentially "Indian," is much more incompatible with his understanding of biochemistry than is Yoga. Yoga, one might say, provides much more conceptual space for interpretation.

Explicit references aside, Dr. Karandikar's concern with ethereal perfection on the cellular level relates very clearly to the embodied logic of *dhātu* transubstantiation. This process is concerned directly with the process by which food is incorporated into the body and then how the body is progressively distilled down from that which is most gross, to that which is most refined and subtle—semen and *ojas*. *Ojas*, which has all of the attributes of ether, is the essence of vital energy—that illusive essence of man making. Dr. Karandikar's theory of cellular health seeks to locate the power of *ojas* in the nucleus of every cell. Defining what may be considered as the "classical" and "textual" rationale for this modern theory, Feuerstein points out the "yogin's claim that [*ojas*] permeates the whole body" (1990: 244).

Although it would be justified—since *ojas* is very closely linked to semen and semen has a certain bearing on man making—space does not allow for a detour into the domain of *ojas*, as the function of *ojas* in the body corresponds, in many ways, to Dr. Karandikar's theory of yogic biochemistry. However, a brief excursion will demonstrate exactly the extent to which the etherics of *ojas* can be used to explain how it might be that Dr. Karandikar's theory has significant popular appeal among those who "think with" modern Yoga.

After pointing out that in the Āyurvedic literature there is some disagreement on the elemental status of *ojas,* S. K. Ramachandra Rao argues that

> the prevailing idea . . . is that even as the bee makes honey collecting nectars from different flowers, *ojas* is formed from the essences of the seven *dāhtus* (cited in Cakrapāni-datta['s commentary on the] *Carakasaṃhitā,* 1,30,7). Therefore *ojas* being essentially indistinguishable from the *dhātus*, cannot be regarded as a separate *dhātu,* or as an *upadhātu.* Besides, the seven *dhātus* support the body (*dhāraṇā*) as well as nourish the body (*pośaṇa*), while *ojas discharges only the former function.* (1987: 219, emphasis added)

The way in which *ojas* supports the body is particularly significant insofar as it can be conceptualized in immunological terms. Rao points out, for example, that *ojas* is that which is in the body that counteracts disease, and that even if "all of the *dhātu* are alright," if *ojas* weakens then the body manifests rather drastic symptoms. Pathology begins as *ojas* is dislodged from the heart, leading to "loosening of the bone joints, numbness of the limbs, wasting of flesh, dislodgment of the *doṣa* from their natural centers, and disinclination to engage in normal activities of body, mind and speech" (1987: 220). Although *ojas* is vital energy, the way in which it manifests this energy is not as narrowly circumscribed by semen—or sexuality—as might be expected. In many respects *ojas* is to the Sāṃkhyan yogic body what cells are to the Cartesian body—the smallest structural unit of an organism that is capable of independent function. In Sāṃkhyan terms, however, it is the other way around. *Ojas* is the most subtle substance in the metabolic structure of subtle anatomy, and its elemental functional role is integral to the health of the organism as a whole. It is on this level that therapy is designed to work.

Although B.K.S. Iyengar's method of therapeutic Yoga is highly refined, Dr. Karandikar is of the opinion that it must be modified for use by sick patients. As he points out, "this is done with the help of different props or by modification of postures which [soothe] the stretch reflex" (n.d.a: 5). In other words, props such as ropes, chairs, bolster pillows, folded blankets, and straps provide support to counteract gravity. The stretch reflex maximizes the relaxed stretching of the muscles as a group—and of each individual spindle within each group—thereby producing chemical equilibrium and improved cell function.

The use of props is not at all indiscriminate, and Karandikar's method is a systematic elaboration of Iyengar's use of equipment such as chairs and pillows to assist beginners and children. What distinguishes Karandikar's method is that every *āsana* is "technology dependent." This defines it as therapeutic. Whereas many people prescribe Yoga as therapy, they tend to instruct patients in the performance of "classical" *āsanas*. Thus, in effect, the idea is to cure disease by turning sick people into disciplined practitioners of Yoga. This, too, is ultimately Karandikar's goal. But whether consciously designed to or not, his innovation allows for a subtle but profound shift in the process of medicalization, insofar as Yoga is not just broken down into discrete postures. It is Yoga that "can be done to the body of sick people" by means of an interventionist technology—much as physical therapy entails various apparatuses. But it also further fragments the body in a manner similar to the fragmentation caused by pharmaceutical technology and surgery. This is the difference between being someone who becomes a practitioner of Yoga—a yogi, in both the classical and the modern sense of the term—and having Yoga "done to you" in a clinical setting.

Although what might be called cosmic biochemistry provides the theoretical basis for Karandikar's method of therapy, the efficacy of various prop-assisted postures is explained in terms that are at once more general and more specific. For example, in a pamphlet entitled *Yoga Therapy in Diabetes Mellitus* (n.d.c) Dr. Karandikar provides sketches illustrating a series of prop-assisted poses that are therapeutic. There are twenty discrete postures, of which a description of one, taken from his publication *A Life Saver* (1997), will serve as an illustration.

> *Equipment:* Bolster, pillow, 3-layered blanket, cotton belt.
> *Procedure:* Arrange equipment and sit in front of the bolster [upon which the pillow and folded blanket have been placed] as in *suptavīrāsana.* Bend your knees and arrange both feet so that the soles touch each other. Try to touch the back of your thighs to the floor. If this is not possible rest your knees on a pillow or blanket. Holding the bolster with both hands, slowly lower your body down as in *suptavīrāsana.* Rest your lower back, upper back, neck and head as in *suptavīrāsana* on the bolster. Keep both hands at right angles to the body, palms turned towards the ceiling and elbows on the ground. Hold this position for five minutes; then, raise both knees, bring your knees to your chest, turn to the right and get up.
> *Note:* By fixing both thighs, feet and lower back with the cotton belt, the posture is more stable.
> *Effects and Benefits:* (1) Keeping your body parallel to the ground reduces the gravitational force; (2) it helps bring breathing and the action of your heart to within normal limits; and (3) it improves the health of the pelvic organs. (1997: 5)

Significantly, this and the other nineteen "post-yogic" postures prescribed for the treatment of diabetes are said to be effective in five ways: "They improve blood supply to the pancreas, old and deteriorated cells are effectively destroyed, dormant cells are stimulated to function, active cells are motivated to produce better yields [and the] reproduction of new, healthy cells is encouraged" (Karandikar n.d.c: 1).

On a day-to-day basis Sunderraj Yoga Darshan, housed in the Parakh Saheb Maharaj Smriti Bhavan, functions through the support of volunteers who serve as trainers. Although many institutions have volunteers, a volunteer in the sense of a *swayamsevak*—a person who gives of and through him- or herself—takes on a particular character with reference to RSS ideology. The volunteers who work at Sunderraj Yoga Darshan are, in a profound sense, invested in what they do on the level of the embodied self in service. They are invested with reference to both Yoga and RSS ideology.

Although patients can and do use the props by themselves, in many instances assistance, direction, and support are required. Volunteers help to cinch each patient's feet toward his or her groin by pulling a cotton strap tight in the back to apply a *suptabaddhakonāsana*. Volunteers help in suspending patients from ropes in various inverted postures. They assist patients in being laid flat in *bhiśmāsana* on eight small rectangular blocks positioned at specific points on the body. Many if not all of these volunteers, most of whom dress in a tee shirt sporting the institution's name and logo, are former patients. There is a clear and profoundly important sense of community and common purpose among all of those involved. The ground floor of Smriti Bhavan is referred to as a *gurukul,* meaning a "traditional" institution of learning where a *guru* imparts knowledge to his disciples. Although difficult to label using English terms, the *gurukul* has the atmosphere of a gymnasium, physical therapy clinic, and temple all rolled into one. The primary connotation of *gurukul,* however, is of a community of disciples, and clearly this is how the term is used by Dr. Karandikar.

In many respects the sense of community is similar to that among the participants in the daily morning regimen of the various chapters of the Bharatiya Yog Sansthan, an organization that grew directly out of the RSS and involves a structured program of Yoga exercise performed in public parks throughout India (Alter 1997). The main difference—apart from the props and clinic-based work—is that the sense of community in Pune hinges on the fact that onetime patients become trainers who then work to heal others. As in the case of Dr. Karandikar himself, a large percentage of the twelve thousand patients treated are heart patients, and there is a clear sense in which those who have suffered a heart attack, but have recovered their health through Yoga, are bound together through shared testimonials concerning the efficacy of Dr. Karandikar's technique. The sense of community and common purpose is integrally linked to the medicalization of prop-based Yoga as a technology of palliative care based on a theory of biocosmic engineering—although one can achieve self-realization on one's own, one must have the space between one's shrinking joints expanded by an experienced and committed therapist.

Yoga International Institute: Psycho-Physical Therapy, *Sūkṣma Vyāyām*, and Yoga Purification

While conducting research in New Delhi one morning in mid-February 1994 I discovered a listing for the Yoga International Institute for Psycho-Physical Therapy (YIIP-PT) in the phone book. Employing what is both the most basic and the most profound methodology of my discipline, I dialed the number. A man by the name of Dr. Kumar Pal answered the phone, and after a brief exchange in which I indicated my research interests I asked if I could speak with him in person. Although leaving shortly for Haridwar, he said I was welcome to come over that morning. His address in Lajpat Nagar was not far, and I arrived shortly after 10 o'clock.

Dr. Pal appeared to be in his late seventies or early eighties. He lived in a house with one large all-purpose room, a small kitchen, and a toilet. He graciously invited me in. As we started to talk he explained that he had just completed the manuscript for a 350-page book on Yoga theory and practice. All but the last six pages needed to be printed before it could be published. The printer, however, had left him in the lurch by changing careers. Dr. Pal was nevertheless hopeful that the project would be done shortly after his return from Haridwar in a few days. He pointed out that this book "would tell me all I needed to know about Yoga," but that I could interview him on specific points after I had read it.

In fact the book has not yet been published, nor was I able to see the manuscript, but I subsequently took "psycho-physical therapy" lessons from Dr. Pal and was able to interview him at length on several occasions. At other times he and I engaged in lengthy conversations.

It soon became clear to me that the YIIP-PT had become, by the mid-1990s, little more than a name. Dr. Pal laughed when I told him how I had found his phone number. The telephone had been registered to the institute in the early 1960s but had been used only as a private line for many years.

One of the first things Dr. Pal told me was that the YIIP-PT used to have a large campus "able to accommodate groups of forty or fifty from

Australia and all over the world." However, as he pointed out with obvious resentment, a large part of the campus was forcibly occupied "by a third party." This party had since died and Dr. Pal was eager to follow through on a long-standing court case to reclaim what he felt was rightfully his. Whether on account of this forcible occupation and subsequent court case or not, the YIIP-PT had, by 1994, clearly lost its status as an international center for psycho-physical therapy.

By his own account, Dr. Pal was interested in Yoga from early childhood. Although he engaged in practice as a young man—during which time he was also a wrestler—he decided to pursue an academic career. In 1940 he received an M.A. in philosophy from Banaras Hindu University, where he studied with Dr. B. L Atreya. Eventually he earned the title of *Sarvadarśanacārya,* Master of All Systems of Indian Philosophy. After several years he submitted his Ph.D. thesis, "A Comparative Study of Yoga and Psychoanalysis."

Relocating from Banaras to Delhi, he established the Yoga Health Center in Lajpat Nagar in 1955. Here he put into practice a kind of therapy combining *āsana, kriyā,* and *prāṇāyāma* as well as isometric and cardiovascular exercises. This center soon began to attract a great deal of interest and was renamed the Yoga Institute for Psycho-Physical Therapy. As a brochure promoting the services of the YIIP-PT describes:

> Several foreigners came to study Yoga and were imparted training. A good number of patients suffering from psychosomatic stress disorder and nervous troubles were also treated. The President of the International Society of Sophorology stayed in the institute for a long time. Groups of Russians, Germans, Americans, Australians, Fins, Swedes, Japanese, Koreans, Thais and other Europeans, and Arabs have been trained. Madam Papova, the Soviet Minister for Social Welfare, and Mr. Walter Scheel ex-President of West Germany visited the Institute and appreciated the work. (Pal n.d.a: 1)

In 1966 the institute became affiliated with the Dr. Bhagwan Das Memorial Trust. It was operated and administered within the framework of the Bhagwan Das Seva Sadan, which included an eighty-bed hospital, a gymnasium, a hostel for trainees, a canteen catering to the dietary needs of practitioners, and a library. At this time "International" was added to the official name and thereafter it was known as the Yoga International Institute for Psycho-Physical Therapy. Although functioning as an institute, the YIIP-PT was designed as an association bringing together practitioners of Yoga therapy from around the country and the world. There were set fees for annual and life membership, as well as a special fee for patron status.

During the late 1960s and early 1970s the YIIP-PT was involved in four main activities: (1) running a clinic for the application of therapy for the treatment of psychosomatic disorders, functional and nervous disorders, headaches, tension, high and low blood pressure, insomnia, neurosis, morbid fears, anxieties, and chronic diseases such as asthma, rheumatism, arthritis, diabetes colitis, constipation, obesity, pleurisy, and paralysis; (2) organizing Yoga camps at various locations where lecture demonstrations on specific topics were given to the public; (3) offering a series of courses on various aspects of Yoga ranging in duration from one to three months; and (4) providing free-to-the-public early morning classes in Haṭha Yoga. Collectively these activities were designed to produce "a message of perfect and positive health for the desperate, drug-soaked world of today" (Pal n.d.a: 2–3).

What distinguishes Dr. Pal's system of yogic exercise from other similar systems is the degree of emphasis placed on what he refers to as *ghāṭā śuddhi* or "purification of the body," on the one hand, and his innovative program of *sūkṣmạ vyāyām* or "subtle postural exercises," on the other. As indicated in a schematic pamphlet delineating eleven categories of therapeutic practice (Pal n.d.b), *sūkṣma vyāyām* was an integral feature of the YIIP-PT program in the 1960s. It was also used as the basic model course for the sessions in which I participated.

To begin our sessions, Dr. Pal would assume that everyone had defecated, urinated, carefully brushed his or her teeth, and cleaned eyes and ears. *Jal neti,* using pure tepid tap water, was performed by pouring water through each nostril with a specially designed pot. As I found out, these "*jal neti* pots" are readily available from stores that sell copper and brass household utensils. I was also instructed to buy a narrow-gauge rubber catheter from a pharmacy, or purchase a packet of waxed cotton threads from an *āśram* near the main post office. These were used to perform *sūtra neti* two or three times a week. Dr. Pal pointed out on a regular basis how important it was to clean the sinuses thoroughly, and advocated massaging the sinuses and "blowing out all traces of water, dirt, and mucus" by vigorously tensing and relaxing the muscles around the eyes, nose, and forehead. This cleaning would ensure that all of the *nāḍīs* were purified. As I was told on numerous occasions, "purity is the way to gain control of the body."

Kunjal, using four to six large glasses of tepid tap water, was required about once every week. Given the option of vomiting out the water either in the sink or in the garden—with the insertion of three fingers down the throat to the base of the tongue—my preference was for the garden. Instructions were given by Dr. Pal on how to churn the water in the stomach by performing *agnisāra prāṇāyāma,* a kind of billows-like abdominal breathing exercise. The principle here was to clean the stomach so as to completely purify the *nāḍīs*. Dr. Pal did not have us perform either *vastra dhauti,* where a long narrow cloth is swallowed to "swab" the stomach and throat clean, or the more comprehensive cleaning of the whole alimentary canal by means of *śaṅkh prakṣālan,* although these techniques were part of the more comprehensive program he advocated.

The next stage of the program involved the performance of twelve distinct *prāṇāyāma* exercises designed as "breath regulation for nervous purity and control." *Prāṇāyāma* was preceded by a deep and long intonation of the sound *OM,* "starting with the sound 'a' formed at the base of the spine and, by increasing tone and reshaping the mouth and throat to articulate a series of sounds between 'a', 'o', and 'um,' moving it upward to the top of the head and letting it reverberate there so as to produce an 'overall health benefit.'" A similar kind of internalized brain humming was "prescribed for mental illness," since, according to Dr. Pal, "vibration of the cortex helped to stimulate the nerve channels leading to the brain." This intonation was followed by a recitation of the *gāyatrī mantra.*

In Dr. Pal's regimen the type, number, sequence, and duration of *prāṇāyāma* exercises performed vary according to the seasons of the year. For example, the cooling *śītalī prāṇāyāma* is cut from the sequence in winter and extended in duration during the summer. *Kapālabhāti,* translated by Dr. Pal as "sinus draining," is always practiced regardless of the season and tends to be regarded as more important than a range of *prāṇāyāma* exercises referred to as "glandular massage, murmuring, mouth cleaning, and intestinal massage." Although technically a *kriyā* technique, *kapālabhāti* was treated by Dr. Pal as a *prāṇāyāmic* extension of *neti kriyā,* and reflects his overall concern with the purity of the sinuses. On one occasion a question on why so much attention was being given to this aspect of Yoga—asked by one of my session mates, a *sannyāsi* with the title Yogi Shanti Swaroop, who regularly refused to perform *kunjal, jal neti,* or *sūtra neti*—prompted a lengthy discourse by Dr. Pal on the anatomy of the face and bone composition.

The last and final part of the routine, which usually lasted half the allotted time of one and a quarter hours, was devoted to *sūkṣma vyāyām.* Although this involved *āsana*-like postures, strictly speaking it did not incorporate yoga *āsana*s as such, other than those identical with various kinds of toe-touching. The *vyāyām* period begin with the performance of *sūrya namaskār*—which Dr. Pal referred to as a kind of exercise invented by the Raja of Aundh (see Alter 2000a)—that incorporates modified *āsana* postures linked together through fluid, step-by-step movement accompanied by rhythmic breathing. The core of the *vyāyām* session involved the performance of modified physical training drill exercises, running in circles and various forms of rhythmic arm swinging. These rather sedate cardiovascular exercises, if done in conjunction with *prāṇāyāma,* were said to "stretch the veins and arteries so that cholesterol would eventually be flushed out."

After the *sūkṣma vyāyām,* the routine was devoted to the performance of eighteen "sitting poses," six "lying on stomach poses," twelve "back poses," four "special poses," and finally nine *mudrās* referred to as "neuromuscular postures," all done in a precise sequence. The sequence of performance is important, since each posture leads into the next, and the sequence itself thus becomes an integral part of the routine insofar as the movement from one fixed posture to the next is part of the exercise routine. For example one moves from an inverted shoulder stand to the plough pose by bending at the waist and lowering one's legs down in front of one's head. Included as part of the neuromuscular poses are a series of *bandha*s, referred to by Dr. Pal as "anal lock," "stomach lock," "chin lock," and "tongue lock," each of which is designed to block and then release the flow of *prāṇa.*

In most general terms, Dr. Pal's ideas about health and healing can best be appreciated in terms of a discussion he had with Yogi Shanti Swaroop as we neared the end of one morning's routine.

> If someone is ill then a posture or exercise can be prescribed and they can do it for ten minutes or more as therapy. But anyone can do the same exercise for a minute or so and benefit from it. Like the humming exercises—the male and female bees—which vibrate the frontal brain and the cortex and are used for the treatment of neurosis and psychosis. If one is just doing these for maintaining good health, then a few minutes of practice is sufficient, provided you do them with a happy mind; in a state of *mastī* so that tension is released. The idea is to purify all of the *nāḍī*s so as to flush out the system. For cleaning out the arteries *apānaprāṇa prāṇāyāma* is particularly useful. Locks are placed on all key points of the body so that air from above is sacrificed on the fire of the lower air, which is moved upward from the *mūlādhāra cakra.*[18]

Dr. Pal and the Politics of Yoga

In my conversations with Dr. Pal I was struck by the extent to which he seemed to embody a tension between Yoga as philosophy, Yoga as physical fitness, and Yoga as cultural politics. For example, although he staunchly advocated his modern program of psycho-physical therapy, in one of our first conversations he indicated his personal preference for what he called "classical" Yoga: "I now devote four hours of every day to Mahā Yoga and Kuṇḍalinī Yoga.[19] This practice is responsible for my good health. All of my wrinkles have disappeared and I only need these glasses to read fine print. Here, look at my arm. See how firm and strong it is? I used to have four teeth that were loose, but they are now strong and firm again. All of this is through the energy activated in the *mūlādhāra cakra.*" Dr. Pal's life story, as it was narrated to me, provides an interesting perspective on how he has come to embody a form of practice that reflects his ambivalence about the relationship between Hindu philosophy and the purity of culture, on the one hand, and the practical value of creative modern innovation, on the other. With much less critical self-reflection—and some might even say reactively defensive fanaticism—this ambivalence is also reflected in the training regimen of the RSS, with which Dr. Pal has been directly affiliated.

Kumar Pal was born in a village near Rohtak, in the Punjab, around 1915. While studying in school in 1928 he was heavily influenced by Gandhi's *swadeshi* campaign and one day took all of his Western-style clothes and burnt them. This created some tension between him and his family, not on account of financial concerns—as they were "quite wealthy"—but because his family was secular and apolitical. Nevertheless he persisted in wearing only *khādī* and also took a vow of celibacy, following to the letter all of the prescripts for a *brahmacārī,* including wearing wooden sandals, a seamless one-piece garment, a *laṁgot,* and a long *cutiyā.* Thus he tried to cut the figure of a traditional Brahmin student.[20] He refused to live in the same house with his mother and sisters and built himself a retreat in the garden near his home, closing his eyes whenever female relatives brought out food. He would practice Yoga in the morning and "sleep with a single brick as a pillow during the night."

Early on Kumar Pal's father tried to arrange his marriage. He had gone so far as to accept Rs 5000 as part of the dowry payment before his son found out and ran away from home, taking refuge at Gurukul Kangri in Haridwar. This action served to make his point and the marriage was called off. Following this Kumar Pal returned to his family home in Rohtak.

During his student days Kumar Pal seemed to move away from his Gandhian inspiration and, along with friends, "became a revolutionary, killing many tyrants, both Indian and foreign." After leaving Rohtak he enrolled at Hindu College in Delhi, where he received his B.A. in philosophy. At this time he was still dressed as a *brahmacārī,* and wore his "uniform" to class. If "modern boys," as he referred to them, teased him, he would physically fight back until left alone. By his own account, Kumar Pal was a tough young man with militant views and strong opinions.

Impressed with his intellectual aptitude, the faculty at Hindu College wanted him to stay there to complete his M.A. But, as he put it—with a clear sense of masculine bravado—"I told them that I had read all sixty-seven of the books they wanted to assign, and that I wanted to go to the center of philosophical learning and study at Banaras Hindu University (BHU)."

After moving to Banaras he supported himself by serving as the accounts manager for the school canteen at Kashi Vidyapeet (a school for Sanskrit studies) as well as by contracting book orders for various libraries. With this financial security he was able to study, "with all of the great swamis of Banaras."

During this time he was still a strict *brahmacārī* and had built himself a secluded retreat on the grounds of a lemon orchard. Here he did Yoga in the morning, studied all day, and then practiced wrestling at a gymnasium in the evening.

He was at the point of becoming a *sannyāsi* by receiving *dīkṣā* from his *guru,* when he experienced a profound, life-changing event just six days before his initiation. He was doing Yoga when a low-caste family came into the orchard under contract to harvest and pack the ripe fruit. As Kumar Pal put it: "They were poor, each with only a thin *gamcā* to wear as clothes, and yet they were all happy. I thought to myself, this family, all full of joy and happiness, does not look as though it is weighed down with responsibility and trouble." Dwelling on this, Kumar Pal began to reconsider his own lifestyle, and in particular his vow of chastity. As fate would have it, the next day a friend serving as a go-between approached him with a proposal from a "very wealthy Marwari cement mogul" to marry his daughter. He agreed to meet the family and ultimately got married. Kumar Pal's father-in-law, it seems, shared many of his son-in-law's ideals, and this was the basis upon which the match was made. Later in life he too "renounced the world" and, as Kumar Pal pointed out, with a twinkle in his eye, his brothers-in-law had to go to court to prevent their father from giving all of his wealth away to charity.

After getting married, Kumar Pal taught history and political science at Kashi Vidyapeet and continued studying with both Bhagwan Das and B. L. Atreya. In 1955 he returned to Delhi and got his Ph.D. from Delhi University. Atreya was a professor of philosophy and Sanskrit literature at BHU, as was Bhagwan Das, and both men had a significant influence on Kumar Pal's intellectual development. The critical scholarship and modern philosophy of the latter have been incorporated into RSS ideology.

During the late 1960s Dr. Pal was associated with the Rashtriya Swayamsevak Sangh and came into contact with a group of men who founded the Bharatiya Yog Sansthan (BYS). His introduction to the BYS came when he was approached by two men who wanted him to explain to them the tenets of Hinduism in basic terms so they could pass this information on to their sons, who were studying in England. As they explained, their sons kept being asked about Hinduism, but were unable to articulate the basic principles of their religion. According to Dr. Pal, later these men went on to found the Vishwa Hindu Parishad, a nationalist organization similar to, and affiliated with, the "Mother Organization," as the RSS is often called.

It was following this meeting that the idea of the Bharatiya Yog Sansthan was conceived in terms of promoting "knowledge about Hinduism" through Yoga. Dr. Pal was one of a small group of men who started this organization under the auspices of RSS. As I have discussed elsewhere (Alter 1997), the BYS extends the idea of nationalism into the global language of "universal brotherhood." In terms of practice the *śākhā* model is used in an effort to turn all public neighborhood parks in India into *yoga sādhan kendra*s (centers for Yoga practice).

At some point, probably in the late 1960s or early 1970s, Dr. Pal became disillusioned with the "fanatical" *pracārak*s (literally propagandists, regional leaders) in the RSS. He also became critical of some members of the new BYS leadership, who he claimed were simply out to secure power and wealth and had turned Yoga into "a half-hour workout." Although he did not say so explicitly, my sense is that the growth and development of the YIIP-PT occurred as he disassociated himself from both the RSS and the Bharatiya Yog Sansthan and directed his considerable energy and talent to building up this institution. As he put it, he came to realize that the basic philosophy of the RSS was incompatible with Yoga, since Yoga "is universal and not limited to Hinduism."

When I first met with Dr. Pal I was introduced to a young man I will call Harish, who worked, with his brother, for a travel agency in Lajpat Nagar. Harish's avocation was Yoga. He also taught Yoga. But, as it turned out, in a very different way from Dr. Pal. An account of how Dr. Pal and Harish worked together—somewhat ambivalently—sheds light on the creative tension between philosophy, physical fitness, and cultural politics in Dr. Pal's program. It also sheds light on the problem of fanaticism and, in fact, on the problem with all forms of uncritical, unself-conscious faith that are at the heart of both nationalism and the embodied soul.

As I noted in my field journal, Harish epitomized the kind of person who is most often characterized as a fraud or charlatan, and not just by those who are skeptical of Yoga as such, but also by those who are vested in the discursive field of Yoga itself.[21] I made an effort to not deal with him as such. Rather I sought to engage with him as an honest broker of knowledge about Yoga. Soon after we were introduced and I indicated my research interest in "modern Yoga" Harish adamantly pointed out that there is no such thing as "modern Yoga." In his view the Yoga being practiced in modern India is the same as the Yoga of Patañjali. Moreover, he pointed out, there can be no understanding of Yoga through education, since Yoga itself is an encompassing system of education.

As a practitioner of what he called Mahā Yoga or Kuṇḍalinī Yoga he explained that the only way to learn Yoga was to experience it. Pulling a piece of copybook paper out of his pocket with a drawing of a stick figure surrounded by circles, he said that he would show me what he meant. Explaining that the circles were the penumbra through which enlightenment could be experienced, Harish told me that he could show me these "sheaths" with my "third eye" after only three days of concentration. Both he and Dr. Pal agreed that there was no magic involved: "it is simply a natural process which the body experiences during Yoga."

Two of the semi-regular participants in my morning sessions with Dr. Pal were a couple from Vietnam studying Yoga in India. They were primarily working with Harish, but had been advised to take lessons from Dr. Pal in preparation for reaching higher states of consciousness. I interviewed Harish in his office one evening while we waited for his disciples to arrive. As we talked, he picked up on a theme of the previous day. "I can give you information you will not be able to get anywhere else in India. You can bring all kinds of doctors if you want. They will see. I can stop my pulse. No pulse! Nothing. No brain waves, even." On the last claim, I gave him the benefit of the doubt.

Harish claimed to have been initiated into Yoga after twenty-five years of study with a tantric *guru* "who hung upside down from a tree for three years before achieving enlightenment." He explained the process of Kuṇḍalinī Yoga as very simple, and directly opposite to religion, "which has complicated and corrupted everything." Kuṇḍalinī Yoga, he went on to explain, provides a perspective on one's own self, and this is the only real benefit it has for society. As Harish described it, the energy of *kuṇḍalinī* is like "an inverted umbrella covered with lights. Once you see these lights the 'throat *cakra*' turns back the tongue onto which drips the nectar of pure bliss. Once this nectar has been consumed, one experiences ecstasy and can see every organ and *nāḍī* in the body quite clearly."

Without a hint of self-consciousness, Harish claimed that he could train people to reach *samādhi,* the final goal of Kuṇḍalinī Yoga, after only about thirty or forty-five minutes of practice. With an attitude of extreme pride and confidence he explained that the Vietnamese woman he was working with had achieved *samādhi* in "a matter of minutes, and had then returned to her normal state of being with a sensation of bliss and a pervasive lightness." To help convince me of this he produced two manuscripts he had written, one entitled "Knowing the Self by the Self in the Self through Simplified Kuṇḍalinī Awakening" and the other "Eternal God—Transitory World." The claim made in the first of these manuscripts is only somewhat more modest than what he claimed in the interview.

Harish was as critical of most other practitioners of Yoga as he was sure of himself, claiming that "99 percent of all self-proclaimed *gurus* are false, and end up spending the energy of their enlightenment on sex with their disciples." Dr. Pal made a similar statement about a very well known international swami, whom he referred to, sarcastically, as a "modern master of Yoga, who smokes cigarettes and wears western suits and boots." For all his grand claims, therefore, Harish shared with Dr. Pal a sense of the way in which Yoga has practical value as a medium through which to achieve social reform in a corrupt society, but also that Yoga can be easily and radically perverted. "Society is currently only living up to 10 percent of its potential," he pointed out. "If the remaining 90 percent could be tapped and channeled, just imagine how much better society would be. There would be no jealousy, anger, frustration, and greed." In other words, Harish conceptualized Yoga with reference to the overarching problem of modernity and imagined a future in which the power of enlightenment would fully factor into social reform.

Unlike Dr. Pal—whose youthful visions of *mokṣa* had been brought down to earth by marriage and many other things, including the realpolitik of the RSS system—Harish was dubious about the healing potential of Haṭha Yoga as a mechanism for enhancing social welfare. He was a staunch idealist. "One can live in the world and practice Yoga," he said. "There is no mystery or magic in that. But no one can cure diabetes with Yoga *āsanas*. That is nonsense! Yes, breathing problems and indigestion can be treated, but not chronic diseases." It was clear, however, that while Harish was critical of applied Yoga therapy—just as Dr. Pal lampooned the half-hour workout of the BYS—his own simplified Kuṇḍalinī Yoga was heralded as pure and powerful enough to cure anything. He had even tried to persuade his father-in-law, a "very well known Āyurvedic physician," to give up his practice in favor of direct enlightenment.

Given this perspective, and despite his obvious friendship and respect for Dr. Pal, it is not surprising that Harish was skeptical of Yoga psychophysical therapy and critical of the kind of book Dr. Pal was in the process of writing. He claimed that Dr. Pal "did not take his study of Yoga past the *āsana* stage" and that he was trying to persuade him to do so. In fact, Harish was virtually dismissive of any kind of physical practice associated with Yoga. "Who has two hours a day to spend standing on his head, pouring water in and out of his nose or swallowing a cloth and pulling it back out!? All you need is half an hour for meditation. You don't need to do all of these things they teach at [the Yoga Institute at] Santa Cruz."[22]

As might be expected—early experience as a revolutionary and youthful status as a "muscular" *brahmacārī* notwithstanding—Dr. Kumar Pal was not explicitly critical of Harish and his simplified system of Kuṇḍalinī Yoga. Whether on Harish's advice or not is unclear, but Dr. Pal had turned to the practice of Mahā Yoga, although in doing so he had not at all renounced his own system of psycho-physical therapy. In any case, one morning after the Vietnamese couple had apparently stopped coming to the sessions, Yogi Shanti Swaroop asked what had happened to them. With a laugh and a sense of what struck me as clear sarcasm, Dr. Pal said, "Oh, they have decided that *āsana* and *prāṇāyāma* are not necessary for what they want to achieve."

Neither the Yogi nor I responded to this. For my part I continued to concentrate on performing my *sūkṣma vyāyām* routine. So did the Yogi, although I do not know what his reaction was. Unlike me, he had not come to learn about modern Yoga and write about its cultural history. He was not trying to prove anything by producing manuscripts of the sort that both Harish and I do. He was studying with Dr. Pal as part of his work for the Shri Raghavendra World Peace Institute and the World Constitution and Parliament Association, in order to "achieve one world government on this earth." In this sense I guess you would call him a transnationalist. He gave me a copy of his curriculum vitae before leaving for his headquarters in Haridwar. In it he claims to "travel to other spiritual planes with his astral body." But since he was there on the floor of Dr. Pal's living room doing jumping jacks, leg lifts, and running in circles around the table with the rest of us, he was also trying, in some way, to effect a more complete link between his physical and his astral body.

In the course of one of my interviews, Dr. Pal pointed out that the RSS *pracāraks* use ideology to secure power and that many are ignorant of the basic precepts of Hinduism and of the true meaning of Hindutva as articulated by Savarkar, an ideologue of the organization, and Bhagwan Das. He himself, however, was clear on the nature of these precepts. His perspective on Hinduism in general reflects, in more than just a metaphoric sense, his integrated practice of Yoga as a modern form of subtle, synthetic physical fitness that purifies the body and society—if not the whole world—in grounded rather than "astral" terms. Although problematic in its own way, the following statement may be read as a different kind of "man making," a different kind of "character molding" from that which is institutionalized by the RSS. But it is, nevertheless, one that is intimately linked to the body and to society. Just as *sūkṣma vyāyām* is a different kind of yoga from the "purebred" yoga of Patañjali, Dr. Pal's understanding of purified Hindu masculinity provides an altogether different kind of theory from the different-but-not-completely-different theory of innate birth-ascribed purity.

> The question of who is a Hindu is a very live question. I follow Bhagwan Das in holding that the basis of Hinduism is found in the four *varṇa* categories and in the four stages of life. On some level anyone who is a Hindu believes in the laws of Manu. But although the distinctions Manu makes are right, they are distorted by the idea that they are ascribed by birth. It should be that a child's *guru,* in consultation with his parents, can decide what the *varṇa* of that child should be, so that the son of a Dhobi can grow up to be a Brahmin. This is true Hinduism.

What is striking about Dr. Pal's life work as a teacher of yogic psychophysiological health is precisely the fact that it is profoundly "Hindu" but with hardly a trace—rhetorical, iconographic, ritual—of what would typically be regarded as Hinduism. There is also hardly any reference made to pan-Indian unity, structured social reform, or selfless voluntary service to the nation. And yet, what is of central importance to Dr. Pal is what is also of central importance to the RSS—the structured purification of bodies and the inculcation of organized, healthy self-discipline into the life of every individual. But whereas the object of RSS discipline is the Hindu body, and the bodies of Hindu men in particular, Dr Pal takes the body as such and subjects it to a modern "Hindu" regimen.[23] In doing so he has come to recognize, very clearly, that Yoga's definition of universal truth is simply beyond belief, and that the embodiment of what is beyond belief—however gross its subtle manifestations may seem—does not make sense as a nationalist project.

Man Making and Purification in Modern India

Arguably, cultural purification is a large part of what nationalism is all about. One need only think of Nazi Germany to appreciate the extent to which concerns with purification and the body merge with ideas about the purity of culture, pure masculinity, and the purification of society, in terms of both social reform and genetically based systems of social engineering of the crudest kind. The RSS seeks to instate a pure Hindu society. To do this, it trains Hindu men to become powerful, disciplined, and well organized so as to purge the nation of all that makes it impure—among other things, secularism, corruption, self-interested consumerism, Christianity, and, of course, Islam. In many articulations of nationalism a key link in the transposition of body and society is between men, muscles, and the motherland.

It is clear that RSS nationalism is based on the presumption of a kind of ineffable, emotional bond between Hindu men and the idea of Bhārat

Mātā, Mother India. This is thought to be a deeply felt bond, and there is much in RSS rhetoric that seeks to articulate what is virtually inexpressible and incomprehensible about it. Naturally, every attempt to describe the essence of this bond reinforces its quasi-mystical, indescribable—and thereby powerful—nature. Poetry, of course, captures the ineffable, inadequately verbalized feeling of this patriotic spirit. To read the lyrics of songs that are written to be sung during *śākhā* sessions (Anonymous 1992a; n.d.b) such as "The Nation Is Calling to You," "Onward Hindu Soldiers," "Mother Your Child Adores You," and "Never Lose Courage" is to gain a sense of powerful attachment to the substance of a national past, a sense of feeling brought on, for example—and the most powerful examples are always intimately biographical—by the smell of the earth after the first monsoon rain. This attachment is, therefore, effected through extremely personal, evocative memories that make the "idea of cultural tradition" so powerful as to be beyond the need for logical and rational comprehension. This "idea of cultural tradition" is, therefore, very much like Yoga insofar as experience counts for everything. And yet it is very unlike Yoga—perhaps the most antithetical thing to it—insofar as emotion and one's visceral attachment to the nation are what counts as real and what defines the meaning of truth. As it reifies and institutionalizes desire, nationalism is virtually a parody of *māyā*, the web of illusion.

But emotions, however deeply felt, are only really powerful when they are not just sensed but physically embodied. Quite apart from its pragmatic concern with martial training, *śākhā* drill is designed to produce a body that is "Indian to the bone," although this very Cartesian metaphor would be much more apt if construed as follows—Indian to the embodied soul. And it is precisely in the aptness of this metaphor that the problem lies.

Given the emotional and profoundly visceral character of RSS "traditionalism"—which is, in fact, extreme modernism—it is striking the extent to which the RSS and those whose views intersect with RSS philosophy conceive of the problem of modernity as an embodied problem and of social problems as problems of health. Although there is much more to the RSS than is encompassed by the body, the body does seem to define a locus point for the development of many things. Thomas Bloom Hansen makes note of this and quotes M. S. Golwalkar, probably the most influential RSS thinker: "The first thing is invincible strength. We have to be so strong that no one in the whole world will be able to overawe and subdue us. For that we require strong and healthy bodies. [But] character is more important. Strength without character will only make a brute of man. Purity of character as well as the national standpoint is the real life-breath of national glory and greatness" (Golwalkar 1966: 65–

66, in Hansen 1999: 82). In this respect the *śākhā* functions as what Christophe Jaffrelot refers to as an ideological *akhāṛā* (gymnasium) (1996: 34–35). Speaking of the RSS's founding principle, Hansen summarizes the intent of *śākhā* organization very well.

> The guiding idea was to inculcate a national spirit as the ultimate and supreme loyalty and to build up a strong fraternal bond between the volunteers, the swayamsevaks. Hedgewar wished to create a "new man"—patriotic, selfless individuals, loyal to the Hindu nation and the RSS—physically well trained, "manly," courageous, self-disciplined, and capable of organization. The RSS swayamsevak was to be the kshatriyaized antithesis to Gandhi's nonviolent, "effeminate" bhakti-inspired Hindu. The ideal swayamsevak was supposed to be a selfless activist dedicated to lifelong service of the nation, but not only preoccupied with a search for truth and perfection of the soul, as were the traditional yogis. (1999: 93)

Along these lines—and given what has been said about modern Yoga in the previous chapters—one would think that physical Yoga of the sort developed by Kuvalayananda could be directly and easily integrated into RSS practice. It could provide a kind of ready-made, "authentically Indian" philosophy of biomorality and character development that would fit directly into the ideology of Hindutva. Clearly the RSS has used Yoga, and a mutation of Yoga and RSS philosophy has inspired people like Dr. Karandikar, Dr. Pal, Harish, and members of the Bharatiya Yog Sansthan to creatively imagine Yoga's modernity. But to pick up on the latent tension—and perhaps critical ambivalence—reflected in the RSS's flirtation with the practice of "traditional yogis," and to thereby bring the analysis around, I would like to follow through on Dr. Pal's observation that Yoga is antithetical to the nationalist ideology of the RSS.

There are many different aspects to this. The two I will discuss here have to do with gender and religion.

Yoga as a form of cultural practice can be linked to Hinduism. Even a cursory glance at various works of academic scholarship shows how "impacted" yogic ideas are in works that have come to define the structure and content of neo-Hinduism. To make this link meaningful, however, requires that the body be extended beyond the realm of *dharma,* but in such a way that it does not disconnect the relationship between *dharma* and Hindutva. Thus to make Yoga relevant to the cultural politics of Hindutva involves a profound contradiction—it must, somewhat ironically, be modernized and turned into a form of physical education, with explicit and clearly explicated social implications, while in cultural terms still be used to invoke Patañjali, among others. It must be Hinduized in spirit but declassicized in practice, and clearly the physical form of Haṭha Yoga helps in this regard. But then, on this level—where jumping jacks and *tāḍāsana*s merge—RSS drill becomes virtually identical to the kind of modern Yoga that has taken on global scope and significance. It is this—where Yoga's modern, transnational scope and truly global appeal threatens to make a provincialized farce of nationalistic Hindu pretense—that makes it extremely difficult for the RSS to do with Yoga what it has done so well with military drill in the guise of physical training exercises. To distinguish Yoga as nationalistic Yoga from decultured "secular" Yoga, the RSS would have to infuse it with an ideology of Hindu man making that is intimately physiological. The logical dissonance created by this is such that you can feel—in your bones, so to speak—the nationalistic tension manifest in trying to do "*āsana*s" that produce muscles of steel.

Beyond this it is the incipient universalism and self-oriented focus of Yoga, along with its primary concern with the physiology of transcendence, which has made it much less important in the scheme of RSS training than it would otherwise be if all it were was a "traditional system of Hindu physical education." In the *śākhā* regimen it is much less important than so-called traditional sports, stave training, and other martial arts, even though in other contexts Yoga and its various permutations have been regarded as central components of organized mass drill. Where the RSS has balked, so to speak, the central government of India has made great strides in the nationalistic production of mass drill Yoga.[24] Given the precept of nonviolence in Yoga, it could be argued that this is obvious. After all, it does not take a great deal of thinking to understand how stave training and "manly sports" like kabaḍḍī (Alter 2000b) fit with the militant ideology of the RSS, whereas Yoga's apparent gender neutrality and nonviolence are much more amenable to the pastoralism of state governmentality.

As I have argued elsewhere (Alter 1994), however, stave training is not only designed to promote organization and discipline. It is man making in an explicit, uncomplicated mode. It is man making much in the way that modern body building is man making. A great deal of drama, discipline, and structured representation of the body is involved, but not much by way of an ethics of embodied masculinity beyond the principle of mass, might, and proportion. In stave training, choreographed, rhythmic, mass drill involves the summing of individual bodies into the collective body of a single-minded, well-organized militant group. In this regard stave training does not contain its own theory of personhood and identity any more than does "callisthenic Yoga." For either one to be "Hindu man making" requires the poetics of visceral nationalism.

Along with the kind of rhetoric about military drill training and the "bodies of steel" this kind of training is thought to produce, many articles in the RSS *Organizer* quote Vivekananda as a proponent of muscular

Hinduism: "You will understand the *Gītā* better with your biceps, your muscles, a little stronger. You will understand the Upaniṣads better and the glory of the *Ātman* when your body stands firm upon your feet and you will feel yourselves as men. What I want is muscles of iron and nerves of steel inside which dwells a mind of the same material as that of which the thunderbolt is made. Strength, man-hood, *kshatriya-vīrya* plus *brahm-teja*" (Anonymous 1947: 11). It is difficult to know what Vivekananda meant by this—or the extent to which he was being literal and programmatic rather than metaphoric—but it is quite clear what the RSS takes him to mean. *Lāṭhī* (stave) in hand, its understanding is profoundly literal.

It must be remembered, however, that Vivekananda was a key figure in the Yoga Renaissance. Invoking him invokes Yoga as well as a complex mix of nationalistic ideas that involve religion in different ways, thereby confounding any simple strongarm attempt at appropriation (S. Basu 2002). In this regard it was not so much the body itself that concerned the missionary monk of neo-Vedānta as the critical metaphysical relationship between *ātman* and the body.

Yoga is man making in a metaphysical mode, and involves the self only as a meta-Self. Therefore Yoga is, in a sense, proto-individualistic, profoundly asocial, and infused with a kind of potent, pervasive sexuality. Although clearly linked to semen—and perhaps because it is too clearly linked to semen—yogic sexuality is very difficult to construe as masculinity, at least of the man-making kind. Simply put, the quote from Vivekananda would make no sense whatsoever if it included the *Yoga Sūtra,* along with the *Gītā* and the *Upaniṣads,* as texts to be understood by "feeling oneself to be a man" with muscles of iron and nerves of steel.

There is an enormous space of knowledge and practice between the message of the *Gītā* and the *Yoga Sūtra* on the one hand and steel nerves and iron muscles on the other, and the Haṭha Yoga literature does not fill this space any better than a Vedāntic reading of Patañjali. As reflected most clearly in Savarkar's *Hindutva* (1969), Golwalkar's *Bunch of Thoughts* (1966), and Upadhyaya's *Integral Humanism* (1991), the RSS recognizes the importance of trying to define the nature of this embodied space, but it is Dr. Karandikar and Dr. Pal—among others—who have engaged the moral substance of this space on the embodied terms it demands. Mahatma Gandhi did as well.

From the perspective of the RSS, Gandhi's problem was that he embodied the power of nonviolence as an effete principle based on a catholic interpretation of Hinduism and human values. For different reasons, and as the result of a different history—along with the fact that it is a cultural entity and not the product of a singular, distinct charismatic personality—the practice of Yoga presents the same problem. Given the Orientalist structure of RSS thinking, Yoga problematically carries with it precisely the image of the effete Indian that was integral to various dimensions of colonialism. It is as though Yoga is all too easily able to stand for almost everything about masculinity that the RSS was established to counteract. Beyond any number of points that could be made with reference to tantric literature, consider, as simply one example, the following passage from Eliade's *Yoga: Immortality and Freedom,* which describes the embodied transcendence of the phenomenal world: "It is the coincidence of time and eternity, of *bhāva* and *nirvāṇa;* on the purely 'human' plane, it is the reintegration of the primordial androgyne, the conjunction, in one's own being, of male and female—in a word, the reconquest of the completeness that precedes all creation" (1990: 271). Quite apart from being able to say, from a psychoanalytic perspective, that the deeply affective bond between mother and son is an articulation of this same yearning, the embodied idea of androgyne is most certainly anathema in the domain of muscular Hinduism.

Although there is no need to synthesize all of the various ways in which different people have engaged with the embodied space between nerves of steel and an understanding of the embodied self—the "*nāḍī*ed self," it might be said, to be metaphorically symmetrical—it is interesting to note that as muscles recede in significance, in the context of nationalism the problem of purification and purity comes to take center stage on a number of different levels. This is quite clear in the case of Gandhi, as manifest in his concern with fasts in particular and hygiene in general (Alter 2000a). It is also reflected in Dr. Karandikar's concern with the biochemical "purity of cells," and the organization at Kabir Baug that was established by him—with unfortunate and probably unintended eugenic overtones—"for the purification and development of human kind." Similarly, Dr. Pal's *ghāṭā śuddhi*—"purification of the body"—is the cornerstone for his yogic program of psycho-physical therapy.

Although McKim Marriott and his students are right in having directed attention away from the dichotomy of purity and impurity as structural principles in Hindu South Asia (1990; Daniel 1984; Raheja 1988), purity as such has tremendous power and persuasive force as a cultural ideal in modern India.[25] Purity and purification are integral to the embodied realization of *paramātman,* and a pure body is, in a very literal sense, a powerful and supremely strong body. What is significant in this is that the difference between the metaphorical connotations of purity as an ideal and its apparently material, organic, phenomenal denotation is not extreme, or not nearly as extreme as in the case of muscularity. Consider what Feuerstein says: "The path of realization (*sādhana*) is . . . couched in terms of purification (*śodhana*). In fact the very process of *kuṇḍalinī* arousal is understood as the progressive purification of the constituent elements (*bhūta*) of the body—earth, water, fire, air, and ether. It is known as *bhūta-śuddhi*" (2001: 357). Of note is the relationship herein between power and purity: "Metaphysically speaking the *kuṇḍalinī* is a microcosmic manifestation of the primordial Energy, or *śakti*. It is the universal Power as it is connected with the finite body-mind" (Feuerstein 2001: 356). It is, therefore, no accident that the integration of Yoga into nationalist projects is relatively easy and meaningful in terms of purity and health, but difficult and relatively meaningless with respect not just to muscle building and masculinity—which is fairly obvious in any case—but to any reified notion of the body as a distinct, finite thing. To be sure, purity and muscularity can both be deployed against the perceived threats of modernity, but as an issue that involves everything from cells and sinuses to immortality and freedom—and everything from earth to ether—purity reflects a kind of power that muscles simply mimic.

Set against the murky obscurity of muscular, regimented masculinity, it is perhaps apropos to quote one of the many references to purification and selfless "character building" that suffuse the classics, and that thereby inform the practice of at least some modern Indian visionaries who reflect on the Self and look both directly at and beyond the limits of a Hindu nation: "When the mind-*sattva* (*buddhi*), whose nature is luminosity, is freed from [the effects of] *rajas* and *tamas*, and has a steady flow without any veiling contamination of impurity, that is, the lucidity . . . has occurred, there is clarity in the inner being of the yogin, which is a progressively clearer and more brilliant light of knowledge of the object as it really is" (Vyāsa, quoted in Whicher 1998: 235).

PART 3

CONCLUSION

Indeed every table of values, every "thou shalt" known to history or ethnology, requires first a physiological investigation and interpretation, rather than a psychological one; and every one of them needs a critique on the part of medical science . . . something, for example that possessed obvious value in relation to the longest possible survival of the race (or to the enhancement of its power of adaptation to a particular climate or to the preservation of the greatest number) would by no means possess the same value if it were a question, for instance, of producing a stronger type. The well-being of the majority and the well-being of the few are opposite viewpoints of value: to consider the former a priori of higher value may be left to the naiveté of English biologists. —*All* the sciences have from now on to prepare the way for the future task of the philosophers: this task understood as the solution of the *problem of value,* the determination of the *order or rank among values.*

Friedrich Nietzsche, *The Genealogy of Morals,* trans. Walter Kaufmann (1968: 492)

PART

CONCLUSION

6

AUTO-URINE THERAPY—THE ELIXIR OF LIFE: YOGA, ĀYURVEDA, AND SELF-PERFECTION

He who takes *śivambu* (one's own urine) daily and excludes salty, sour and bitter foods from his diet acquires divine accomplishments quickly. Freed from all ailments, and possessing a body comparable to that of Śiva himself, he deports himself like the gods in the universe for an eternity.

Ḍāmara Tantra, Śivambu Kalpa, śloka 30, 31

Fortified by my faith in what I thought to be the correct interpretation of the text [Proverbs 5:15, "Drink water from your own cistern"], I fasted for forty-five days on nothing but my own urine and tap water—and this despite the doctor's assertion that eleven days without food was the limit to which a human being could go! . . . At the end of the treatment I felt and was "an entirely new man." I weighed 140 pounds, was full of vim, looked about eleven years younger than I actually was, and had skin like a young girl's.[1]

J. W. Armstrong, *The Water of Life* (1971: 29)

The Water of Life

A CONCLUSION IS designed to summarize and distill down the essence of an argument, but it should also indicate the direction in which a line of reasoning—if not a stream of consciousness—might flow. The point of departure for this, the first of two concluding chapters, is the fact that in yogic practice there is a procedure called *amarolī* which involves drinking one's own urine.[2] It is described in the *Haṭhayogapradīpikā* as follows: "One should enjoy the middle flow of one's own urine, discarding the first part since it increases bile and the last part because it has no essence" (III: 96).[3]

Clearly, then, J. W. Armstrong was not the first person to use his own urine in order to try to solve the "problem of the body," and to try to solve the problem of human suffering manifest in death, disease, and decay. But it is fair to say that he invented auto-urine therapy as a system of alternative medicine. In 1918 he advocated the exclusive use of one's own urine to cure all ailments, developed specific therapeutic regimens, and, most significantly, treated "tens of thousands" of patients. By his own account many of these patients were cured.

Armstrong's book *The Water of Life: A Treatise on Urine Therapy,* published in 1944, had a profound impact on Raojibhai Manibhai Patel, a Gandhian social reformer. After recovering from a heart attack and curing himself of hypertension—and curing, by his own account, hundreds of people—Patel published his own book, entitled *Manav Mootra: Auto-Urine Therapy.* Full of testimonials and easily followed, step-by-step procedures, *Manav Mootra* has been translated out of Gujarati into both Hindi and English. Originally published in 1959, the Gujarati edition is now in its tenth edition and has sold thirty-nine thousand copies. The Hindi version is in its seventh edition and has sold thirty-five thousand copies. Now in its third edition, the English translation has sold twelve thousand copies.

In a previous publication I have pointed out that auto-urine therapy makes almost perfect sense in terms of Mahatma Gandhi's expansive, inclusive, and inherently somatic understanding of the principles of self-rule (Alter 2000a). Having earlier examined some of the political implications of this in the context of postcolonial nationalism, my concern here is to focus on the structural logics—with an emphasis on the plural—underlying auto-urine therapy. What is involved when a body consumes part of itself to make itself better? I will argue that a principle of self-perfection, and the inherently self-sufficient and somatically introverted logic reflected in the idea of drinking one's own urine, transforms a fluid body subject to constant change through contact with the environment into an extremely fluid—but insulated and "immunized"—body whose fluids are recycled.

Although conceived of by Armstrong in terms of the relatively static principles of a mechanistic, Cartesian, biological body, the idea of gaining better control over the cause and consequence of flux by self-regulating the body's fluid nature—which is what auto-urine therapy entails, regardless of how physiology is understood—made perfect sense to Patel, who read Armstrong with a different kind of body in mind, and a different understanding of nature. On the one hand, he and his readership found in auto-urine therapy a practical solution to the problem of dualism and the body's objectification as this was reflected in the increasing hegemony of biomedicine in modern India. On the other hand, however, the development of auto-urine therapy as a distinctively modern Indian practice of alternative healing provided a logical—though perhaps not easily accepted—solution to the enigma of humoral balance and the paradox of perfect imperfection manifest in the *doṣic* epistemology of Āyurveda (Alter 1999). First published in India in 1971, and extensively quoted, always paraphrased, and sometimes flagrantly plagiarized in the forty or so books published on the subject in Hindi, Gujarati, Marathi, and Bengali, Armstrong's book is now in its fifteenth impression. Elsewhere it is out of print.

In an earlier work I have analyzed the conjunctural structure of Yoga and Nature Cure in terms of the practice of the friction sitz bath (Alter 2000a). The argument put forward there—as it is germane to this case—was that the friction sitz bath enjoyed widespread popularity in early-twentieth-century India because it made sense on both an ontological and an epistemological level, even though, given its somewhat masturbatory connotations, it made no formal cultural "sense" at all. The apparent "senselessness" of rubbing one's own genitalia with a wet cloth, and integrating this into a public discourse on public health—with an emphasis on the "public"—was rendered meaningful and significant through the friction sitz bath's translation into the language of *prakṛtic* transformation.

In the early part of the last century the subtle, elemental structure of Yoga physiology was increasingly made the object of gross manipulation in terms of the logic of German Nature Cure. The friction sitz bath, developed by Louis Kuhne, was understood by Indian Nature Cure physicians as particularly effective because it fit into their understanding of nature through association with the fifth element, ether. In fact, one might say that the friction sitz bath was more "at home" in modern India than in Germany, because there it could be firmly grounded in the embodied ontology of *prakṛti* rather than linked, loosely, to a somewhat dislocated, modern theory of nature. In the hands of Indian Nature Cure physicians the friction sitz bath was made to make more sense in terms of the manipulation of subtle *ākāśa* than in terms of calming and cooling the nerves through the gross mechanics of rubbing the penis or vagina with water[4]—as Kuhne had intended—even though the action itself remained exactly the same. Thus the convergence of "ethereal" Yoga and "mechanical" Nature Cure opened up a logical space in which the relationship between subtle and gross attributes could be radically reconceptualized.

My concern here is not, however, the history of auto-urine therapy's incorporation into the plurality of medical practices in contemporary India. Nor am I concerned, as I have been elsewhere, with the politics of this event. My concern here is with the structural logics that emerge out of the mixing of Sāṃkhya metaphysics, reflected and operationalized most clearly in Āyurveda, and auto-urine therapy. I am interested in the convergence of the specialized, rather marginalized, often maligned—and problematically categorized and classified—"branches" of Yoga, Āyurveda, and Nature Cure, and the way in which urine, a natural product of the body, is understood to be a substance with supranatural power.

The focus here on the relationship between Yoga and Āyurveda is designed to be, at least in part, a critical commentary on the rather uncritical blending of Yoga and Āyurveda in contemporary New Age practice.

Unlike the friction sitz bath, which was a completely new idea that emerged out of a transnational conjuncture of ideas and practice, drinking one's own urine was practiced in India long before Patel adapted J. W. Armstrong's technique. In the case of the friction sitz bath there was an interesting shift in meaning and an extension of structural logic whereby water and nerves translated into semen, ether, and *nāḍī* physiology. It was possible to "rub the penis" and almost completely disassociate the act from sex itself. In the case of auto-urine therapy however, it is almost impossible to disconnect urine as abstract signifier from the signified substance that is both produced and consumed by the body. With apologies to the poet, urine by any other name would smell, taste, look, and feel the same way. This has led, I will argue, to the paradoxical situation wherein the popularity of auto-urine therapy in India can be explained in terms of Āyurvedic and yogic principles but where the "indigenous" literature on the subject is not regarded as authoritative or even very good.

Ḍāmara Tantra: A Problem of Textual Authority

In *Manav Mootra* Patel makes passing references to the use of human urine as prescribed in the "Āyurvedic" medical literature. In particular he quotes extensively, in a short chapter dealing with the "Eastern tradition," from the *Śivambu Kalpa* section of the *Ḍāmara Tantra,* which he refers to as an Āyurvedic text "belonging to the Puranic age." The *śivambu Kalpa* is a short treatise containing 107 *śloka*s or stanzas dealing exclusively with *śivambu*—pure water, or one's own urine. Although it does not appear in Ram Kumar Rai's translation of an early, undated, Bengali version of a Sanskrit text entitled *Ḍāmara Tantra* (1988),[5] R. B. Athavale of the B. J. Institute of Learning and Research claims that he was given a copy of the manuscript from the archives of the Shankaracharya of Dwarkà (Karlekar 1972: 30). Patel, writing in 1959, does not give citations, but it seems unlikely that he was working with the same manuscript Athavale was given "by a friend" in 1967. In any event it is clear that the *Śivambu Kalpa* is not a text in wide circulation. It is presently most easily available appended to contemporary books on auto-urine therapy. In quoting from this text Patel makes the point that it is inherently mythological, rather than scientific—that it is full of exaggerations, and also that it makes reference to "various concomitant recipes" called *anupāl*[6] that should be regarded as "not pertinent" to the practice of auto-urine therapy (1991: 9–10; see also Mithal 1979: 17).[7] Nowhere does Patel draw on the *Ḍāmara Tantra* as a practical guide. Rather it is used simply to point out that "urine therapy is not a new discovery, [that] it was prevalent in India hundreds of years ago, [and that] it has curative as well as preventative value" (1991: 9).

A more recent book, published anonymously by "an experienced physician" and titled simply *Auto-Urine Therapy,* follows this same pattern. The bulk of material is drawn from personal experience and from both Armstrong's and Patel's work, but the book also contains a short two-page section quoting single passages from various Āyurvedic sources. Even though the *Śivambu Kalpa* is published as an appendix to this book (see also Hiralal 1988: 57, ślokas 1–21; Karlekar 1972: 150–61; Mishra 1998: 98–117), it is never used as a resource for the development or refinement of therapy per se. Ambiguously—and in sharp contrast with Patel—the author of this book points out that the *Śivambu Kalpa* is important precisely because it provides *anupāl* recipes for mixing one's own urine with herbs, elements, and minerals to effect specific cures. But in keeping with the purist tradition of Nature Cure as reflected in most Indian books on the subject (Gotham 1988: 48–72; Mithal 1979: 41; Shaha, Shaha, and Dholkiya 1997: 38–121; Agarwal 1992: 21–32; Thakkar 1997), the anonymous physician does not make use of this information and advocates the exclusive use of unadulterated urine (see Hiralal 1988: 167–68).[8] The issue is further complicated since the "experienced physician" goes on to claim that "what is most important [about the *Śivambu Kalpa* is its discussion of] *kayākalpa,* a complete regeneration and revitalization of the whole body" by means of urine therapy (Experienced Physician n.d.: 8–9).[9] There is a clear sense in which Armstrong, Patel, and others believe that urine promotes strength, energy, fitness, and longevity, but again not in terms of the specific *kayākalpa* techniques outlined in the *Ḍāmara Tantra,* even though, in India, the authority of the *Tantra* is invoked to bolster the claims of those who advocate auto-urine therapy.

Although the *Ḍāmara Tantra* is most clearly regarded as the single most important source of information about the South Asian system, Patel and others do cite other sources, most notably the *Vayavaharsūtra,* composed by the Jain Acharya Bahadrabahu, where it is said that one should drink one's own urine when fasting or taking a *pratimā* vow (Patel 1991: 10–11; see also Experienced Physician n.d.: 9; Mishra 1998: 119–20; Mithal 1979: 17–18). Most sources also go on to note that "Buddhist monks and lamas" were able to perform extreme penance and live to the age of 150 years or more by drinking only their own urine (Hiralal 1988: 55; Mishra 1998: 120; Shaha, Shaha, and Dholkiya 1997: 9). Patel, paraphrasing Armstrong (1971: 16), claims that Sir Morris Wilson discovered this when on his expedition in the Himalayas. By drinking his own urine he was able to withstand the discomfort of cold and altitude sickness while climbing Mt. Everest (Patel 1991: 11). In many respects Hiralal's book *Vijñānic Svāmūtra Cikitsā* contains the most comprehensive—though eclectic, dislocated, and anecdotal—account of where and by whom auto-urine therapy has been practiced. Expanding on Armstrong, and following Patel closely (1991: 13–17), he quotes from *Soloman's English Physician,* published in 1665, and refers to seven different uses for urine found in *One Thousand Notable Remedies,* an early-nineteenth-century English text (1988: 47–64).

The question, then, is what is the relationship between *śivambu* and auto-urine therapy? Since Armstrong was influenced, simply, by his grandmother's and mother's use of urine to cure toothaches and bee stings, and the generous interpretation he gave to the biblical passage "drink water from your own cistern" to mean drink your own urine, it seems to be a rather coincidental and ironic accident of history that auto-urine therapy, as a permutation of Nature Cure, should become popular in India. It is, you might say, akin to the mistake of taking coal to Newcastle. But it is only coincidental to a degree, since the larger argument against institutionalized medicine, which runs as a constant refrain through Armstrong's, Patel's, and almost all other books on the subject, helps to explain why the putatively Āyurvedic basis of *śivambu* was viewed as problematic—it is specialized, arcane, and technical whereas auto-urine therapy is designed to be the antithesis of all that. Moreover, even though Nature Cure is, by definition, natural, the discourse and practice of Nature Cure in both Europe and India is suffused with the language, technology, and culture of modernity. Although radical in form, and therefore maligned by the medical establishment, the claims Patel and Armstrong made were based on reason, reason that took shape as a truly "natural" science of the whole body. This was seen as an alternative to the particulating, atomizing, and reductionist sciences of biology, physiology, and anatomy. As Patel points out, the *Ḍāmara Tantra* spoke with the hyperbolic authority of mythology, not the rational logic of objective proof based on direct experience. He and Armstrong did that, albeit in slightly different ways and with reference to different bodies of knowledge.

Śivambu and the Principles of Āyurveda

As historians of the subject are well aware, in studying Āyurveda—and many other things as well—one is often confronted with the problem of what is or is not legitimately part of the system. One could, very easily, imagine an Āyurvedic physician turning his nose up at the very idea of auto-urine therapy and dismissing the *Śivambu Kalpa* as tantric quackery.

I am sure that arguments could be made that the text is marginal at best, if not completely over the top. The practice itself would appear much more convincing if Suśruta, Vāgbhaṭṭa, and Caraka had incorporated and integrated the practice of *śivambu* into the mainstream of Āyurvedic thinking instead of making only rather vague references to it. Even a cursory glance at the primary texts of the corpus shows that these authors were much more concerned with classifying animal urine into very distinct pharmaceutical categories than in delineating the quality of human urine as such.[10] Almost every book on auto-urine therapy quotes the same three passages: one from the *Suśrutasaṃhitā* stating that human urine is the antidote to poison, a second from the *Bhāva Prakāśa* where human urine is said to "destroy poison, give new life, purify the blood, and clear up skin ailments," and a third from the *Harit* which points out that human urine "destroys diseases of the eyes, makes the body strong, improves digestion . . . destroys coughs and colds [and is] basic, bitter and light" (Gotham 1988; Mishra 1998: 7–8, 36–37; Mithal 1979: 13–14; Satyananda Saraswati 1981: iv; Shaha, Shaha, and Dholkiya: 1997: 2–6). Only Hiralal's 240-page-long treatise contains a short, three-page section entitled "Āyurveda and Urine Therapy," which deals with the dominant theme of zoological and ecological classification. Gotham's book is the only one I have seen that seeks to link auto-urine therapy with cow-urine therapy (1988: 73–104), but only rather tenuously in terms of Āyurveda (1988: 77).

There is also the problem that the *Śivambu Kalpa* appears to be a yogic text rather than one that is Āyurvedic since it refers to the practitioner as a *yogi* or *mahāyogi*. Under the guise of *amarolī*, modern auto-urine therapy is also proclaimed by some to be primarily yogic in nature (Satyananda Saraswati 1981; see also Mishra 1998: 120; Mithal 1979: 14–17; Patel 1991: 10; Thakkar 1997:35), at least when combined with *vajrolī*, a purificatory practice wherein water is drawn into the bladder and then expelled (*Haṭhayogapradīpikā* 3: 96–97). The objection to this argument, as Satyananda Saraswati's own treatise on the subject reveals, is that beyond the single, rather cryptic reference in the *Haṭhayogapradīpikā*, which enjoins practitioners to "partake of the middle stream," there is no distinctly yogic elaboration on the techniques and procedures of *amarolī*. Satyananda Saraswati invokes the authority of the *Ḍāmara Tantra*, and an interesting selection of scattered references in the *Yoga Ratnakar*, *Bhāva Prakāśa*, and *Gyānarnata Tantra*—where no comment is made on what is Āyurvedic and what is yogic. In the body of the book, however, he reports on modern research conducted at the Bihar School of Yoga in order to "present a scientific, objective view of *amarolī*—assessing all the points of kidney, urine and its uses—in order to approach the subject with adequate understanding and a more balanced perspective" (1981: 15). The report itself is based largely on personal experience, a few experiments, and the work of modern Indian practitioners such as Patel and Karlekar. However, neither of these two men conceived of what he was doing in terms of Yoga, at least as Yoga is commonly understood.

Even so, one could argue that the *Kalpa* is more like the *Haṭhayogapradīpikā* than the *Carakasaṁhitā* or the *Suśrutasaṁhitā* and should be read as an elaboration of *amarolī*. The problem is that the *Kalpa* makes no reference to any yogic practice other than "partaking of the middle stream." There is also the problem that the yogic text is coincidentally medical, whereas the *Kalpa* is thoroughly medical and concerned with the pharmaceutical nature of urine, rather than with the use of urine as a replacement for water in the practice of various *kriyās*.[11] In many respects, therefore, the *Kalpa* is much more like the treatises on *rasāyana* therapy in the *Carakasaṁhitā* and the *Suśrutasaṁhitā*, with the added paradox that Lord Śiva, the archetypical mahāyogi, and source of all *siddhis*, appears in the text in guise of a supreme *vaidya* giving careful instructions on *anupāl* decoctions. It is along these lines that R. B. Athavale, with a degree of Armstrong-like rhetorical flourish, refers to *śivambu* as "the mother of all Āyurveda" (in Karlekar 1972: 19).

Sidestepping the problem of chronology, strict classification, and maternal metaphors, the perspective taken here is that, as an ancient text radically modernized by Armstrong's reading of the Bible, the *Śivambu Kalpa* has come to be located somewhere betwixt and between Āyurveda, Tantra, Siddha, and Yoga. It makes sense in terms of an image of the perfected body that derives from Sāṃkhya and it employs the logic of Siddha and Yoga, but its principles find clearest expression in the grounded language of Āyurvedic medicine. As we shall see, in Armstrong's therapy urine is understood to be a distillate of natural elements, a derivative of the body that can strengthen and cure by setting up a closed circuit of recovery. In the *Śivambu Kalpa* urine transforms the very nature of the body and thus sets in motion a spiral toward perfection, or, to use better imagery, a sequence of progressive condensation, purification, and refinement.

Śivambu and the "New Man"

The *Śivambu Kalpa* text itself is in the form of a dialogue between Lord Śiva and his consort Pārvatī and begins (*ślokas* 1–4), with a delineation of the types of container in which one's own urine should be collected. Although almost any material can be used, copper is regarded as the best. Before collecting one's own urine in a copper bowl, one must abide by a regimen of self-preparation. Although not particularly detailed or delineated, the prescription is that one should eat light meals of unsalted and nonbitter foods, get plenty of rest, sleep on the ground, and control one's senses (*śloka* 5). Then one should wake up before dawn, after three-quarters of the night has elapsed, and, leaving the first and last portion, collect the middle portion of the morning's first flow in a bowl. The stream of urine is likened to a serpent, the head and tail of which is poisonous. But, with regard to the middle stream, Śiva explains to Pārvatī: "*Śivambu* is heavenly nectar, which is capable of destroying senility and diseases. The practitioner of Yoga should take it before proceeding with his other rituals" (*śloka* 9).

Ślokas 10 through 21 may be regarded as a distinct set, since they outline a twelve-year course of tonic-based metabolic self-development. Also, this set precedes a larger section dealing with *anupāl* pharmaceutical decoctions, and is distinct in exclusively prescribing the unadulterated middle stream as heavenly nectar. After explaining that the collected urine should be drunk in the morning after cleaning the mouth and evacuating the bowels, Lord Śiva charts the effects of the course of therapy along a timeline that may be tabulated as follows:

One month—brings about "purification"
Two months—"stimulates and energizes the senses"
Three months—"destroys all diseases and frees one from all trouble"
Five months—produces "Divine vision and freedom from all disease"
Six months—produces "high intelligence and proficiency in the scriptures"
Seven months—gives "extraordinary strength"
Eight months—imparts "a permanent glow like that of gold"
Nine months—"freedom from tuberculosis and leprosy"
Ten months—"makes one a veritable treasury of luster"
Eleven months—"purifies all the organs of the body"
One year—produces "radiance equal to the sun"
Two years—gives "power over the element earth"
Three years—gives "power over the element water"
Four years—gives "power over the element light"
Five years—gives "power over the element air"
Seven years—gives "power over pride"
Eight years—gives power "over all the important elements of nature"
Nine years—gives "freedom from the cycle of birth and death"
Ten years—produces the ability "to fly through the air without effort"
Eleven years—the ability to "hear the voice of one's own soul"
Twelve years—bestows the power to "live as long as the moon and the stars last; immunity from the danger of animals and the poison of snakes; an inability to be burnt by fire; and the ability to float on water just like wood."

Curiously no mention is made of what happens after the sixth year. Logically the continued consumption of *śivambu* would, by this point, produce power over the element ether. Quite obviously, the logic employed here is the same as that in *kuṇḍalinī,* where the raising of the serpent power is cognate with the reintegration of the five primary elements. It is perhaps significant that the sixth year is only the midpoint of the regimen. It would seem to make more sense if it were the apex, producing, in effect, power over all five *prakṛtic* elements. What else, one might ask, is possible or necessary? What else would even make sense? And yet the list continues, with *svāmūtra mokṣa* achieved in the ninth year, after having conquered pride, but—oddly it would seem—before being able to fly, becoming immune to poison and incombustible, and gaining a kind of stellar immortality.[12]

I will return to this regimen in a moment, but it is first useful to look at the rest of the *Śivambu Kalpa*. Although not delineated as such, *ślokas* 22 through 33 constitute a second set, insofar as they precede a section dealing with massage. Each *śloka* prescribes *anupāl* pharmaceutical additives to the middle stream. The *ślokas* in this section are also linked together to the extent that they express themes dealing with the conquest of death and disease, the development of hyperstrength, and various kinds of immortality. These appear to be the type of "exaggerations" to which Patel makes dismissive reference in *Manav Mootra*. Here are a number of examples.

> Powdered *harītakī* (*terminalia chebula*) should be taken assiduously with *śivambu*. This combination destroys senile degeneration and all diseases. If this practice is continued for a year, it makes one exceptionally strong. (*śloka* 23, 24)
>
> One gram of sulphur should be taken with *śivambu* every morning. He who continues this practice for three years will live as long as the moon and the stars. His urine and feces will whiten gold. (*śloka* 25)
>
> The powder of the *kośta* fruit should be mixed properly with *śivambu* and taken in the prescribed manner. If this practice is continued for twelve years, one's body will be free from the ravages of old age such as wrinkles on the skin and whitening of the hair. One acquires the strength of a thousand elephants, and lives as long as the moon and the stars exist. (*śloka* 26)

In some instances the decoctions are quite complex and detailed, as are the symptoms for which they are prescribed.[13]

> The essence of mica and sulphur should be taken along with *śivambu* and a little water. This cures all disorders caused by the malfunctioning of the digestive system and all disorders caused by the humor *vāta*. He who takes

this mixture regularly becomes strong, acquires a divine radiance, and can escape the ravages of time. (*ślokas* 28, 29)

A mixture of equal parts of sulphur, powdered *āmvla* (*phylonthus emblica*) fruits and powdered nutmeg (*myristica beddomci*) should be taken first and then followed by *śivambu*. This will eliminate all diseases. (*ślokas* 37)

He who takes rock salt mixed with an equal quantity of honey every morning, and follows it up with *śivambu* comes to possess a body with Divine attributes. (*ślokas* 36)

Śloka 44 marks a significant point in the *Kalpa,* since it introduces the practice of urine massage, which is developed clearly through to *śloka* 55 and then appears intermittently throughout the rest of the text, usually as supplemental to the consumption of various *anupāl* decoctions.[14] Unlike *śivambu,* which must be drunk fresh, one's own urine has to be aged in order to be used for massage. Through the aging process three-quarters of the liquid evaporates, leaving a condensed residue which, when massaged into the body "nourishes the limbs and cures all disorders" and imparts flexibility and unrestricted, fluidlike movement. It also bestows "the strength of one thousand elephants and the ability to digest any food" (*ślokas* 48, 49).

There does not appear to be any discernible pattern to the text from *śloka* 55 through the end, where most passages simply catalog the way in which drinking *śivambu* with one kind of herb, element, or animal product in conjunction with massage will produce phenomenal results. A few examples will be illustrative.

Oh dear one! He who is unyielding in his practice of taking roasted grams with jaggery, drinking *śivambu* and massaging his body with it for six months acquires the ability to see clearly things situated at great distances, to be able to smell things from great distances; he is not subject to ailments, and his body becomes light and supple. (*śloka* 55, 56)

He who sedulously drinks *śivambu* after taking equal parts of the powders of *amṛta, triphal, kady,* dry ginger, cumin seeds and the roots of piper longum, and keeps a diet of only rice and milk, will . . . within three years acquire great strength and valor; he becomes a veritable god on earth. He becomes omniscient, acquires all spiritual attainments, can expound even the scriptures and sciences which he has not studied, and all the three worlds are visible to him (*ślokas* 60, 61)

If he massages his body with *śivambu* three times in every period of a day and night he will be strong in his body and in all the joints of the body, he will constantly be in a state of ecstatic happiness, he will always have friendly feelings for all, and his body will shine with a golden luster. (*śloka* 120)

Mūtra Mokṣa: Soma, Svāmūtra, and the Logic of Rejuvenation

Although the procedures are quite different, and the regimen much simpler and self-contained, it is worth considering the suggestion that *śivambu* builds on the idea of radical rejuvenation as reflected in the therapeutic procedures associated with Āyurvedic *rasāyana*.[15] More specifically it is useful to think of one's own urine—as quite distinct from someone else's—as comparable to *soma*, as *soma* is understood in the medical literature to produce immortality by "killing off" the body prone to aging, disease, and death and replacing it with a flawless reproduction (see D. White 1996: 10–11, 26–29). It would, of course, also be possible to see urine as directly comparable to mercury in the tradition of Siddha alchemy, and to understand *śivambu* as a kind of *rasa-rasāyana* (Hiralal 1988: 56; Rao 1985: 80–82; D. White 1996: 52–57). Clearly the mythology and magic associated with *tantra* is directly relevant (see Rao 1985: 9–12). And as David White points out—with reference to the multivocality of *rasa*, for example—the difference between *soma*, mercury, semen, and the moon is not always sharply marked. The reason to stick with, or at least start with, the terminology and therapeutics of Āyurveda is because it is here where the structure and function of physiology is most clearly worked out and empirically based.

Both Caraka and Suśruta provide detailed accounts of *rasāyana* therapy, which is, in effect, a means by which to prevent aging and embody immortality. I have discussed the implications of this regimen elsewhere (Alter 1999), and good, clear accounts are available in several secondary sources (notably Wujastyk 1998: 171–77). In outline, however, *rasāyana* therapy lasts for several months, during which time the body of the "patient" is decomposed and than recomposed through a combination of *soma* nectar consumption, massage, herbal rinses, and a carefully regulated diet. The decomposition and recomposition of the body is described in clinical detail by Suśruta. On the fourth day, for example, the body swells and then exudes worms. By the seventh day the patient is "fleshless and has become mere skin and bone," and on the eighth day, after a second dose of *soma*, "his flesh begins to fill out, his skin splits open and his teeth, nails and body hair fall away" (in Wujastyk 1998: 173). Recomposition appears to start on the tenth day, and is facilitated by penetrating massages, rinses, and, most significantly, by a third dose of *soma*, the first two doses of which had precipitated the body's dramatic decomposition. The third and final dose seems to have an opposite effect on the body, for from day ten through sixteen the skin gets progressively firmer. Day seventeen marks the beginning of a series of dramatic changes which are described by Suśruta with great rhetorical flourish: "On the seventeenth and eighteenth days his teeth appear, sharp, smooth, even, firm, strong and as bright as diamond, beryl, or crystal . . . [On the twenty-fifth day] his nails appear, shining like coral, as red as a ladybird, or like the rising sun; firm smooth, full of good signs. . . . And his skin shines like a blue lotus, like white flowers of flax, or beryl" (in Wujastyk 1998: 174). Throughout the course of treatment attendants carefully nurse the patient, and each phase of transformation is followed by a series of specific procedures involving the use of all kinds of different organic substances—milk, penetrating oil, a decoction of white cutch tree, barley porridge, grains of mature rice, cuscus grass paste, sandalwood, black sesame, mallow oil, white dammer tree paste, soups, broths, embolic juice, and liquorice, among many other things. The patient's movement, mood and exposure to the outside world is carefully managed. The description given by Suśruta of "the new man" is noteworthy in the context of both the epigraphs to this chapter and the specific problem of making sense of *śivambu* and the modern Indian practice of auto-urine therapy.

> The visionary man who makes use of the king of plants, *Soma,* wears a new body for ten thousand years. Neither fire nor water, neither poison, blade nor projectile, are powerful enough to take his life. He gains the strength of a thousand well-bred, sixty-year-old, rutting elephants. . . . He is as beautiful as the god of love, as attractive as a second moon. He is radiant, and brings joy to the hearts of all creatures. He truly knows all sacred knowledge, with all its branches and sub-branches. He moves like a god through the whole world, with infallible willpower. (in Wujastyk 1998: 176)

Although it may seem perverse to suggest that *soma* and *śivambu* are analogous, my argument is that despite formal incongruity—and golden color notwithstanding—it is worth considering why they seem to occupy the same conceptual space, as it were, in the logic of medicalized rebirth and embodied immortality. It would be tempting at this point to embark on a purely symbolic analysis, with Freudian overtones. *Soma,* after all, is replete with symbolic significance: it is golden in color, it grows in tandem with the waxing and waning moon, and it exudes a milky liquid when pierced. To extract the juice one must pierce it with a golden needle. As David White has argued in convincing detail, *soma* and semen are homologous substances. Writing about *rasāyana,* he says, "It is here, at the level of the replenishment and maintenance of vital fluids, and most particularly the vital fluid that is semen, that the disciplines of Āyurveda and *haṭha yoga* intersect . . . semen is the raw material and fuel of every psychochemical transformation the yogin, alchemist, or tantric practitioner undergoes, transformations through which a new, superhuman and immortal body is 'conceived' out of the husk of the mortal, conditioned, biological body" (1996: 27).

How much easier it would be if the *Śivambu Kalpa* were concerned with the consumption of semen rather than urine! Everything would seem to fall almost perfectly into place. And there is even a tantalizing "model" for this possibility. As White points out, there is a sense in which Haṭha Yoga is built around a model of how semen is channeled up through the body to the "cool" cranial vault, where it is transformed into *amṛta,* the consumption of which bestows immortality. In the imagery of *kuṇḍalinī,* the seminal nectar of immortality drips down onto the tongue of the adept. Of critical significance here, however, is the relationship between semen and digestion, for if semen is left in the lower abdomen, the fire associated with this part of the body will cause it to flow. The flow of semen is a key process in the sequence of aging, disease, and death, in terms of both physiology and the extended logic of procreation. Only when semen is channeled up and "cooled" by the antithesis of fire does it transubstantiate and become that which drips down onto the tongue of the adept. Thus it would seem that while it would make perfect symbolic sense to drink one's own semen, it makes no sense whatsoever in terms of the underlying physiological principles of Āyurveda and Yoga. It would be burned up in the stomach. Here the structure of metabolism trumps the symbolism of substance.

On a related note it would also be tempting to follow the logic of a different homology and point out that the penis performs the dual function—and a seemingly contradictory one at that—of elimination and procreation: the excretion of a waste product, on the one hand, and the channeled flow of the body's most pure, powerful, and life-giving substance, on—and sometimes with—the other. This dual function might, following Lévi-Strauss, be reduced down to the opposition of life and death. And Śiva's metaphoric reference to the first and last flow of urine being like the head and tail of a snake evokes not only possible Freudian interpretations—as does the phallic Lord himself—but the entire corpus of serpent lore and snake mythology, culminating, perhaps, in the image of the tail-sucking oroborus snake who churned the ocean to create life, and upon whom the whole universe rests.

Beyond this there is the curious fact that in mythology in general and tantric mythology in particular there is a direct correlation between the figure of the serpent and the residual precipitates of time. This is linked to the way in which a snake sheds its skin and appears to re-create itself, an image that is apparent in the skin-splitting birth of the new man through *rasāyana* therapy. What is important here is that the snake itself is thought to be "composed of the dregs, the calcinated residue of past creations" (D. White 1996: 215). Therefore, in essence, the snake's endless regeneration is based on the recycling of residual precipitates. With auto-urine therapy in mind, David White's analysis of Śeṣa Nāga mythology is particularly apropos: "In this way, Śeṣa, the cosmic serpent who ever renews himself from one cycle to another, remains the same serpent even as he is reconstituted from a new mixture of recycled elements. As such his body is an endless source of raw material for renewed creations. For this reason he is also called Ananta, 'Endless'" (1996: 216). From these associations it would be a relatively simple move to say that *śivambu* imparts life by means of a cognitive slight of mind wherein urine is symbolically purified through association with semen and the snakelike organ of elimination/procreation. Insofar as this purification entails the power of life over death, the consumption of one's own urine could be seen, like the snake biting the tail of its own residual body, as a means by which the cyclic time-governed duality of birth and death is replaced with the monistic, timeless eternity of youth. The only problem with this compelling logic is that it is purely symbolic and does not engage with the logic of medical practice.

Piss, *Pitta*, *Ojas*, and Other "Waste" Products

An interpretation that goes beyond simplistic symbolic correlations must consider the nature of *mala*, as *mala* are linked to the body's metabolic structure. *Mala* derives from the root *mṛj*, which means to purify or clear out. It is usually translated as waste product. However, as S. K. Ramachandra Rao points out, it is important to keep in mind that *mala* are "waste products of body metabolism," which are eliminated *through* feces, urine, and sweat. The *mala* are, therefore, very much part of the body, as the body constantly reproduces itself through the metabolic processes of digestive cooking. As Rao puts it:

> [*Malas*] employment in the context of the main triad of life and health (the three *doṣas*, the seven *dhātus* and the *malas*) suggests a wider connotation. It is an essential ingredient of the living organism, an indispensable activity in the living body, viz. production not only of material which needs to be eliminated from the system (for which the expression *kitta* is used) but also of material that can be utilized to support the body (hence called *dhātu*).[16]
>
> It is also usual to refer to *mala* as "polluting agents" (*malinīkaraṇat*), which, unless expelled from the body, would render the body impure (viz. unhealthy, diseased). But it is important to recognize that what are called *mala* are actually by-products of the digestive process, and that as long as they are in proper proportion they do not cause any disorders in the body,

> but, on the other hand, sustain the body and facilitate its efficient functioning. It is therefore why they are called *mala-dhātu,* which may sound paradoxical. (1987: 116)

I would suggest that if one is a practitioner of *śivambu* or auto-urine therapy, this begins to sound less and less paradoxical. Even a cursory glance at the contemporary literature, starting with Armstrong and Patel, shows that advocates of auto-urine therapy are adamant in their belief that urine is the pure basis of life rather than excrement (see Agarwal 1992: 17–21; Experienced Physician n.d.: 20–21; Gotham 1988: 12–13; Mishra 1998: 129–31; Shaha, Shaha, and Dholkiya 1997: 30). Hiralal puts it succinctly when he points out that a child's urine is the distilled essence of mother's milk, and "urine is the pure, filtered juice of digested food and drink" (1988: 82). Consider what Dr. G. K. Thakkar, founder and chairman of the Bombay-based Water of Life Foundation, says: "In this polluted world the only unpolluted thing is our own urine. In all the passenger vehicles there is an emergency exit. In the same way, the merciful, all loving and caring God has put one panacea in our body at the time of birth (Even before birth the foetus in the mother's womb floats in and drinks amniotic fluid which is 90% urine)" (1997: 36).

Although *mala* is used in a commonsense way to signify feces and urine, it is perhaps more useful to think of these gross body substances as first-order excrements. They derive from the primary digestion of food into *anna-rasa* during the *prapāka* stage of digestion, which is not metabolic but simply what takes place in the gastrointestinal tract when food is liquefied.[17] During the *jātharāgni* stage of digestion, *rasa* is broken down into *sāra* "nutrients," on the one hand, and urine and feces, on the other. The *sāra* is then transported to the heart, which is the locus point for metabolic transformation. The production of second-order *mala* is linked to the internal process of *dhātu* transformation from *rasa* (digested food juice), through *rakta* (blood), *māṁsa* (flesh), *medas* (fat), *asthi* (bone), and *majjā* (marrow), to *śukra* (semen). The sequence of transformation occurs through the action of the *dhātvagni* (constituent fires), such that at each of the seven stages of "cooking" the *dhātu* in question itself undergoes a transformation from subtle to gross, and this produces two other aspects: the subtle form of the next *dhātu* in sequence and *mala* by-products as a kind of residue from the endless metabolic transformation of gross into subtle *dhātu.* This is how the body maintains its structural and functional integrity. Thus looking at the first three *dhātu* alone produces an interesting configuration of "waste" products. As chyle is cooked by the chyle fire it changes from its subtle, functional aspect into its gross structural form and produces subtle blood and *kapha* as *mala*. As subtle blood is cooked it takes on the structural attributes of gross blood and produces subtle flesh and *pitta* as *mala.* As subtle flesh is cooked it becomes gross flesh and produces subtle fat and—contrary to what one might expect, given the sequential production of *doṣa*—not *vāta,* but secretions from the nose, ears, eyes, and penis.

Rather than see these *mala* as waste products, with primarily negative connotations, it is worth considering that they are more like precipitates in the sense of being compounds which derive from the biochemistry of gross-into-subtle-into-gross transformation. Of interest is the fact that semen, at the top of the *dhātu* chain, so to speak, is cooked but produces *ojas,* which is purely and simply subtle energy—and is not a *dhātu* as such. Rao is somewhat inconsistent on this point, stating at one place that the process of semen-cooking produces no *mala,* and at another indicating that *ojas* itself is *mala* (1997: 59).

Curiously urine is not mentioned by name as *mala-dhātu,* but would seem to be classified along with secretions from the nose, ears, and eyes. That is, it would seem to be on the same order as tears, ear wax, and snot. On the level of metabolic *mala-dhātu,* feces and skin derive from marrow. Sweat is mentioned as it precipitates out from the *medagni* cooking of fat into bone during the *dhātvagni* process. Whereas sweat stands alone, and would appear to be the same on both the cutaneous and the subcutaneous level of *dhātu* cooking, on a metabolic level there is what appears to be on odd pairing of urine and tears, and feces and skin. At the very least, therefore, one is left with a perplexing situation in which that which has come to be regarded as quintessentially excrement is ambiguously classified both as gross excrement and as *mala* on the level of *dhātu,* whereas two out of three humors—the integral constituents of the body—along with *ojas,* vital energy itself, are classified as *mala-dhātu.* Obviously the meaning of *mala* is far more complex, inclusive, and implicated in the body's integral transformation than the English gloss "waste product" would allow.

It is noteworthy that first-order feces and urine are the product of first-order digestion, and do not seem to be the residual by-product of the body's metabolic transformation as manifest in either *bhūtāgni* (elemental digestion) or *dhatvagni* (constituent digestion). As Rao points out, they both are the specific "waste product" of *anna-rasa,* as *anna-rasa* is the nutritive essence of food before it is assimilated into the body. To understand this process—and to understand what seems to happen when urine is ingested—it is necessary to briefly examine processes of digestion as they are linked to fire in general as *agni* and *jātharāgni* in particular: the internal fire which sustains life by, in effect, cooking the body as a whole.

All thirteen of the body's fires derive from a single source, solar heat, but *agni* itself, according to the Nyāya-Vaiśeṣika perspective reflected in this aspect of Āyurvedic theory, has two different dimensions, one permanent and the other transient. Permanent heat is located in "extremely minute, partless units of matter that are beyond the range of sensory perceptions" (Rao 1987: 20). Transient heat is constituted by impermanent aggregates of these minute particles and is reflected in things that can be sensed. Directly related to this distinction is the agency of *pāka* (cooking), which is manifest in, and the basic force behind, such things as growth, decay, transformation, and action. As Rao points out: "The Nyāya-Vaiśeṣika school of thought recognizes two kinds of cooking: conversions that occur in the nature of things as a result of the combination and recombination of the ultimate elements (*pīlu-pāka,* a term that roughly denotes chemical changes) and [those] involving a change in the very nature of the thing (*piṭhara-pāka,* a term that may roughly mean physical changes)" (1997: 20). It is difficult to know what exactly the difference is between these two, since the term "nature of things" is rather vague, but it is clear that the first cooking has what might be called a "mixing" effect whereas the second is more of a self-contained transformation.[18] In any case, both kinds of cooking are manifest in the body. If he is using the terms consistently throughout, Rao seems to suggest that the elemental and constituent fires cook by mixing and bring about a conversion in the nature of things, whereas the stomach fire produces a physical transformation in the nature of food as it becomes *rasa.*

In the case of *śivambu* what is significant is the way in which the consumption of one's own urine has a kind of mutating effect whereby the *jātharāgni,* which is normally responsible for a kind of cooking that is nonmetabolic, becomes a kind of cooking that is more inherently "chemical" in nature, like the cooking done by each of the fires associated with *bhūta* conversion and *dhātu* transformation. Although urine is not food, and therefore does not break down into *rasa,* like all organic matter it is constituted of the five elements. Significantly, the process of metabolic digestion as a whole, including *jātharāgni, bhūtāgni,* and *dhātvagni,* is understood as a process that breaks material down, first into tastes, and then into the five primary elemental units. These five elements are then absorbed into the corresponding elements of the physical body. Thus in some sense, digestion is a process that produces organic correspondence, and as this correspondence is rendered more and more direct and efficient, the overall health of the organism—measured in terms of the balanced flow of *doṣic* humors—increases until you have a perfect correspondence between the structure of nourished and nourishment; digestion and digested. What you get is a situation in which the body is not so much nourished as alchemically transformed, and where the body itself may be understood as a kind of particulate by-product of well-cooked—in the sense of being remetabolized—urine.

Although it is admittedly only a logical conjecture, it would seem that one's own urine, as it changes the nature of the *jātharāgni*—the first effect of which is extremely violent—subsequently moves through a circuit of ingestion and elimination and is progressively refined and rendered more and more subtle as are each of the *dhātu*, until finally one is drinking a nectar that is as pure and powerful as semen. Digestion, rather than simplistic symbolic homology, is what transforms urine into an *ojas* like elixir.[19]

Along these lines it is interesting to note that in the *Śivambu Kalpa* as well as in Suśruta's description of *rasāyana* rebirth, considerable attention is given to the way in which therapy has a profound effect not only on the body as a whole but on the skin, fingernails, teeth, and hair in particular. These are all parts of the body that can or need to be removed and are, therefore, in some sense by-products. Applying the useful ambiguity of the term *mala*, one might well think of skin, fingernails, teeth, and hair as embodied waste products produced as the body outgrows itself.[20] But when the body undergoes a chemical transformation these apparently "dirty," impure by-products are refined and become permanent physical features as the process of growth and physical change becomes self-contained self-consumption. *śivambu* and *rasāyana* are completely different insofar as what substance is ingested, but they are the same in changing the way in which the body cooks itself. Growth, and aging as the long-term effect of growth, is a symptom of imperfect health. Perfect health is achieved when the body no longer grows or changes in a physical sense, but only meta-metabolizes by remixing its own self-contained constituent elements—and this can go on for eternity.

Beyond Āyurveda

Admittedly, Āyurvedic theory only allows one to take this argument to a certain point. Moreover, most of the literature on auto-urine therapy is rather vague on the details of metabolism and physiology, with one notable exception. In his book *Vijñānic Svāmūtra Cikitsā,* Dr. Hiralal develops a novel argument concerning the nature of urine in relation to the body's elimination of waste. Using the analogy of juice from crushed sugarcane and oil from pressed nuts, he says that urine is to feces as the juice of cane is to the dried, discarded—but still compostable—stalk (1988: 82–83).[21] If one follows this argument it provides a possible missing link in the logic of refinement. As one drinks and then redrinks one's own urine, its refinement is predicated on the progressive elimination of some quantity of waste. This takes the form of feces. Except in the case of some extreme forms of Aghorī practice, fecal material is never consumed.[22] In Hiralal's logic it would also not make sense to consume it, since it would simply pass in and out of the body in the same form, effecting no transformation in the process, as does happen in the case of urine.

In a different context Hiralal engages in logical speculation about the relationship between urine and mother's milk, both of which can be considered refined, filtered by-products of blood.[23] Interestingly, he supports this claim by comparing the nutritional and chemical content of each as measured in terms of biomedical criteria (1988: 81). But he concludes by citing an Āyurvedic principle that a person should only consume medicines that are the product of the land in which he or she was born. Giving this—which is the same kind of broad metaphorical interpretation that Armstrong gave to the key biblical passage, "drink water from your own cistern"—he points out that most intimately the "land" in which one is born is one's own body.[24] Thus milklike urine is the best and most appropriate medicine (1988: 82).

Although Hiralal's theories are unorthodox—but, then again, that is the domain we are in—one can appreciate the extent to which a philosophically driven medical system such as Āyurveda might postulate a purely theoretical basis for auto-urine therapy. At the same time, however, Āyurveda is characterized by a high degree of empirical pragmatism, and an epistemology grounded in curing disease and maintaining the best possible health in a world of chronic pain and suffering. The theoretical seductiveness of *śivambu* therapy, as it is presented in the *Ḍāmara Tantra,* becomes clearer when looking at it in the more general terms of Sāṃkhya philosophy.

Above all else, to drink one's own urine is to consume a part of oneself. It is, therefore, an essentially self-oriented act of self-containment and self-sufficiency. In the Sāṃkhya tradition that most directly influenced Āyurveda and Yoga, the self is not pure consciousness separate from nature. Rather, the self is directly linked to the *tattva* categories, *prakṛti,* and the *vikāra*s that together constitute the person as a fluid whole. As Rao points out: "The self somehow gets related in a characteristic manner to the elements mentioned above and renders them organized, integrated, enlivened, and patterned. And consciousness emerges *sui generis* from this organization which is described as the phenomenal self or the heap-person [*rāśi puruṣa*]" (1987: 8–9). What is significant about this notion of the relationship between self and consciousness is that it is fundamentally materialistic and sense driven; "it is a quality that emerges as incidental to the involvement of Self in the phenomenal mass" (1987: 9). Locating consciousness in the field of direct human experience made it possible for Sāṃkhya philosophers to think in terms of the development and growth of consciousness. As is well known, however, this development and growth were understood to be a progressive devolution into more impacted states of ignorance and error produced by the illusory sense of static continuity projected onto the conglomeration of categories that constitute the person as a shifting heap. Growth and development on both a universal, cosmic level and on an individual level happen as a consequence of a disruption of unmanifest equipoise in the primal *guṇa* constituents. That is, reality and the perception of reality are both predicated on the creative force and latent energy manifest in the endless struggle for ascendancy between the destabilized *guṇa*.

Although self-expression most often takes the form of engrossed phenomenal involvement, what is significant here is that Sāṃkhya philosophy allowed for the theoretical possibility of a materialist search for self-expression that would work against the grain of *pariṇāma* evolution. This was effected by means of isolation and discrimination through the involuted "dissociation of the Self from phenomena" (1987: 10). Rao captures the dynamic contrast between pain-provoking evolved self-expression and the search for primordial preconsciousness when he writes that

> evolution is an onward process of progressive differentiation and proliferation, greater and more complex structuring, multiplication of coordinates and dimensions, and projection of more planes of experience. It is a spreading out and hence called *prapañca*. The method that the Sāṃkhya indicated (and the Yoga developed) is an involution, a backward process of gradual attenuation, closing in and concentrating the consciousness into an undifferentiated mass (*samādhi*). (1987: 14)

Elaborating on this, he points out that "the systematic and progressive undoing of the evolutionary process (that is to say, the senses, mind and egoity) so as to regress into the original state of 'mere-I-ness' (*asmitāmātra*), undifferentiated, unconditioned, unqualified and non-particular, is the method employed" (1987: 14). Although Yoga has developed as the primary means by which to effect this method through the manipulation of the body/mind complex, it would seem that *śivambu* puts abstract Sāṃkhya theory into applied practice. In some sense the all-powerful immortal body described in the *Śivambu Kalpa* is the incarnate form of *asmitāmātra*—self-unto-itself. The idea that urine can cure any disease and bestow immortality is linked to the idea that perfection is a state of absolute timeless constituent balance.

The Practice of Auto-Urine Therapy in India

There is no question but that auto-urine therapy as it is practiced by people at large in India today—with the exception, perhaps, of self-proclaimed yogic practitioners of a pure *amarolī* tradition—is based on the writings of J. W. Armstrong and men like Raojibhai Patel who translated Armstrong's treatise into terms that made sense to a middle-class Indian audience. Whereas one can make sense of *śivambu* using Āyurvedic theory, it is difficult to find more than a cursory theoretical justification for auto-urine therapy in Armstrong's own writing. He relied, almost exclusively, on the authority of scriptural references, folk practice, contradictory statements made by physicians, and, most directly, on personal experience. Using anecdotes like the following—some of which are, I think, clearly tongue in cheek and intended to be titillating—he tried to prove *that* auto-urine therapy worked, not *how* it worked.

> *En passant,* I may mention that not so long ago one of the most exclusive and expensive toilet soaps was made from the dehydrated salts and fats of the urine of grass-fed cows, and another from the urine of Russian peasants (My informant was a chemist who knew what he was talking about). (1971: 18)

Despite the anecdotal and largely case-by-case logic reflected in Armstrong's book, there are hints about a possible theoretical basis for the practice he devised.

As Armstrong points out, auto-urine therapy is linked to the key principle of Nature Cure, which holds, simply, that any ailment can be cured by the natural elements—earth, air, sunlight, and water. Significantly, however, Armstrong points out that urine is more natural than these elements, since its source is the body itself and not the environment at large. Following from this, he breaks from the inherent logic of Nature Cure by pointing out that "naturopathy, as it is usually practiced does not go far enough, for although it can cleanse the body of its toxins, it cannot replace wasted tissues incidental to such grievous ills as consumption or other diseases of equal gravity" (1971: 11). Unlike most Nature Cure doctors, Armstrong was primarily concerned with the development of a natural therapy that would not just fight against disease but develop the body's natural strength and vitality and restore vigor and health. That is, he was interested in the idea of tonics and dietary supplementation, not simply purgative restoration and balance. As he pointed out, urine is not a product that should be wasted through excretion; like leaves into the soil, grass cuttings into gardens, and manure into fields, it should be plowed back in to promote growth out of the chemicals produced through decay and decomposition (1971: 19–20). Thus he derived his basic theory from a model of natural recycling, and suggested that if the body is natural it should conform to this law of nature as well. Significantly, however, Armstrong went one step further in trying to explain the process.

> Urine, on being taken into the body, is filtered; it becomes purer and purer even in the course of one day's living upon it, plus tap water, if required. First it cleanses, then frees from obstruction and finally rebuilds the vital organs and passages after they have been wasted by the ravages of disease. In fact it rebuilds not only the lungs, pancreas, liver, brain, heart etc., but also repairs the linings of brain and bowel and other linings, as has been demonstrated in the case of many "killing" diseases, such as consumption of the intestines and the worst form of colitis. (1971: 26)

Armstrong does not explain this process in any greater detail, but it is noteworthy that the case histories he gives invariably refer to patients gaining weight, wounds healing with remarkable speed and very little scarring, and people, in the end, looking much younger than they really are. Because the following case study compares so well with the description given by *Suśruta* on the one hand and Śiva speaking to Pārvatī in the *Ḍāmara Tantra* on the other, it is quoted in its entirety.

> The first case of gangrene I ever treated was in 1920. The patient was a lady of fifty-three. She had been in the care of a well-known Bradford physician who was an authority on fasting and dietetics. Anaemia had developed, the lungs showed signs of grave disturbance, and there was a gangrenous condition in one foot, with a number of skin eruptions of varying dimensions on each leg. There was also a jaundiced condition which had turned her complexion to that of an Eurasian, and the whites of her eyes were yellow. Her abdomen was distended and hard, and her body had become thin and scraggy, almost to emaciation.
>
> Although the doctor was quite willing that my method should be tried for at least a month, I was loathe [*sic*] to advise upon the case, for I felt that no period of less than sixty or seventy days would restore the patient to health. . . .
>
> By dint of fasting the patient on her own urine and water, and rubbing urine into her body and applying urine compresses, at the end of ten days the kidneys and bowels were working "overtime," and though the eruptions had increased, they were less irritable. The breathing became normal and easy, the patient slept better, and above all, the gangrenous foot began to show signs of healing.
>
> By the eighteenth day of the fast the foot was quite normal; the urine had formed new skin, and there was no trace whatever of the livid abrasions. The foot had healed without even leaving a scar.

> Yet need we be surprised, once we understand that urine is not dead matter, but so to say, flesh, blood and vital tissues in living solution? (1971: 32–33)

However intriguing in and of itself—and however clearly it may resonate with the *Ḍāmara Tantra*—Armstrong's technique did not simply get put into practice in India. It was subtly, but very significantly, modified by Patel and others. It is to their books to which we must turn.

Patel, Karlekar, and others in India who have followed on and developed their work are, unlike Armstrong, very concerned—or at least worried—about the question of whether or not auto-urine therapy is scientific. That is, they are concerned with the question of why and how auto-urine therapy works. For his part Armstrong conflated medicine with science, and was indiscriminately and categorically critical of both: "But though the autocracy of the clergy in now more or less a thing of the past, unless we are very firm in asserting our democratic rights, we may be faced with an even worse form of autocracy, and that is the autocracy of what goes under the name of Science. And I say advisedly 'goes under the name,' because whilst true Science endeavors to understand the Laws of Nature, false science tries to improve upon Nature" (1971: 134). In Armstrong's opinion the authority of nature is greater than the authority of science, and for him, in effect, the proof was simply in the pudding, even though "good" science could provide some insight into how and of what the pudding was made. A number of contemporary books on the subject published in the United States, Australia, and Germany—where there is some renewed interest if not a revival per se—contain sections giving extensive scientific "proof" for auto-urine therapy based on chemical analyses (Bartnett 1998; Beatrix 1996; Christy 1994: 17–32; Kroon 1996; Lara 1999; O'Quinn 1980; Peschek-Böhmer 1999).

Patel's view is significantly different from these because he subscribes to a position in which nature—and the laws of nature in particular—is the basis for understanding, not the object of disinterested investigation. Thus for him the critical distinction drawn by Armstrong between understanding and improving is moot in light of the fact that nature itself *is* a science. One does not understand nature; one understands and acts in terms of natural laws. In order to abide by the laws of nature, one's intellect must harmonize with those laws. Objective science is, according to Patel, the antithesis of harmony. In fact, he is very clear in stating that in "revealing her secrets" and discovering "new potentialities" science works against nature (1991: 7).

What comes across in Patel's work is not a straightforward critique of medical science based on the laws of nature. Unlike Armstrong he develops an alternative science wherein auto-urine therapy is both the means and the ends of study—the object, subject, and theoretical basis of investigation. At first glance this gross tautology seems illogical, and Patel says as much when he points out that "one who claims that a subject in itself is scientific may not know what science is" (1991: 19). However, he goes on to say that in his experiments on himself, and then on others, auto-urine therapy revealed a truth about health, nature, and the nature of the body that is pure, undistorted and universal.

Just as there is "useful" ambiguity in the meaning of the term *mala*, there is also an intrinsic ambiguity in the way in which various sanskritic terms get translated as knowledge or science. As explained in chapter 2, this ambiguity is most clearly reflected in the way in which the term *Yoga vijñāna* is used to mean both the scientific study of Yoga and Yoga as a science unto itself. The same principle applies to Patel's notion that auto-urine therapy produces an experience or realization of truth, not just knowledge about truth as such. With reference to *vidyā* one knows in terms of that which is known, and what Patel seems to be critical of is the discriminating nature of *vijñāna* science. What he is advocating is a kind *adhyātmic vijñānic vidyā* wherein urine is both *sādhya* (object) and *sādhana* (means). To be sure, Patel is not entirely consistent, for he does call forth as evidence an introductory biochemistry textbook written by Fehren. Citing it he points out that to understand the laws of nature, "we should know the ingredients of urine as found out by scientific methods" (1991: 24). However, Patel is fairly consistent, and also quite clear, about how it is that nature manifests truth and how, through auto-urine therapy, one can go beyond knowledge and embody that truth.

Patel's argument hinges on the logic that God is perfect and that that which he has created must also be perfect, even though it is understood as "harsh, ferocious and meaningless" by imperfect human beings who have become alienated from nature.[25] Alienation from nature produces ignorance, and ignorance makes it impossible to live in harmony with nature. The only way to overcome this is to re-cognize—in the full, transformative sense of the term—one's intimate affinity with every single part of nature regardless of the extent to which it is "imperfectly" ascribed cultural value as good or bad, fragrant or stinky, essence or excrement. As Patel puts it, when "the Creator of the Universe is perfect, every part of the universe must also be perfect . . . nature creates every organism complete and self-sufficient."

By this logic, it is not so much that the universe is in a grain of sand as that the perfection of the universe—if not God himself—is in every drop of urine, and that by drinking one's own urine one can overcome ignorance and experience truth-as-health. This experience is ultimately beyond the range of objective, scientific investigation reflected in the milligrammic tabulation of urea, creatinine, ammonia, sodium, potassium, magnesium, and other ingredients. But for good measure, in his chapter dealing with the analysis of urine, Patel reproduces such a tabulation from Fehren's *Introduction to Biochemistry* (1991: 24).

In this sense, Patel's perspective is more radical than Armstrong's, since it problematizes science as a way of knowing. Significantly, however, Patel's alternative science of auto-urine therapy draws together strands of meaning that derive from both Āyurvedic theory and the principles of Nature Cure. With great rhetorical flourish, and a degree of bombastic self-confidence, Armstrong sets auto-urine therapy above Nature Cure—and then has very little to say about the natural elements—whereas Patel is careful to work out the way in which his Indian practice is more directly linked to the nineteenth-century Continental tradition, and through that tradition back to principles that are in harmony with—if not exactly the same as—some of the basic tenets of Āyurveda.

As pointed out above, however, these links to Āyurveda are not made explicit and, it could be argued, are not even implied. Patel, expressing Gandhi's own view, is as vehemently critical of *vaidyas* as he is of physicians, both of whom have been "blinded" by medical science and have "lost the courage to challenge" that science (1991: 20). Regardless, it is possible to see how auto-urine therapy emerges as a complex and not entirely consistent variation on a theme defined by the harmonic tone produced by the convergence of *prakṛtic* and natural elements. It is interesting that this harmony is made possible by the dislocation of both Āyurveda and Nature Cure from any specific cultural affiliation to either India or Europe. It is remarkable to read, in the relatively inexpensive books and pamphlets written on the subject in various regional languages (Acharya 1978a, b; Agarwal 1992; Gotham 1988; Hiralal 1988; Jagati 1991, Mishra 1998; Mithal 1979; Patil 1996; Sharma 1998; Shobhan 1992), how easily the authors slip back and forth between statements about the *pitta* content of the first urine expelled, for example, and claims—based on science done in San Francisco—about a nitroglycerin-like dilating agent discovered in human urine. Many of these authors make reference to an article in the medical journal of the Integrated Medical Association of Mysore claiming that Dr. T. N. Shivanandiyan had some success curing patients of asthma by giving them urine injections. But it is extraordinary and not just remarkable to read this kind of open-ended amalgamation of data, not because things seem out of place, or mixed up, but rather because of the way in which the authors "bring it all back home," so to speak, and define the practice of auto-urine therapy in India in global, transnational terms. In doing so urine becomes a medicine linked to the body and nature and not to the heritage of India at large, or even to the embodied land of one's birth as is the case in Hiralal's interpretation of Āyurvedic texts (1988: 82). Written about in

Gujarati, Hindi, Marathi, and Urdu, auto-urine therapy does not belong to any cultural tradition. It is therefore reductionist in a totalizing way that allows for a truly holistic integration of elements from all over the world.

Patel's understanding of nature is directly and intimately linked to the body, as the body is a microcosm of the universe. In outlining what he regards as the fundamental principle of auto-urine therapy, he writes:

> The universe is composed of five elements: vis. the earth, water, fire, air and sky. Human body is also composed of the same five elements. Every organism is constituted of all the five elements in appropriate proportions. A person falls ill when the balance of elements is disturbed through his or her own faults. In order to restore health, the balance must be restored. This function can be performed easily by auto-urine only. The proper maintenance of human organism rests on urine just as the earth's balance rests on the ocean. (1991: 18)

Beyond the standard microcosm/macrocosm scenario, the idea that urine is to the body as the ocean is to the earth is a key principle in Patel's thinking, and it is based on the same kind of "recycling" model invoked by Armstrong. Significantly, Patel employs a more explicitly fluid, hydrological logic. Instead of leaves "rotting" and being plowed into the soil, the hydrological model of recycling is based on purification through stages of evaporation, condensation, and flow. It is not simply that life on earth would not exist without the ocean, but that the ocean structures life and maintains order. On a related note Patel makes the argument that water is the most important and most powerful of all five elements, since it can absorb each of the others (see also Hiralal 1988: 162–63; Mishra 1998: 98). Water is also the source of all life, both in the world at large and in the body. Urine, in this scheme, is like water, but, as Patel puts it, it is "far more than mere water and so it acts as the healer of the organism" (1991: 21). One's own urine "is a living solution and contains the substances which build, nourish and enliven the flesh, blood and tissues of the body" (1991: 22). Although Armstrong makes similar general statements, Patel's specific logic—as quite distinct from Armstrong's—is based on the idea of integrated balance and the transformation of elements one into another. In turn this is based on the principle that anatomy and physiology have the same ontological structure as nature. On one level, then, urine, as it is consumed, refined, and consumed again in an endless cycle, becomes an ever more perfect solution—in both senses of the term—to the problem of inherent imbalance. If the human organism is a microcosm of the universe, then urine is a microcosm of the human organism insofar as it "has the power to contain all the elements of the body . . . and restore . . . lost health to the body" (1991: iii).

On another level—and recalling the early stages of *rasāyana* therapy—urine functions as an extreme purgative: "[It] washes out accumulated waste matter, layers of harmful toxins, the injurious substances sticking in the intestines, mucus deposited in the chest, lungs and stomach and other foreign deposits. They come out by way of vomiting, or by loose motions. There is nothing to be alarmed at these reactions. One should think that the poisons deposited in the body are thus coming out and the body is becoming more and more clean" (1991: 35).[26] Overall there is a kind of congruent function involving the dual cycles of purification through fluid flow and balance through stages of progressive refinement. Although not as extreme as the descriptions contained in the *Śivambu Kalpa* and the *Suśrutasaṁhitā*, Patel's statement echoes the logic of purgative purification that is central to these texts. Here again the model of the ocean is significant. Rivers, born of the pure distilled essence of evaporated moisture, pick up and clean out the effluvium of life and wash it out into the ocean, where it is absorbed and purified. *Peśāb*—a colloquial term for urine—employs a verb-tense prefix, *peś*, such that the most appropriate gloss for the term, "piss," does not capture the honorific sense of the Hindi word, which can be said to mean "gift of flowing water." In any case, *peśāb*, as a riverlike stream that flows out of the heap person, is cognate with Punjab—the land of the five rivers that flow down from the Himalayas, to the east and west of Gujarat.

Patel is explicit in pointing out that it was Armstrong's work that inspired him to experiment with auto-urine therapy. The only change he instituted was to selectively drink the "middle stream." He did not consume every last drop, and—speaking of disgust—he did not do as Armstrong did and break his urine fasts by eating raw beef. Although he was aware of the *Śivambu Kalpa*, in his view it was arcane and contaminated with too much "mythological excess" to be of any direct practical value. Moreover, it did not advocate fasting, as did Armstrong and more mainstream practitioners of Nature Cure (Karlekar 1972: 134–36). Thus it seemed to undermine, with the consumption of food—no matter how pure and wholesome—its own logic of self-contained perfection.

Given the profound influence that Patel's work has had on other practitioners of auto-urine therapy in India, it is safe to say that although there may be some who prescribe the kinds of decoctions described in the *Ḍāmara Tantra*, the vast majority of people who practice auto-urine therapy in India do so in terms of its being a so-called rational science unto itself—the penultimate form of nature and expression of nature's law—rather than a branch of Āyurveda. And yet, I think, Patel and his followers have read Āyurvedic and Sāṃkhyan principles into Armstrong's therapy and thereby have engaged in a process of complicated, not always conscious, triangular translation that revolves around the ontology of rebirth, immortality, and transcendence. Karlekar, a contemporary of Patel's, quotes the sage Dnaneshwari when trying to explain the apparently "exaggerated and ridiculous" claims of the *Kalpa*. Dnaneshwari points out that the body becomes ethereal and transcendent as its elements are progressively absorbed one into another. In the end, when air becomes ether, "the body's existence ends . . . what remains behind is atmosphere—the oneness, neither felt nor experienced!" (n.d.: 135). In some ways Patel, Karlekar, and others writing about and practicing auto-urine therapy effect an elemental reconvergence of Āyurveda and Yoga.

Although "exaggerated" and "mythological," the *Śivambu Kalpa* provides the basic logic for understanding how the body produces its own fountain of youth. For his part, Armstrong almost finds the fountain of youth while looking for a cure for common ailments. However, his understanding of the body and nature is not fluid enough to allow for the possibility of perfect health in eternal transformation. Nevertheless he put into common, simple, rational practice what is otherwise uncommon, arcane, and secret. This effectively opened up space—both theoretical and practical—into which the abstract, depersonalized, but very clearly embodied principles of *rasāyana* and *śivambu* could be applied. But these principles could not be put into general practice simply as they were, for they represented the logical extreme and fantastically supranatural manifestation of Āyurveda's more consistent—and consistently restrained—concern with fluid flow, balance, and metabolic transformation. To be sure, the principles of *śivambu* did not need to be watered down in order to be applied. You can, if you so desire, follow Lord Śiva's instructions word for word.

The point is that the underlying theoretical logic of *śivambu* is much more down to earth and empirically grounded than one would assume given the effects the therapy is reputed to have, and Patel, Karlekar, Hiralal, and others have given well-reasoned voice to this logic. They were, in a sense, able to translate Armstrong's and Lord Śiva's equally grand claims not just into Gujarati, Hindi, and Marathi but into a modern language expressing an alternative science of the embodied soul. What they have written speaks to the needs of a significant number of middle-class Indian men and women in search of alternative senses of self, self-fulfillment, and self-control in the alienating, evolved, inherently unhealthy, and intrinsically painful world in which modern India is implicated.

One might say that in misunderstanding the nature of nature as intrinsic to the self, rather than as an extrinsic ecological force—and in seeking a kind of health that is not just good, but gets better and better—Patel came to a refined, consistent, and holistic understanding of the connection between urine, nature, and the body. This understanding brought to light a possible history that could have been categorically Indian—its point of origin being in the mistaken metaphorical entailment of the land-of-one's-birth and body. But this history did not occur. Or perhaps every time it did occur it ended, as the *Kalpa* does, in the end of time. Perhaps this history keeps repeating itself, like *kayākalpa, rasāyana,* or the tail-biting snake, thereby rendering itself meaningless. For his part, Armstrong misread the Bible—for it is impossible to see any metaphorical link between cisterns and bladders in the word of the Almighty God—but clearly he found that drinking his own urine cured him of various ailments. In any event his misunderstanding led to a better understanding of the way in which culture can make unnatural things natural and also a better understanding of the inherent contingency of accepted truths. He also showed how pure nature—that putative ideal that he found within himself and, in another place and time, that Sāṃkhya philosophers located in the primordial heap person—can make it difficult to swallow the truth that culture produces as it transforms nature in various ways.

Since it is ambiguity and misunderstanding—albeit ingenious misunderstanding—which characterizes the history and logic of the middle stream, it is good to end with a statement made by Armstrong:

> Those who read the widely known book *Mother India* may remember some passages therein devoted to the "filthy habits" of the native peoples. Among the health "superstitions" its authoress pointed out, was the belief that the waters of one part of a famous river in North Middle India possesses healing properties. People bathed in and drank its waters. Wondering whether there could be something more than faith in cures effected, she had samples of the water analyzed by European analysts. The healing liquid proved to be nothing more than a weak solution of urine and *aqua pura!* (1971: 125)

While an obliquely ethnocentric and evasively racist statement such as this might well piss people off, who really does have the last laugh? Oh Pārvatī! Is it not the greatest yogi of them all? Is it not the mercurial Lord Śiva—ash-covered, snake-bedecked, blue-throated drinker of the churned ocean's poison—from whose head this "middle" stream, this *Śivambu,* originates?

7

MIMETIC SKEPTICISM AND YOGA: MOVING BEYOND THE PROBLEM OF CULTURE AND RELATIVISM

> The falseness of a judgment is for us not necessarily an objection to a judgment; in this respect our new language may sound strangest. The question is to what extent it is life-promoting, life preserving, species-preserving, perhaps even species cultivating. And we are fundamentally inclined to claim that the falsest judgments (which include the synthetic judgments *a priori*) are the most indispensable for us; that without accepting the fictions of logic, without measuring reality against the purely invented world of the unconditional and the self-identical, without a constant falsification of the world by means of numbers, man could not live—that renouncing false judgments would mean renouncing life and a denial of life. To recognize untruth as a condition of life—that certainly means resisting accustomed value feelings in a dangerous way; and a philosophy that risks this would by that token alone place itself beyond good and evil.
>
> Nietzsche, *Beyond Good and Evil*, trans. Walter Kaufmann (1968: 202)

> The last achievement of all thought is a recognition of the identity of spirit and matter, subject and object; and this reunion is the marriage of Heaven and Hell, the reaching out of a contracted universe towards its freedom, in response to the love of Eternity for the productions of time. There is then no sacred or profane, spiritual or sensual, but everything that lives is pure and void. This very world of birth and death is also a great Abyss.
>
> Ananda K. Coomaraswamy, *The Dance of Śiva* (1956: 140)

Yoga and Relativism: Beyond the Value of Context

BY NO STRETCH of the imagination can Yoga be considered dangerous. If its practice does not in fact bring about enlightenment or relief from stress and ill health, it most certainly does not threaten the well-being of those who practice it. As a cultural system Yoga does not present a threat to the integrity of any other cultural system. One can even say that it places the highest value on life, insofar as life itself is a necessary condition for human enlightenment. Nevertheless, some kinds of yogic practice and some aspects of yogic philosophy—both ancient and modern—must seem to nonpractitioners so strange as to defy comprehension. It is the profound "strangeness" of Yoga—as well as its magical quality—that makes it directly relevant to a consideration of cultural relativism and questions about cultural relativism in anthropological theory. For a concept of the bizarre presents almost as many problems for relativism as does evil itself, and can, therefore, serve as a point of theoretical entry.

For example, consider the following with reference to any one of a number of events, ancient or modern, that seem to incarnate evil: in the context of a discussion of *maithuna*—mystical eroticism in which the bliss or orgasm is cognate with transcendence, and where semen is "immobilized" rather than spent—Eliade, referencing a philosophical point made by Kṛṣṇa to Arjun in the *Bhagavad Gītā* that has become paradigmatic on many levels, points out that

> the tantric texts frequently repeat the saying, "By the same acts that cause some men to burn in hell for thousands of years, the yogin gains his eternal salvation." . . . This, as we know, is the foundation stone of the Yoga expounded by Kṛṣṇa in the Bhagavad Gītā (XVIII, 17): "He who has no feeling of egoism, and whose mind is not tainted, even though he kills (all) these people, kills not, is not fettered (by the action)." And the *Bṛhadāraṇyaka Upaniṣad* (V, 14, 8) had already said: "One who knows this, although he commits very much evil, consumes it all and becomes clean and pure, ageless and immortal." (1990: 263)

By recalling some of the radical examples of Yoga in practice, the problem can be put this way: you can understand everything from Dr. Udupa's experiment on rats doing *śirṣāsana* on the one hand to *maithuna* on the other from the perspective of an insider—although, to be sure, it would be impossible to know what the rats inside the test tubes thought they were doing. You can understand, from an insider's perspective, the discourse of Himalayan sages as well as the idea put forward by Patañjali that our perception of reality is an illusion—that killing is not killing and that sex is not sex. Although, again, it is impossible to know what the sages really know. In other words, you can understand what Kṛṣṇa said about war to Arjun by contextualizing it to a point at which killing comes to make sense, even though the context in this case is that everything is ignorance and illusion. But what, if anything, does a cultural perspective on Yoga provide beyond a relativist understanding of human ingenuity and creativity? What is it worth beyond being a contextualized understanding of a different kind of philosophy?

In this concluding chapter my purpose is to develop what might be called a yogic theory of mimetic skepticism in order to reflect further both on Yoga as a modern phenomenon, and on the way in which an analysis and understanding of Yoga's physical philosophy can provide insight on anthropological theories of culture. My argument is that doubt about the meaningfulness of Yoga as the embodiment of Universal Truth can be extended—through a consideration of the logic of relativism—into analytical skepticism about the claim, both anthropological and popular, that cultural reality itself is the defining basis of human experience. Yoga's key perspective on the contingency of perceived reality, and on the way in which cognition is linked to misperception, can, I think, be translated out of a context within which cosmology and philosophy hold sway, and into the domain of social history.

I take Yoga to be the product of human intelligence, not a condition of enlightened being. Therefore, the idea of transcending the self and achieving immortality and freedom is a cultural idea located in the time of human experience and in the spacial matrix of the material world. It is not a universal truth. Yoga reflects a fetishistic desire for the experience of something beyond human experience. As such it must be subject to the same sociological and philosophical critique as religion. It is often easy to lose sight of this since Yoga is rooted in the natural world of experience and practice, rather than in the domain of the purely supernatural. But it is precisely on account of this—this easy-to-lose-sight-of materialist metaphysics—that Yoga provides the logic for a more profound and encompassing critique of culture and society than does the social facticity of religion as spirituality qua spirituality. It is this logic I wish to pursue.[1]

This book has so far engaged directly with the theory and practice of modern Yoga. In this final chapter I will continue along these lines, but more obliquely and more by way of anecdotes than in previous chapters. More important, the argument developed here is informed by certain aspects of Yoga philosophy, as this philosophy enables an engagement with contemporary social theory. To a degree, but only to a degree and not completely, the perspective taken here is reversed from that taken in the previous chapters so as to reflect Yoga on questions of anthropological significance and to take anthropology as a "cultural" subject. Therefore the focus on cultural relativism may seem to direct attention away from Yoga as such, but in an important sense mimetic skepticism is a kind of yogic social theory. I ask my reader to allow for a degree of strategic blurring between theory, philosophy, and "ethnographic" subject matter. Relative to my own discipline—humanistic social science, if not hard science or pure philosophy as such—I am putting myself in the shoes of Kuvalayananda, Udupa, Karandikar, Pal, and, of course, Patel.

Textbook Terminology—Understanding Difference

In an environment where education, like Yoga, is increasingly commodified, and knowledge often perversely reified and fetishized, there are reasons to be nervous about using undergraduate textbook definitions of key terms as a point of departure for a critical reevaluation of analytical methods in a discipline. However, to start with these definitions—as it has been necessary to start with simplified definitions of yogic concepts found in "popular" books—is to recognize the extent to which certain terms have become iconic, and therefore have come to stand for more than their specific analytical usefulness. They have come to mean more than what they directly signify. In anthropology the significance and meaning of cultural relativism extends well beyond what that term denotes.[2] But what the term denotes is captured in a number of standard textbooks. For example, calling it a "fundamental research tool of anthropology," Serena Nanda and Richard Warms define cultural relativism as "the notion that a people's values and customs must be understood in terms of the culture of which they are a part" (1998: 10).[3]

The logical problem with cultural relativism is well known. Sooner or later one is confronted with a problem of where to draw the line between the meaningfulness and legitimacy of cultural differences—cannibalism, foot binding, and female circumcision, for example—and some universal standard of human rights. This is directly related to the only slightly less problematic question of whether or not all forms of cultural expression are equally meaningful and legitimate. If it is appropriate to pray for world peace, is it or is it not appropriate for anyone to do anything else that will bring about the same end? People with absolute faith in a specific god will say it is not—or perhaps only ignore the fact of difference—whereas others will say yes to almost anything, including yogic flying and the Maharishi Effect, as alluded to in the introduction. And then there is the question of whether or not those who take a relativistic stand on the Maharishi Effect simply are being tolerant and analytically curious, or believe, in fact, that yogic flying can effect world peace. At some point relativism is confronted with narrowly configured cultural beliefs—a willingness, or lack thereof, to step beyond the suspension of doubt and embody difference.

Although the debate between advocates of cultural relativism and advocates of human universalism has tended toward dogmatic, ideological positionality, many anthropologists and cross-cultural sociologists have taken a compromise position, holding that methodological relativism and the analytical understanding of difference do not entail an abdication of one's human responsibility to discriminate between what is right or wrong, just or unjust, moral or immoral (Herzfeld 1997; Salmon 1997, 1999; B. S. Turner 1993; T. Turner 1997). Thus one can understand, and even develop a degree of analytical empathy for, the practice of genocide, while still condemning it as immoral and inhuman. In fact it could—and should, I think—be argued that the strength of one's moral and human conviction is directly proportional to one's ability to develop a degree of empathy, or what Schultz and Lavenda call "sympathy" (2001: 25), for "the native's point of view."[4] To be able to condemn slavery, the Holocaust, or foot binding—or even to point out the fallacy of both the Maharishi Effect and prayer—one must first be able to understand the cultural context of these practices from the inside out, regardless of how the inside is defined.[5] Historically, at least, this has been part of the justification for anthropology.

A key term in this debate seems to be "understanding." Both judgment and meaningful analysis are based on the principle of making sense. Understanding goes to the question of what culture is, and the relative positionality of one's perspective on being human. For this reason the proposition put forward here is that cultural relativism is analytically, politically, and morally problematic not because of arguments made by universalists in the name of some standard of human kindness, but because the principle of positionality is inherently untenable. Relativism depends on the perspectivity of positionality. This raises and redirects many questions, perhaps the most basic one being not only how to understand difference, but how to understand difference in light of our common humanity.

The argument here is that to understand difference in nonrelativist terms one must extend the radical logic of relativism beyond culture and approach the question of human rights—and what counts as being human, which is a key aspect of the ontological question in Yoga—from a perspective that may be called mimetic skepticism.[6] Using Yoga as a frame of reference, mimetic skepticism is intended to question the basic assumptions of the debate on cultural relativism and thereby provide a perspective on the problem of being human—a problem of "being" that is prior to, but also central to, the question of human rights. I realize, of course, that many whose primary focus is on serious human rights issues will regard this as facile intellectualism and rhetorical sophistry. They will ask, pointedly, are not intellectual questions of a philosophical nature mooted by the immediate need to stop genocide, terrorism, and violence of all kinds? To a degree, yes. But I think that anthropology, if it is to be worth anything, must first be intellectually informed.[7] It must address itself to the level of the question that concerned Arjun. It must interrogate the logic and cognitive politics of mootation, whether cosmic or more mundane.

In most textbook definitions of relativism there is a tacit assumption that culture, no matter how open ended and subject to interpretation, is a thing to be experienced as bounded on some level.[8] Otherwise the question of relativism—this in relation to that—would not make sense. The concept of culture evokes a sense of possessive belonging and situated being. It presumes dialectical difference as a fact of life, albeit one that may not easily be located as such. Most definitions also presume that knowledge is local and produced by the subjectivity of a specific cultural experience. The relativity of relativism is inherently perspectival and based on a phenomenological subject position.

Developments in anthropological theory since the publication of Geertz's *The Interpretation of Cultures* (1973) have made it clear that culture is not a thing and that cultural perspectivity is not fixed. In light of these developments the idea of cultural relativism is something of an anachronism. And yet, as every textbook points out, the idea is central to anthropological analysis. This may well indicate that there is something fundamentally wrong with the intellectual coherence of the discipline as a whole—that there is logical inconsistency in the relationship among methodology, analysis, and theory. Unless one reverts back to Lévi-Strauss's, Leach's, or Linton's conception of culture, it is no longer possible to say that what any given person says is an articulation of some predefined, or even definable, cultural whole. Culture is constructed. But rather than see this as an opportunity to discard an anachronistic concept, perhaps an analytical recognition of the constructedness of culture makes the problem of perspectival relativity much more interesting, engaging, and challenging. And perhaps an engagement with the challenge can provide a somewhat different way to think about questions that have been raised about the analytic utility of the culture concept.

A range of scholars have critically focused attention on the concept of culture and the crisis of cultural representation precipitated by the publication of *Writing Culture* (Clifford and Marcus 1986) and *Anthropology as Cultural Critique* (Marcus and Fischer 1986).[9] It is not my purpose here to review this literature, or to directly engage in the debate about whether or not the concept of culture continues to be analytically useful (see Brightman 1995 for a comprehensive review and Brumann 1999 for an attempt at salvage). Rather, my purpose here is to use the moral, political, and logical problem of relativism as a mechanism by which to gain a critical and skeptical—rather than holistic, interpretive, and constructionist—perspective on human experience. By framing the problem of culture in terms of relativism it is possible to develop a skeptical perspective that recognizes the power of, but does not get lost in, the cynical logic of negative deconstructionism.[10] Thus I seek to engage directly with the problem of nihilism. This is done proactively—in the mode of neo-yogic philosophy—in order to develop a framework for an anthropology that is focused on the future condition of being human rather than on the logic of culture either as a thing or as a logical mode of meaningful production and reproduction.[11]

Yoga philosophy may be interpreted to provide a theoretical basis for an engagement with the reality of nihilism, although the term "nihilism" is relevant and appropriate only to a "cultural" understanding of Yoga.

> It is here, in this fundamental affirmation (more or less explicitly formulated) that the cosmos exists and endures because of man's lack of knowledge, that we can find the reason for the Indian deprecation of life and the cosmos. . . . From the time of the Upaniṣads India rejects the world as it is and devaluates life as it reveals itself to the eyes of the sage—ephemeral, painful, illusory. Such a conception leads neither to nihilism nor pessimism. *This* world is rejected, *this* life depreciated, because it is known that *something else* exists, beyond becoming, beyond temporality, beyond suffering. (Eliade 1990: 9–10)

Yoga becomes nihilistic only when and if "the possibility that something else exists" is denied, but when the value of that "something else" is dependent on the devaluation of everything other than that.

As a consequence of the Orientalist legacy—in which value of any kind is defined with reference to spirituality and mysticism—in contemporary scholarship there is a degree of nervousness in attributing to Yoga a "negative" perspective on the world. Nevertheless, it is quite clear that Yoga is based on the fundamental assumption that human experience, both good and evil, profound and mundane, is the product of *avidyā*—ignorance. Knowledge is not the opposite of ignorance, for knowledge is not based on duality and the endless change that duality implies. Rather, true Knowledge is that which is beyond all experience—*puruṣa*.

Most significantly—both for Yoga as such and for the development of a social theory based on Yoga—there is a mimetic relationship of extreme subtlety that enables the conscious apprehension of *puruṣa*. Paradoxically, consciousness as such cannot have any relationship to the absolute, since it is above all experience. As Eliade points out, the key to this paradoxical situation is that "the most subtle, most transparent part of mental life, that is, intelligence (*buddhi*) in its mode of pure luminosity (*sattva*), has a special quality—that of reflecting Spirit. Comprehension of the external world is possible only by virtue of this reflection of *puruṣa* in intelligence" (1990: 26). Thus it may be said that in and of itself luminous intelligence has no value other than being able to reflect *puruṣa*.

If one accepts that Yoga is a cultural construct, a philosophy of consciousness but *not* transcendence itself, then it is possible to find—in the "key to the paradox," so to speak—the elemental basis of being: a desire for something beyond experience, but the recognition that experience constructs the very idea of something beyond itself. Culture, at least in part, is spun from the webs of this paradox, this flawed understanding of the relationship between experience and truth. The flaw in Yoga is the desire for there to be no flaw in reflection. But it is precisely this flaw that enables a recognition—a critical remembering—that human intelligence conceived of *puruṣa* as an idea in the first place, and thus conceived also of the idea that all other ideas and experiences are an illusion. In fact, however, it is logical to assume that a conception of cultural life as flawed and imperfect—disgust with *saṁsāra,* as Eliade puts it (1990: 40), but also the more commonplace experience of pain, suffering, sickness, and death—gave rise to the idea of *avidyā*. In turn this gave rise to the desire for a reality other than that which is grounded in everyday life.

Paradoxically this desire for transcendence is dependent on experience. As Eliade puts it:

> In other words, one cannot free oneself from existence (*saṁsāra*) if one does not know life concretely. Herein lies the explanation of the paradoxical teleology of creation, which according to Sāṃkhya and Yoga, fetters the human soul and at the same time urges it on to liberation. Thus, the human condition, although dramatic, is not desperate, since experiences themselves tend to deliver the spirit. . . . Indeed, it is only through experiences that freedom is gained. Hence the gods (*videha,* "the disincarnate")—who have no experiences because they have no body—are in a condition of existence inferior to the human condition and cannot attain a complete liberation. (1990: 40)

In some respects, a grounded, experiential philosophy of *avidyā*—devoid of its transcendent analog and thereby brought firmly down to earth—provides a solution to the conundrum of relativism, and provides a perspective on human experience that is *reflected* in history rather than in culture. As Yoga makes clear, reflection is what matters, and reflection—this in that, that in this—is integral to mimesis, as mimesis constitutes the experiential nature of human being. Ironically mimesis is what fouls up the logic of relativism, since relativism is based on the illusion that something can make sense unto itself by means of self-referentiality. A perfect reproduction of the self through self-reflection is duplication. And duplication is a kind of reflection that is not reflection.

Relativism and Culture

As Geertz made clear a number of years ago (1984), Melford Spiro's work has come to define that branch of anthropology concerned with the discovery of universal patterns manifest in the full range of cultural variation. As an advocate of empirically grounded comparative studies of culture, Spiro is an antirelativist (see also Kuper 1994; Reddy 1997; Sangren 1988; Tilley 1998; Valjavec 1992; Wrong 1997). In responding to Geertz and making a case against the interpretive, hermeneutic turn in anthropology, Spiro has done one of the most comprehensive analyses of exactly what is meant by "cultural relativism." The distinction he makes between descriptive, normative, and epistemological relativism clears up many misconceptions and is extremely useful in understanding both the history of the discipline and how the concept relates to different levels and kinds of analysis (1992: 3–52).

The internal logic of Spiro's argument against relativism is impeccable, as impeccable as Geertz's interpretive critique of the discourse and academic practice of antirelativism. The critical point of disagreement between Spiro and Geertz is about what culture is. As the first footnote in his essay makes clear, and as references throughout demonstrate, for Spiro culture is a thing; statements people make refer to this thing, as culture belongs to groups of people (1992). For Geertz this is not the case. Culture is a construct; it is a process generated in public through human interaction. It belongs to no one, and everyone has a hand in its construction.

If culture is a thing that can be isolated and studied as a coherent, self-contained—but changing and flexible—unit, then Spiro is correct. From this perspective Geertz's anti-antirelativism is simply a powerful statement in defense of what Spiro would call strong descriptive relativism and epistemological relativism. In Spiro's view Geertz and those who follow his line of thinking focus on the limitlessness of cultural diversity and refuse to make generalizations about human culture on the basis of the incommensurability of cultural forms. But if cultural forms reflect an open-ended, inconclusive conversation, and take shape as texts, then the representation and interpretation of meaning becomes an end in itself rather than a means by which to understand culture as a thing. This has generated a great deal of debate—sometimes nervous, sometimes wistful, often dogmatic—on the question of anthropology's scientific status, and the paradigmatic coherence, or lack thereof, between the subfields of the discipline. (See Borofsky 1994; Carrithers 1990; Spiro 1996.)[12]

All of this is well known. The point here is not to rehearse the science/antiscience debate. Nor is the point, *pace* Geertz, to develop an anti-antiscience argument, although one is tempted to ask not whether anthropology is or is not a science but whether, given its history, it cannot but be one. To engage in the debate circuitously by refining the perspective of relativism would, in essence, be to use the language of epistemology to communicate insights on hermeneutics. The purpose of rehearsing this debate is to point out that since the basic misunderstanding about relativism has to do with paradigmatically different conceptions of culture, a different analytical perspective is required on what makes us human. This sounds very grand, but any perspective that seeks to escape the conundrum of relativism must encompass everything, but also account for the possibility that anyone can say anything about whatever he or she wants, and mean it.

Meaning, as Spiro indicates in his essay, is the crux of the issue, and he is quite right in pointing out that anthropologists before Geertz were concerned with it. Indeed it may well have been the rather awkward relationship among meaning, function, and structure manifest in the work of midcentury American cultural anthropology that inspired Geertz's interpretive move. Nevertheless, meaning is at the center of the culture concept because it defines a kind of intrinsic principle of coherence—sense making, in whatever terms and by whatever means: linguistic, mythic, historic, psychic, and social, for example. The question of meaning is all the more central to cultural relativism, because the most extreme form of relativism is linked directly to the principle that something makes sense in and on its own terms, rather than in terms alien to it. The most extreme form of antirelativism holds that only universal truths are meaningful. But what is this principle of coherence? By what logic can things be said to make sense?

Culture, however one chooses to define it, is an encompassing analytical abstraction designed as a way to think about being human. As such it has become reified as a thing, albeit a conceptual thing. This is clearly so when one thinks about the idea of Japanese, Hawaiian, or Indian culture, for example, but also in terms of more constructionist understandings. In terms of a constructionist framework, culture is a dynamic, dialectical, open-ended process. But for all its polysemic multivocality, a dialogically oriented constructionist framework presumes a degree of underlying coherence and anticipates the production of meaning as a logical entailment. Even when, for whatever reason, people who have nothing other than their humanity in common get together for the first time, what they produce, no matter how fragmentary and inconclusive, is said to be a meaningful cultural text. The longer they converse about more and more things the more full of meaning their conversation becomes, until it begins to define a context for itself beyond what is directly communicated. To a degree the rich thickness of constructed contextual meaning creates an illusion of coherence that belies the fact of cultural inconsistencies and contradiction, just as the apparent inability to communicate—at first contact, so to speak—creates an illusion of incoherence that belies the fact of cross-cultural translatability. Regardless, from a constructionist perspective there is always the assumption that no matter how divergent, polysemic, or multivocal, there is, on some level, a single point of consensus. What gets learned, shared, and communicated constitutes what is real and meaningful about human experience. This would seem to be self-evident.

But is it?—and this simple question, I hope, justifies the somewhat long-winded buildup. What if one takes a perspective that is counter-intuitive? What if the sense of coherence that culture is thought to have does not so much reflect a meaningful world as it does an effort to deploy meaning against the contingency of being human in a world defined by the past?[13] What if the sense people make—of themselves and of others—is not inherently meaningful? What if it is meaningful only to the extent that it obscures that part of the past that does not conform with their assumptions, and selects as history those parts that do? If this is so, then as an analytical abstraction the concept of culture defines a level of human experience that is epiphenomenal rather than phenomenological, and the meaningful worlds people create are, in fact, not webs of meaning but, as Yoga suggests, the ensnaring web of *māyā*. Culture can be made to make sense, either from the inside looking at itself or from the outside looking in. But in making sense is there not another more true-to-the-world reality that is obscured? Think of it this way: the development of language promotes human communication, but the history of languages does not. Perhaps, therefore, the development of language is not what makes us human but that which prevents us from seeing ourselves—and recognizing the importance of so seeing ourselves—as a species of animal, as beings animated by anima: the *jīvātman* of our evolutionary and *saṃsāric* lineage. To see, in this sense, is to see ourselves through the medium of *darśana,* as *darśana* means both profound, visionary insight and very practical and down-to-earth vision. I will return below to the grounded "animal" nature of being human, and to the way in which the idea of history as a visionary reflection—like the idea of *puruṣa* reflected in pure *buddhi*—provides a way to think about the nonsensical relationship between language and languages, and among culture, Cultures, and cultural constructions.

Humanism and Its Entailments

Drawing on the work of Bourdieu and Foucault, anthropologists working in the 1990s have developed powerful arguments for why the concept of culture has lost much of its analytical utility. As Lila Abu-Lughod has pointed out (1991), it is more useful to think about being human in terms of discourse and practice than in terms of culture, regardless of how constructionist one's conception of culture is. In pointing out how anthropologists should write against culture in order to produce anthropological knowledge, Abu-Lughod deals with the nitty-gritty of everyday experience: what people see, say, and do. In writing against culture she makes what is probably a reasonable assumption. People mean what they say, even though they may mean many different things at different times, or even several things at the same time. Ultimately she roots her analysis in the direct experience of people's lives. Her own work is one of the best examples of a kind of ethnography in which individual lives are understood within a framework wherein the humanity of those lives is represented in a meaningful way, meaningful precisely because it strategically blurs and manipulates the boundary between the particular and the general.

Even though the question of what constitutes truth can be debated, as can the question of what counts as representations of truth, anthropologists—in contrast to yogis—have tended to work under the assumption that what people say is truthful and that social life is real. Even the most reflexive field research is predicated on the assumption that meaningful knowledge, anchored in the present, is the product of social interaction. Participant observation is designed as a method to engage in and with the social construction of knowledge, and ethnographic texts are meant to represent meaning. But what if the intentionality of perspective and locus of knowledge is in question? What if what people say and do provides us with a perspective on their lived experience, and is the terms of our dialogic engagement with them, but is understood as meaningless—if the term may be used nonpejoratively, though with a trace of skepticism—in relation to a broader discursive field? What if what people think they are doing is not at all what they end up having done? Therefore, what if what they think they are doing is not at all what is significant about what they are doing in the first place? The elipse of time and logic is critical here.

This may seem nonsensical, but it seems to be a reasonable interpretation of Foucault's perspective on history, and therefore on a history of the present. If the history we create is not what we had in mind, what does this suggest about "what we have in mind"? Anthropologists who have tried to apply Foucault's notion of discursive power to their understanding of being human have not, it seems to me, fully engaged with either the question of how discursive power displaces meaning as a frame of reference for both hermeneutics and epistemology, or the implications of making this question central to social analysis. This is probably because, given the subjective, humanistic nature of fieldwork it is very difficult to maintain "methodological scepticism about both the ontological claims and the ethical values which humanist systems of thought invest in the notion of subjectivity" (Gordon 1980: 239). It is difficult, in other words, to deploy trust as a methodological tool when doubt is considered to be the basis of knowledge. The conundrumic elipse of time, manifest in a history of the present, makes this less difficult, as does a yogic conception of time and knowledge.

With regard to the idea that transcendence is achieved by traveling back through time to the moment before time began, the terminology of Yoga is wonderfully apt—and not just because animals in general and headstanding rats in particular have been invoked. The term is *pratiloman,* which means "going against the fur," the image being that of an animal being brushed the wrong way: against the direction of growth and the smooth, flat, integrated coherence of a pelt. A cow licking its own flank produces this furry, ruptured image of history.

It is significant that history understood in this way—as a kind of intellectual time travel, that is—is dependent on the idea that there is coherence and meaning in the present and in the future, but that this coherence is "ruffed up" by a perception of the passage of time. In Yoga this "furry history" is regarded as the fabric of illusion stretched out over time. The point is to get to a point of origin beyond time. However, it is useful to think of *pratiloman*—which is cognate with *ujāna sādhana* or "going against the current," manifest, among other places, in auto-urine therapy, the "return of semen" in *vajrolīmudrā,* and in the simple form of a *śirṣāsana*—as a means by which to reflect the contingency of history onto the present. The point is to ruffle the feathers of coherence, and take seriously the fact of ignorance, as ignorance and error produce and reproduce a past. This past may have no more meaning than the present, but it is a past that can be understood through reflection as mimesis rather than through the dialectics of relativism. Thereby this past should be taken as the locus of knowledge that is not limited by experience or direct perception.

Mistakes, Misunderstanding, and Meaninglessness

In a short but important essay Johannes Fabian uses mistakes in understanding as a means by which to question the nature of ethnographic representation, and to caution against the uncritical use of context to frame meaning. He poses the question: "Do misunderstanding and understanding relate to each other like error and truth? Perhaps a case could be made for misunderstanding as committing an error, but not for understanding as attaining truth" (1995: 41[42/43]). The thrust of Fabian's argument is to question the criteria that are used to establish understanding—to question what counts as a shared frame of reference. Through a series of examples he points out that "even on the level of interpreting grammatical and lexical meaning . . . translation requires historical background knowledge" (1995: 43). As he puts it: "History, despite expressions such as 'historical context' that come easily to most of us, provides connections that are contingent, unpredictable, and unsystematic and are therefore not really 'con-text' in either the linguistic or literary sense of the term" (1995: 43). Context, therefore, is constructed. It "must be constituted in a practice that is individually and therefore historically situated and determined. Ethnography is biography is historiography—a position that can escape tautology if it rests on a dialectical conception of knowledge. The point of insisting on dialectics is to overcome facticity through overcoming positivity" (1995: 48). A dialectical conception of knowledge holds that knowledge is praxis. It seems to me that the creative potential of this praxis as it creates and recreates the "context" of history is suggested by Fabian's reference to a statement made by Wilhelm von Humboldt (1988: 48): "Nobody means by a word precisely and exactly what his neighbor does, and the difference, be it ever so small, vibrates, like a ripple in water, throughout the entire language. Thus all understanding is always at the same time a not-understanding" (1995: 48).

Understanding that is also not-understanding is a fairly good definition of what I mean by the significant meaninglessness of the present. If we take this perspective and apply it to the problem of relativism, the question becomes not whether all forms of discourse and practice are equally meaningful, legitimate, justified, and significant, but the extent to which what people think is meaningful and significant is only so contingently, and, therefore, with reference to history, not significantly meaningful at all. With reference to the future, mistakes and meaningless contingency cause agency to unravel as time goes on. The point is to redefine the question of relativism in terms of a different understanding of culture. Instead of being a positive, evaluative framework focused on sense making, it should come to reflect a critical and skeptical focus on confusion and misunderstanding, as these conditions are produced by a kind of chronic dissonance between the past, the present, and people's strategic goals for the future. The critical focus of study then becomes the structure of this discursive dissonance.

From this perspective attention shifts away from the question of what is right and what is wrong—as well as away from a classification of everything and anything as contextually "right"—to a deconstruction of all specific oppositions, such as normal/bizarre, that are included within the ur opposition of good and evil. In some manifestations of tantric Yoga—most notably among the Aghorapanthīs—"transcendence" can be experienced through a complete and fearless abandonment of the self to everything that is thought to be abnormal and impure: "These Aghorīs eat from human skulls, haunt cemeteries, and still practiced cannibalism at the end of the nineteenth century. . . . They eat all sorts of refuse and any kind of meat except horse meat. They justify these practices by saying that all of man's natural inclinations and tastes should be destroyed, that there is neither good nor evil, pleasant nor unpleasant, etc. Even as human excrement fertilizes a sterile soil, so assimilating every kind of filth makes the mind capable of any and every meditation" (Eliade 1990: 296–97).

Although qualifications concerning horse meat do, in some sense, cause the whole structure of antistructure to logically unravel, in an important sense the Aghorapanthīs embody "understanding that is also not understanding." Thereby they suggest a theory of culture that is not reducible to the binarism of "meaning-full" relativistic opposition. Here the incipiently comparative framework of pure versus impure is used, in a sense, against itself—and against the binary epistemology upon which it is based—to deconstruct the categorical opposition of good and evil. What is required is not only incessant, unending, reflexive questioning, but a critical examination of what constitutes the ontological question upon which culture and the epistemology of relativism is based. In extreme forms this can mean the complete and unrestrained abandonment of the self to desire. Clearly this is not a charter for direct action, unless one chooses to become an Aghorī or engage in the activities of various other groups such as the Kāpālikas and Lokāyatikas (see Lorenzen 1972). But it is an appeal for a comprehensive politics of knowledge, a kind of praxis that is not lost in the conundrum of relativism and the search for meaning in context. Ultimately it can provide the basis for a politics of action that is just and humane, but where justice and humanity are not defined by a priori assumptions about the cultural form of value.

Fetishism, Mimesis, and Human Being without Culture

Apart from Yoga, inspiration for this kind of thinking comes from an engagement with three distinct but related projects: Arjun Appadurai's orientation toward the world through ethnoscapes, Lila Abu-Lughod's advocacy to write against culture, and, most significantly, Michael Taussig's deployment of the fetish as the subjectobject of critical analysis. Although it is a perspective that might well be characterized as resolutely postmodern, ultimately it is grounded in ethnographic reality. Thereby it is also, *pace* Nanda and Warms, "a fundamental research tool of anthropology." In order to gain a clearer and more anthropologically relevant perspective on mimetic skepticism it is necessary to tack away from Yoga as such, and consider—in conjunction with Fabian's work—certain important aspects of contemporary social theory.

Mimetic skepticism is a way to think about being human in terms analogous to those used by Appadurai to refer to ethnoscapes—deterritorialized, lived experiences that are driven by a globalized imaginary. In advocating a strategy to do anthropology after the crisis of representation, Appadurai writes: "Ethnography must redefine itself as the practice of representation which illuminates the power of large-scale, imagined life possibilities over specific life trajectories. This is 'thickness' with a difference, and the difference lies in a new alertness to the fact that ordinary lives today are increasingly powered not by the givenness of things but by the possibilities that the media suggests are available" (1991: 200). In developing this strategy for a cosmopolitan ethnography, he calls for the construction of genealogies of the present. In trying to get a critical fix on the relationship between global and local, Appadurai points out that "the most appropriate ethnoscapes for today's world, with its alternative, interactive modernities, should confront genealogy and history with each other, thus leaving the terrain open for interpretations of the ways in which local historical trajectories flow into complicated transnational structures" (1991: 209).

Appadurai's perspective provides a helpful way to think about the present in relation to the contingency of intersecting histories, and he is assiduously aware of the extent to which these intersecting histories create conflict, confusion, and misunderstanding, along with the more commonplace dissonance of multiple perspectives. But there is a sense in which Appadurai's radical perspective on global flow nevertheless entails a kind of faith in what might be called grounded—albeit deterritorialized—coherence. It is not so much that his arguments resolve into coherence, for that is a universal phenomenon—at least of good scholarship—but that a presumption of ethnographically locatable coherence dogs his skepticism about the bounded, coherent nature of culture.

This is also reflected, perhaps more clearly, in Abu-Lughod's critically self-conscious invocation of "tactical humanism" as a strategic position from which to write about being human while writing against culture. In Appadurai and Abu-Lughod's work, coherence and meaning are not manifest, primarily, on the personal level of everyday life. If that were the case, the concept of culture would do just fine. Rather there is a sense in which whatever it is that you write about when you write against culture does intrinsically make sense, and that the object of the exercise is to make anthropological sense of the sense it makes. Similarly, in Appadurai's analysis ethnoscapes are exceedingly complex, distorted by changes in scale, and characterized by shifts in meaning, but nevertheless "what is real about ordinary lives is . . . real in many ways that range from the sheer contingency of individual lives and the vagaries of competence and talent that distinguish persons in all societies to the 'realisms' that individuals are exposed to and draw upon in their ordinary lives" (1991: 199).

In both Appadurai and Abu-Lughod's work there is what seems to be a degree of contradiction between an epistemic stand focused on the contingency of human life and an implicit ontological assumption about the continuity of experience as real and meaningful on a phenomenological level. This contradiction seems to displace, but not resolve, the problem of relativism. If there are multiple realities you must represent those realities as meaningful in and on their own terms, regardless of how global and discontinuous the flow of ideas and things, and regardless of the constructed nature of reality. Meaningful reality demands some kind of direct representation that, in grating against the contingency of history, transforms a genealogy of the present into a singularly nervous, unstable exercise.

Appadurai's focus on the intersection of genealogy and history to gain a perspective on the deterritorialized, cosmopolitan present is extremely useful. But its analytical value is blocked by the conundrum of relativism and cannot be fully realized until the ontology of realism is sent packing along with the epistemic significance of the culture concept as a representation of reality. Dislocated critical skepticism is directed against a kind of residual hope—as dialectically defined by hopelessness—that meaningfulness has somehow survived anthropology's critique of culture. If it has, it should not have.

However it may seem, this is not negativism. It does not make sense in terms of a dialectical mode of thinking. Therefore, in this regard—and with help from the nondualist philosophy of Yoga—I depart from Fabian's line of reasoning. Dislocated critical skepticism seeks to put into perspective an analytical attitude that derives from Deleuze's interpretation of Nietzsche's concern with the nonbinary transmutation of negation into active creative affirmation (1983: 147–89). But for anthropology, rooted as it must be in the material world of human experience, if not also—as some of us might continue to hope—in the domain of Marxist praxis, the best way to realize this, and to develop the principle of active creative affirmation as a purposeful perspective on the human condition, is by means of the fetish, an ideathing which, not coincidentally, is directly implicated in the logic of relativism.

Fetishism provides a useful way to get beyond the contradiction between a belief in ontological contingency, on the one hand, and, on the other, faith in an epistemology of knowledge that either presumes or produces coherence. That is, it provides a means by which to think and act against relativism, antirelativism, or anti-antirelativism by enabling a perspective that is trenchantly critical of what appears to be real, without proclaiming, simply, that there are multiple meaningful realities. In forcing the question of signification and meaning back on itself, fetishism defines difference in terms of both not making and making sense, as both of these operations are coeval and consubstantial. The principle of fetishism refines an attitude that is critically dislocated into one that is mimetically skeptical.

Although there is a considerable literature on fetishism and representation in cultural studies, feminist theory, and literary criticism, much of which is useful, Taussig's anthropological work is of particular value precisely because it is resolutely materialist in a way that ethnography demands, and unambiguously concerned with a kind of human dignity that is otherwise compromised by the dialectics of culture and relativism. This human dignity, made visible through the refraction of fetishism, is very much an emergent principle rather than a kind of absolute point—primordial or utopian—reflected in the ideology of liberal humanism. It is the product of contingency. Significantly, Taussig's discussion of fetishism provides a critically new perspective on the nature of culture as a thing, and the reification of that thing as an object of anthropological knowledge; the point being not to unmask culture or cultural process to discover what is really meaningful, but to engage with the fetish form of culture as both a concrete thing and a conceptual abstraction. This kind of engagement is iconoclastic, much as Abu-Lughod's admonition to write against culture is self-consciously iconoclastic, except for the fact that to write against culture is a methodology of representation bent on the production of meaning from meaning whereas an engagement with the fetish form of culture entails a kind of historical perspective on the depersonalized present.

Fetishism is central to Taussig's critical analysis of capitalism and colonialism where he shows how violence and reason, curing and killing, faith and disbelief are impacted in and extracted from one another in various complex and consistently inconsistent ways. In "Maleficium: State Fetishism" (1993a: 217–47) his concern is as much with the fetishism of society in sociology as it is with the fetishism of the state in politics. Consequently it is an argument that is directly relevant to the reification of culture in the context of anthropological debates about relativism, and the reification of relativism in the context of anthropological debates about culture.

Taussig makes a convincing argument against the standard interpretation that holds that Durkheim disentangled social facts from individual action, thereby enabling the scientific study of social life. In pointing out the extent to which the objectification of social facts as suprahuman things made empirically minded social scientists nervous about the relationship between ideas and things, Taussig writes:

> My argument, of course, is that [the brilliance of the *Année Sociologique* school] was not the result of a step-by-step development from social fact as thing to social fact as moral web and the fetishization of Society (as *deus*), but instead, it was the result of a specific epistemic tension within the very notion of the Social as both thing and godly at one and the same time. In other words, far from being an unfortunate side effect, it was Durkheim's very fetishization of "society" that provided the intellectual power of his sociology. (1993a: 229)

Taussig is adamantly critical of a perspective that holds that social science triumphed with the successful and complete abstraction of "society" and the "individual." Instead he employs the nervous rationalization of scholars like Radcliffe-Brown, Evans-Pritchard, Parsons, and others to critically reproblematize the relationship between what is natural and what is supernatural: things and God.[14] As Taussig makes clear, it is possible to reify society and the individual, and regard them as distinct and inanimate things, but the fetishization of society necessarily entails what is referred to as "the formal mechanism of fetishism . . . whereby the signifier depends upon yet erases its signification" (1993a: 225). It is this "dependent erasure" that renders meaningfulness rather mysterious and paradoxical, directing attention away from the engaged agency of self-determining individuals to the problematization of praxis: "the subject making itself through making the object" (1993a: 225). Developing this idea as an alternative to a bland social constructionist view of reality, Taussig defines what he refers to—in terms that are strikingly yogic—as mimetic excess.

> Mimetic excess as a form of human capacity potentiated by post-coloniality provides a welcome opportunity to live subjunctively as neither subject nor object of history but as both, at one and the same time. Mimetic excess provides access to understanding the unbearable truths of make-believe as foundation of an all-too-seriously serious reality, manipulated but also manipulatable. Mimetic excess is a somersaulting back to sacred actions implicated in the puzzle that empowered mimesis any time, any place—namely the power to both double yet double endlessly, to become any Other and engage the image with the reality thus imagized. (1993b: 255)

Keep in mind here a few images—Yogeshwaranand disecting the orb of the heart, as discussed in chapter 2; Kuvalayananda discovering the Madhavdas Vacuum, as discussed in chapter 3; *bīṛī*-smoking ex-addicts performing *prāṇāyāma* in the slums of Delhi, as discussed in chapter 4; Dr. Karandikar devising a technique to tap into the power of ether by manipulating scapulas, as discussed in chapter 5. And then, of course, there is the elixir urine. Mimesis provides a way out of the conundrum of relativism manifest in a constructionist view of reality as really made up in a multitude of equally meaningful ways. Mimesis holds that differences are not differences in kind, but differences as mutually implicated one in the other. Thus there is no context for things to make different kinds of sense—they make sense only relative to one another (see Taussig 1993b: 249), and the sense they make is in terms of a reconstruction of the endless process of engaging "the image with the reality thus imagized." Mimetic excess is a kind of remembering that is required as a consequence of the fact that to live in society we must regularly—minute by minute if not second by second—forget that meaning is constructed and act as if it is natural, bounded, and whole. Thus in Taussig's formulation, mimetic excess plays remembering and forgetting off of each other with a kind of synergy that produces an understanding of what is inherently paradoxical if viewed in parts. Mimetic excess is an emergent process of understanding rather than a means by which to arrive at a conclusive understanding. It is, therefore, characterized by "endless mobility one step ahead of interpretive discharge" (1993b: 249).

The analytical power of mimesis, revealed in the form of fetishized things, provides a means by which to get beyond the concept of culture and find a solution to the problem of relativism by undermining the relevance of contextual meaning to understanding.

Although in principle Taussig is absolutely right, I am nervous about the extent to which the praxis of mimesis is dependent on images, and the juxtaposition of images—carved icons, pictures, films, decoys, sculptures, texts, "classical anthropology," phonographs, Cuna *molas,* money, fingerprints—to the exclusion, it seems, of people proclaiming what they believe to be absolutely true, apart from things. Is it possible "to live subjunctively as neither subject nor object of history but as both, at one and the same time," without running aground on someone else's subjunctivity or mistaking your own subjunctivity as the same as everyone else's?[15] It is, I think, but first the concept of "agency" must be sent packing along with the notion that cultural constructions are rendered meaningful by context.[16] The concept of agency undermines the synergy of mimesis by confusing the relationship between forgetting and remembering. It imagines actors to be inherently creative. But, as Taussig points out, "no matter how sophisticated we may be as to the constructed and arbitrary character of our practices, including our practices of representation, our practice of practices is one of actively forgetting such mischief each time we open our mouths to ask something or make a statement. Try to imagine what would happen if we didn't in daily practice thus conspire to actively forget what Saussure called 'the arbitrariness of the sign'" (1993b: xviii).

From a slightly different angle, then, agency can be understood as the form of a mistake or a self-conscious "conspiracy" of misunderstanding. To focus on agency as the basis upon which social reality is experienced is, ironically, to immobilize the power of mimesis; and it is out of this immobilization that the problem of relativism emerges and reemerges. It would seem then that mimetic excess must be dislocated from any notion of the person as meaningfully self-determining, and relocated in public space, as that space is defined purely by the intersection of perception.

If this can be done, then the space of intersection becomes a place where lives are lived subjunctively and where it is possible to take seriously everything and nothing anyone says about himself or anyone else. This makes no sense whatsoever, unless one is willing to accept—to extend and adapt Taussig's adaptation of Benjamin—that Truth is only truth insofar as it does justice to misunderstanding. When it seeks to make sense of things, it falls into the conundrum of relativism.

The problem is that while this perspective might allow for an archaeology of the present dealing with material objects and things and their relationship to one another, does it enable an ethnography of the present based on what people say and do?[17] The things people say are "things" of a kind, to be sure, particularly when they end up in notebooks, interview transcripts, or survey questionnaires. But statements about the nature of truth are often made with conviction. How can one be skeptical of conviction without undermining the kind of trust that, on some level, must be part of field research? Perhaps it should be put this way, *pace* Marcus (1998: 1–29): could a graduate student—or even a middle-aged professor—write a grant to conduct interviews in the space of intersection? If so, would the natives therein, bent on making sense of themselves and of representing themselves as sensible, hold tight to their masks? Presenting themselves as unambiguously real and meaningful, would they refuse a mimetic intervention and simply force the problem of relativism?

The only way into this is to do ethnography. Multisited ethnography of ethnoscapes, to be sure. But ethnography must become history through representation so that one is not just writing against culture, but writing against the apparent meaningfulness of the present and the continuity between it and history. Historically mediated ethnography is a representation of being human rather than an account of culture. Stop making sense so as to understand what-has-become-history-through-ethnography on its own past-tense terms. The issue of context-specific accountability is thus categorically displaced. Needless to say, this is not an ethnographic approach that is "sympathetic" to people's belief in themselves. And this may be the most difficult thing to accept about mimetic skepticism. It is, in a sense, the very enemy of rapport, as rapport—a concept that is, I think, perverse on many levels (see Alter 2000c)—pretends to articulate truth in the intimacy of shared knowledge.

Remembering the Forgetting of the Arbitrariness of the Sign

For ethnography to become this kind of history does *not* entail the passage of time. It entails a perspective that is not delimited by the present tense. This is what I think Taussig is getting at by the notion of subjunctivity. Subjunctivity is reality that is based on creatively destructive hypothetical action. At any given moment in time this is nonsensical. And to even view history as moments in time is to make sense of nonsense. But to make ethnography as history involves—if I may twist Taussig's phrasing quoted above—imagining what has happened as a result of our daily conspiracy to forget what Saussure called the "arbitrariness of the sign" (1993b: xviii). History, viewed in this way, does not take shape as a fetish—although that is always possible. It takes shape as a kind of chain reaction set in motion by fetishization—the signifier endlessly depending upon yet endlessly erasing its signification. In part, at least, relativism resurrects the moribund problems of the culture concept, and to escape these problems entails a different attitude toward the relationship between lived experience and past experience: the present and the past. Anthropology, it seems to me, should be directed at what might be called the ever-present slipstream of fetishized reproduction, or the residual traces of the shibollithic moment. It should be directed at what von Humboldt conceived of as the ripple of understanding as not understanding that vibrates through language.[18]

Here a useful perspective can be gained on what might otherwise appear to be recursive nihilism by working through, but then upending—in the manner of a *śirṣāsana*—the philosopher W. V. Quine's thesis of the indeterminacy of translation as it relates to field linguistics.[19] As a thought experiment Quine posits a language, "Jungle," that can be translated into English only in the same way a child might learn Jungle growing up: through direct observation and strategic participation in speech situations.[20] The goal of the field linguist would be to develop linguistic proficiency through the construction of a manual of translation. An independent field linguist engaged in what Quine calls radical translation would proceed from simple, single-word observation sentences to more complex sentences by asking for or responding to positive and negative reactions from a native speaker.

> We readily imagine the translator's ups and down. Perhaps he has tentatively translated two native sentences into English ones that are akin to each

> other in some semantic way, and he finds this same kinship reflected in a native's use of the two native sentences. This encourages him in his pair of tentative translations. So he goes on blithely supposing that he is communicating, only to be caught up short. This may persuade him that his pair of translations was wrong after all. He wonders how far back, in the smooth flowing antecedent conversation, he got off the beam. (1992: 47)

Of note here is that the act of translation, which is also the act of learning any language, produces a reality that is inherently inconclusive, incomplete, and tentative. Significantly it is also inherently corrective, and creatively "backward" looking, in a way that is designed to move forward, but without any real sense of reaching a conclusion. We all, even native speakers, are always learning our own language by recalling the mistakes we make. In and of itself, radical translation highlights the constructed, unbounded nature of culture, albeit with an emphasis on epistemology rather than on hermeneutics.

Quine's more radical contribution is in terms of what happens, as is always the case, when there are two or more translators working independent of one another in their effort to produce comprehensive manuals of translation, and, most significantly, how one compares these manuals to each other. As he puts it:

> These reflections leave us little reason to expect that two radical translators, working independently on Jungle, would come out with interchangeable manuals. Their manuals might be indistinguishable in terms of any native behavior that they give reason to expect, and yet each manual might prescribe some translations that the other translator would reject. Such is the indeterminacy of translation. . . .
>
> The thesis of indeterminacy of translation is that these claims on the part of two manuals might both be true, and yet the two translation relations might not be usable in alternation, from sentence to sentence, without issuing incoherent sequences. Or, to put it another way, the English sentences prescribed as translation of a given Jungle sentence by two rival manuals might not be interchangeable in English contexts. (1992: 47–48)

Here then one has a multiplicity of truths; but truths that get tripped up, so to speak, when an effort is made to repatriate them. The act of reflexive retranslation undermines the incipient sense of coherence in the mother tongue of the field linguist. Although the manuals are both true relative to Jungle, relative to each other they produce incoherence. This becomes all the more clear when Quine makes the following point: "I have directed my indeterminacy thesis on a radically exotic language for the sake of plausibility, but in principle it applies even to the home language. For given the rival manuals of translation between Jungle and

English, we can translate English perversely into English by translating it into Jungle by one manual and then back by the other" (1992: 48).

It is useful to focus, with an analytical attitude made possible by the power of fetishism and yogic *avidyā,* on the so-called perversity of this exercise in translation. It is precisely by learning Jungle as a speaker of English and then turning English back on itself through recursive translation that provides the means to develop a critically skeptical perspective on the inherent misunderstanding that is embedded in all acts of communication. Compare what Quine says about language with what Taussig says about fetishized ideathings: "Mimetic excess is a somersaulting back to sacred actions implicated in the puzzle that empowered mimesis any time, any place—namely the power to both double yet double endlessly, to become any Other and engage the image with the reality thus imagized" (1993b: 255). Quine's conclusion about becoming "any Other and engag[ing] the image with the reality this imagized" is this: "What the indeterminacy thesis is meant to bring out is that the radical translator is bound to impose about as much as he discovers" (1992: 49). But not only this, it seems to me. What gets imposed is not so much an ethnocentric value judgment, however benign, as a profound misunderstanding of the self as ontologically real. What Quine refers to as "ontological relativism" has less to do with the categorical choice of manuals one makes, than it does with the emergent realization that one must creatively remember what gets lost, or misconstrued, in translation.

The argument here is very general, but it is not very abstract. Therefore, any given case should be as good as any other to make the point that being human is to live through the present to make history—to take action in order to produce history rather than to be invested in the value of that action unto itself. This signals an inherently changing or shape-shifting reality. To match this shape shifting requires—somewhat ironically—disembodiment, to the extent that history cannot be located in the person of any given person even though it might very well be inscribed on specific, individual bodies. The point here—to once again, at least obliquely, reference Arjun's yogic discourse in the *Gītā*—is that the possibility that absolute power can be made sense of in terms of relativism both essentializes power and reifies the notion of freedom and free will. This undermines the creatively destructive potential of a history that feeds off of the way absolute power endlessly depends upon yet endlessly erases freedom. To understand this history you can no more believe a person who articulates a position of absolute power, or—and this is much more difficult—believe a person who is subject to that power but aspires to freedom as a reified ideal. You cannot define what is good in terms that universalize that ideal as a principle of human action in relation to others, which is what provoked Arjun to ask Kṛṣṇa the question. The problem is with belief; and with belief as a material fact of conscious being. Belief forces cultural understanding into either a dialectical mode or a straightforward choice. To again invoke textbook examples, the question of who is right, slave or slave master, and whose view of the world makes better sense, is a recursive question even when the meaning of each perspective has been radically and reflexively imagined as a decentered, polyvalent construction.

In terms of situational activism, which remains problematic in other ways, clearly everyone must act in terms of his or her contingent beliefs. On this front, on this level, I am more than willing to say unambiguously what is right and what is wrong—and here Kṛṣṇa is no more an authority than any other *videha*. However, to locate the ethical basis of action in cultural understanding is to credit anthropology with unwarranted moral authority, as religion has been ceded that authority in the context of other disciplinary divestments of will. Analytically it is necessary to disconnect belief from analysis and replace conviction with skepticism. Otherwise answers define questions. What is required is not so much to write against culture in order to reconstruct belief as to write beyond good and evil. I take this to be very close to what E. Valentine Daniel means by a "counterpoint to culture" necessitated by the moral, ethical, and theoretical problem of representing violent ethnic conflict (1996: 194–212). In some sense belief itself, and a kind of faith in a definitive representation of reality that belief presumes, is the locus of the problem. What is required, as Daniel indicates, following Celan, is to be true, through one's faithlessness, to pain, suffering, and loss.[21]

In standard textbooks, such as the fourth edition of *Cultural Anthropology: A Perspective on the Human Condition* (Schultz and Lavenda 2001), twentieth-century genocide in Germany is used as an example of the "extreme case" where cultural relativism can be applied. The extermination of one race by another—which, of course, can never be justified in any meaningful terms—is understood as a "meaningful way of life" and "system of beliefs," as this system of beliefs is defined holistically, contextualized historically, and explained without recourse to cultural determinism.

But hatred, prejudice, and killing is one thing. What about peace, nonviolence, and the valuation of life above all else? Can we—indeed must we—not agree that, differences aside, "all people are created equal," and mean it? And mean it not just in principle but as so self-evidently true as to be sacred? Is this not the only possible position to take against crimes against humanity? In the present, at any given moment, of course. But the problem is that faith in an ideal of humanity incarnates the crimes against it and makes it necessary to savage the savagery, regardless of the form of action—terrorism, legalism, policy, pastoralism, or police action. To get beyond the dialectic of good and evil, as it is reproduced by any absolutist position, it is necessary to think of the impossible possibility that what appears to be equality can be made to appear as, and be, inequality. But the key point is that it is necessary to out-absolute the absolutists and force the issue of mimesis into those areas where there would seem to be no problem with perspectivity, and, indeed, where it would seem that there are dangerous consequences to questioning an ideal. Is this not what Yoga has done?

In conclusion I would simply like to explore, in a provisional and exploratory way, one direction in which mimetic skepticism might lead when unleased in the domain of Universal Truth.

Provisional Conclusions: Yoga and the Animal Nature of Being Human

One of the most enigmatic artifacts that has come to occupy a space in the history of Yoga is the so-called *pāśupati* terra-cotta seal—which is not a *mudrā,* but a seal in fact, as a real thing used to mark and seal things—dating to the period of the Indus civilization (2600–1500 B.C.E.). The relief of the seal shows the figure of a person with large, somewhat stylized horns seated on a low seat in a posture that looks somewhat like a *gorakṣāsana.* It is difficult to tell, but the figure appears to have an erect penis. Located around the figure, on a smaller scale, are four animals: a tiger, an elephant, a rhinoceros, and a buffalo. Beneath the figure are a pair of antelopes. For this reason the figure has been identified as Lord Śiva—or an archaic proto-Śiva deity—who has been designated as *pāśupati:* Lord of the Animals. While naming the figure on the seal "Pāśupati" is somewhat arbitrary (and recall here the arbitrariness of all signs), it is logical and suggestive of various possible logical entailments, most directly linked—if one is permitted to leap, shamanlike, across the span of two thousand years—to the Pāśupata tradition defined and elaborated by a second-century ascetic named Lakulīśa and codified several centuries later by Kauṇḍinya in the fifth century C.E.

Without going into detail, there are two interesting features to Pāśupata philosophy and practice that relate to the issue at hand, and to the connection among the *pāśupati* seal, Yoga, and the animal nature of being human. With respect to practice, the Pāśupatas can be said to have consciously rejected culture in toto, and to have embodied a kind of life set against the most elemental features of cultural being. They babbled, snorted, walked in ways that perverted the civilized motility of upright posture, made odd gestures with parts of their bodies that were no meant to be used for gesturing, crudely flaunted their sexuality, and in general went out of their way to act as though they were not human, and to bring disapproval and condemnation on themselves for doing so. The goal was to transcend good and evil by embodying absolute dispassion. Pure, absolute dispassion seemed to entail the rejection and perversion of everything that counted as being human.

With this in mind, it is important to understand that Pāśupata philosophy is radically theistic. Śiva is conceptualized as an all-knowing, all-powerful God whose nature is completely distinct from and independent of the law of karmic integration that defines the universe as such. It is on this level that Śiva, as *pāśupati,* is lord of the beasts, for the beasts—human and animal alike—"are none other than the fettered souls that, in birth after birth, are forever recycled in the great ecology of Nature—unless they experience the grace of Śiva" (Feuerstein 2001: 261). Śiva is not only *pāśupati,* he is also the archetypal yogi.[22]

The *Gheraṇḍasaṁhitā* contains an interesting reference that helps to explain, at least in the discourse of modern practitioners, why so many postures are named after a certain class of "fettered souls"—animals. The second chapter begins by pointing out that there are 8,400,000 postures, and that this number is equivalent to the number of different kinds of living things in the universe. A quick review of the shorter list of postures that are said to be of use for "mankind in this world"—one wonders, immediately, what other postures, other creatures, elsewhere, in other worlds, are doing for the benefit of their own species—reveals that there is a lotus posture, a lion posture, a fish posture, a peacock posture, a cock posture, a tortoise posture, a tree posture, and postures named for eagles, bulls, locusts, dolphins, camels, and snakes. Mimetically speaking, Yoga embodies the whole organic universe. In other words, *āsana*s are inherently fetishistic in a fairly straightforward way. Consider two examples:

> Sitting on the ground, cross the legs in the *padmāsana* posture. Push the hands and arms between the thighs and the knees. Stand on the hands and support the body on the elbows. This is called the cock posture.
>
> From the navel down to the toes touch the body to the ground. Place the palms of both hands on the ground and lift the upper part of the body like a serpent. This is called the serpent posture.

Among the postures, there is not a single one designated "human" as such. But perhaps there are serpents in some other world who perform a person posture? Is this not, on some fundamental level, the simple connection that a person in the posture of a snake is trying to make? And does not a person in the posture of a snake produce the same embodied image as a horned man depicted on a terra-cotta seal surrounded by animals?

As Mircea Eliade made clear over sixty years ago, Yoga is directly linked to shamanism. Even if Eliade was wrong about the specifics of cross-cultural contact in the early historic and prehistoric period of interaction between groups, and even if he was wrong about the relationship between different manifestation of shamanism in various parts of Asia and Oceania, there is no question but that he was right to link the yogi's concern with the dissolution of the body, magical flight, mastery over the elements, and "the ability to assume animal forms" (1990: 320) to the shaman's initiation through dismemberment, death, and resurrection; his ability to become invisible, fly, and cure people; his mastery over fire; and his ability to assume the form of animals. Beyond this, Yoga and shamanism are concerned with a kind of power that is both natural and supernatural, human and nonhuman. Recognizing the problems inherent in overgeneralization—one in particular being that such generalizations become meaningless—there is some sense in which the "shamanic complex"—including Yoga—defines a kind of truth that is universal on a cosmic scale, rather than definitive of truth on a scale that is configured by the global diffusion of cultural traits manifest as different from one another—but only relatively so—the more they have become disconnected by movement across space and through time.

All claims to Universal Truth that purport to transcend the domain of culture are seductive. But because these claims always emerge from situated social and time-bound knowledge they are, in many ways, based on a profound contradiction. Social science is designed to study the manifestations of this contradiction on different levels, and in different forms, by coming to understand all knowledge as a social construct. However, the unself-consciousness of claims to Universal Truth found in religion and science are of particular interest as forms of knowledge, because they provide a means by which to engage in critical social analysis on a scale that extends beyond situated knowledge and the cultural form of any given construction.[23]

Although similar to science and religion in this respect, Yoga is somewhat unique. It claims to articulate a kind of truth based on universal laws that extend "beyond" nature and beyond the attribution of power to God. Yet the experience of these laws through the medium of the embodied self is extremely "personal" and therefore "local" on a subcultural, purely experiential level. To be sure, every *guru* has a name—Vivekananda, Sri Aurobindo, Madhavdas, Swami Kuvalayananda, Rajarshi Muni, Swami Sivananda, Yogeshwaranand, Swami Rama, Shri Yogendra, Swami Shanti Swaroop—and emerges out of, and usually works within, a social environment. But from the vantage point of ethnographic engagement with "the native's point of view" it is significant that there is no cultural context for making sense of what he or she knows. What he or she really "knows" transcends consciousness and only gets imperfectly reflected in what gets said and done. In a sense the absence of either God or an ontology grounded in materialism—and the fact that *paramātman* is singularly insulated from cultural manipulation and defined in terms that are "beyond" monotheism, polytheism, spirituality, and mysticism—makes it much more difficult to establish the epistemic basis for a social analysis of Yoga than is the case with a social analysis of either religion or science. To be sure, one can undertake a study of Swami Rama and the Maharishi Mahesh Yogi by locating them and their practice in a cultural context. The 1960s counterculture movement comes to mind as one possible context. One can make sense of Swami Sivananda with reference to the cultural context of institutionalized Hinduism in the 1930s and 1940s. As indicated in the body of this book, defining the sociohistorical and cultural context of practice is a necessary point of departure. But Yoga as such stands in a more interesting relationship to "the social" than can be understood within the framework of any given *guru*'s career, or within, and in relationship to, the institution of embodied enlightenment.

Although "coded" to human intelligence and human ways of knowing, Yoga is, in fact, an inclusive philosophy of Life—with a capital "L"—that extends beyond the range of what counts as human. *Saṃsāric* rebirth signals the intimate connection between all living organisms, even though this "intimacy" is regarded as very hierarchical. It is precisely this that Yoga is designed to transcend. Life is an experience of suffering, where suffering defines an ontological plane on par with what are regarded as natural laws in the domain of physics. Nevertheless, what is of critical importance is the way in which Patañjali and his redactors, from Vyāsa up to Taimni, Iyengar, and Whicher, have conceptualized Yoga—correctly, I think, and resiliently against the trend of several thousand years of religious thinking—as the transcendence of Life itself, rather than in much more limited terms as the salvation of humankind as a distinct category of living being: a beast with cultural credentials. There is no agency in Yoga other than that of *ātman*. There is no theology. No ritual. Gods are disembodied and therefore powerless. The possibility of transcendence is dependent on Life itself, as Life is experienced through the body by a person who practices Yoga. If religion is the fetishization of society, Yoga is the fetishization of being. If the festishization of society made modern sociology as such possible, then a consideration of Yoga's relationship to being should enable a new kind of anthropology.

In many respects everything hinges on the shift from singular to plural, and the way in which Yoga reveals the contingency of all plurality in relation to the singularity of being. As an object of social analysis, this singularity of being translates all too easily into a kind of generic universalism that is manifest as human nature. Sociobiology has fallen deeply, fatally, and dangerously into this trap. But if the singularity of being is understood mimetically as the fetishization of Life, then explaining the singularity of plurality—this religion in the context of all other religions, this expression of genocide in relation to all other cases of genocide—no longer need structure the epistemology of social science. Instead one must look at the fundamental disarticulation between a singularity and its plural forms. The simple contradiction that language enables communication, but that languages do not, produces a singularly skeptical perspective on human nature wherein the self-evident significance of language to culture comes into question. This can be extended from the domain of communication to that of value.

Violence and the desire to be in control and dominate others characterize our species. However, equality—or the desire for there to be equality—can be said to be the basis of our collective humanity. By using the term "equality" I mean to evoke the final goal of an ethical position. But as a rudimentary, proto-moral concept, equality is based on the recognition of sameness rather than difference. And this is where to begin. The idea of sameness is, on a fundamental level, linked to ideals of peace and nonviolence. But our common humanity—our species-specific sameness—also defines, rather precisely, the range and scope of "meaningful" violence.

Quite apart from what it means and whether it is justified, the will to control and dominate other people through violence "makes sense" as a cultural concept. But the species-specific sameness that defines violence as meaningful—that on some level, for brother to kill brother can be made to make sense—also produces categorical differences that are understood as para-cultural, and these differences make us—animal organisms—seem fundamentally and unself-consciously different from all other living things. This para-cultural difference has become so profound that in many cases violence is not recognized as violence at all. It "makes sense" for the state to kill a man accused of murder, although it is called execution. As every anthropology textbook makes quite clear, you can "make sense" of genocide. But no one thinks that it makes sense to speak of pesticides as weapons of mass destruction or to speak of their everyday use in golf courses, gardens, and the industrialized fields of modern agriculture as mass murder. Consider the logical absurdity of thinking about water purification—which involves the planned killing of trillions and trillions of micro-organisms—as the destruction of lives not worth living.

What makes us human—a beastly being with culture—is what makes us fundamentally unlike other living things. Or, rather, this is what we have made of ourselves. It is what we seek to remake, with a vengeance, in the domain of religion and also, most certainly, in the domain of anthropology. There is a whole history of savagery in that distinction—a key distinction in the history of culture and the development of civilization, only part of which is reproduced in the history of racism and genocidal violence, or even in the legitimized violence of the state. In this light moral progress and the development of a humanitarian ideal called equality, among other logical outcomes of the Enlightenment, are, in their artifactual—and artifactually inclusive—plurality, a species of violence. The cultural conquest of our animal "instinct"—the ongoing search for meaning in terms that are human—is, in this sense, to reproduce the structural relationship between good and evil.

Yoga is not unique in its advocacy for nonviolence. But it is unique in recognizing that for nonviolence to have any significance it must extend to all manifestations of Life, and that this extension must be materialized and experienced as dispassion. It must encompass human action but neither begin nor end with human beings, where its expression is always compromised. In this sense a consideration of Yoga makes it possible to think around the "problem" of equality-and-inequality—which is a relationship of intimate relativism—to a consideration of what makes us human in relation to all expressions and experiences of life.

When done from the perspective of dislocated mimetic skepticism, anthropology is not concerned with the interpretation of constructed reality. It must proceed as an experimental argument with reality—as an engagement with the very real and serious possibility that nothing is as it seems. This requires belief in disbelief—the shamanic-like power "to become any Other and engage the image with the reality thus imagized" (Taussig 1993b: 255)—rather than the temporary, and therefore somewhat disingenuous, suspension of belief. From this vantage point textbook examples of genocide, slavery, female circumcision, and foot binding are, in a sense, not so much examples of why relativism is either methodologically necessary or morally untenable, as examples of the fetishization of mimetic excess and the illusion created, thereby, that there are categorical truths about human nature. Genocide cannot be explained on its own terms, no matter how broadly or flexibly defined those terms are—for what are they?—or explained away in terms of reason. It is but one of the most spectacularly meaningless and horrifically nonsensical forms of human engagement. But, as such, it is not opposite to anything at all, and—as Kṛṣṇa tried to explain to Arjun—that which is horrifically nonsensical is thereby not categorically evil in relation to some ideal that is not nonsensical. To understand and do justice to the experience of being human requires that compassion, for example, be regarded with the same attitude of skepticism as might be directed, with greater ease and easier rationalization, at the "cultural context" for any given expression of hatred. In this light a perspective on human experience is gained by understanding the "dependent erasure" of life and death. This, in some sense, is *samādhi.*

To argue with reality requires a different kind of empathy than the inherently humanistic, liberal attitude that is the bedrock of most anthropology. Instead of building rapport one must engage with the means by which people engage in their own mimetic reproduction. This kind of anarchy of the will, or belief in disbelief, enables historical representation through a strategic dissimulation of the present. Conversely it enables ethnographic representation through a strategic dissimulation of the past. Perversely, to once again invoke Quine's sentiment of recursive translation—as well as the attitude of the Pāśupatas—an anarchy of the will allows for the dissimulation of dissimulation. If done artfully, this is a kind of magically mythological truth telling. If there is a question of ethics here—as there must, for that is what is at stake in the debate on relativism—it is a question of finding the means by which to represent the present's historicity without reproducing the present in terms of historicism. And the politics of this ethics is in *every* act of representation and engagement with the world, not just in those situations where justice and human rights seem to be most directly at stake.

While the perspective taken here might appear, in many ways, to be the antithesis of what Nancy Scheper-Hughes has called an ethically grounded militant anthropology (1995), that is not what is intended. In defining what she means by "the primacy of the ethical" in a politically engaged anthropology, Scheper-Hughes refers to a set of standards that are directly linked to, and presuppose, the presence of others and one's engagement with them. She speaks of the standards of responsibility, accountability, and answerability to "the other"—on either a global or a more personal level—as "precultural" in the sense that these standards are what make culture take shape, rather than what emerge out of cultural experience. It is noteworthy that Scheper-Hughes roots an argument that admonishes anthropologists to actively and assertively make distinctions between what is right and what is wrong in Emmanuel Levinas's philosophy of meaning and sense (1987). She follows Levinas in saying that ethics are logically prior to, or more primary than, culture, because ethics presuppose all meaning (1995: 419). The fact of mortality—a characteristic we share with all living organisms—does not distinguish us as human, and so our consciousness of mortality should enable an ethics of being.

Scheper-Hughes takes this in the direction of a firmly grounded militant anthropology anchored in a "womanly" ethic of care and responsibility, and then brings it back as a powerful critique of cultural forms. In doing so, however, the implied critique of culture as such is incomplete. Another direction to go, as I am suggesting here, is not opposite to this, but simply to more trenchantly question the condition of our humanity on the basis of an ethics of care and responsibility that might extend beyond cultural forms. To use Scheper-Hughes's own apt phrasing, this requires politically engaged anthropology to "flirt" more explicitly, if still ironically, with the sociobiology toward which her analysis "dangerously veers" (1995: 419). To be an ethically responsible anthropologist, a "witness accountable to history," entails a recognition that all action is political, that action produces history as it is intended to change the future, and that actions reflect the artifactuality of history as much as they reflect the cultural forms and social facts of justice and injustice, violence and nonviolence. Consequently, no matter how "confusing" and "wearisome"—the terms are Scheper-Hughes's—it is necessary to continue to engage with the so-called postmodern critique of representation. To do so is not to discover, through empathy and respect, that what we share with "others" is some basic sense of being human, but that being human is, perhaps, a limited framework for sense making. But this perspective must be achieved, as I think Scheper-Hughes would agree, through a kind of empathy and respect for life itself as a transhistoric precultural principle.

The concept of culture creates the problem of relativism. Therefore it is not surprising that the condition of being human beyond culture begs the question of where, why, and how the line is drawn between our own and other species.[24] This is not so much an evolutionary question as it is a question of radically inclusive animal rights. It is, therefore, also a profoundly ethical question implicated in the politics of knowledge. As such it is an exercise in extending the logic of mimetic skepticism back into the fetishistic structure of the most basic of basic social facts in which "the signifier depends upon yet erases its signification" (Taussig 1993a: 225).

Along these lines—and to return directly to a point raised in the introduction—Donna Haraway's critical feminism provides a useful perspective. She poses the question of what it is to be human in radical terms by showing that, in many instances, the very embodied state of the species is not predefined:

> By the late twentieth century in United States scientific culture, the boundary between human and animal is thoroughly breached. The last beachheads of uniqueness have been polluted if not turned into amusement parks—language, tool use, social behavior, mental events, nothing really convincingly settles the separation of human and animal. . . . Movements for animal rights are not irrational denials of human uniqueness; they are a clear-sighted recognition of connection across the discredited breach of nature and culture. (1991: 152)

Our beings are increasingly constituted of the bits and pieces of other organisms and inorganic material. We are all, to a degree, cyborgs—

recombinant inorganic organisms. In this Haraway sees the potential for a radical politics of being that is not limited to, or by, the all too human features of individual agency or straightforward oppositional struggle.[25] It seems to me that the figure of the human-but-not-human cyborg incarnates a form of mimetic excess that goes beyond race, ethnicity, gender, and class. With the aid of artificial prosthetic technology it defines human justice in organismic terms.[26] The cyborg rewrites history by writing against nature. And so in seeing animal rights as human rights one can engage with the manifest fetishism of nature in culture. To get a fix on this it is useful to entertain the possibility, as Haraway does, that animal sociology is human sociology. Not because there is any truth in sociobiology, but because speciocentric social science seeks to define the truth of life exclusively on its own terms. With this in mind I would agree with Haraway's characterization of a critically skeptical animal sociology as having radical potential, provided we count ourselves and our "fettered souls" as being among "all God's creatures."[27]

> We need to understand how and why animal groups have been used in theories of the evolutionary origin of human beings, of "mental illness," of the natural basis of cultural co-operation and competition, of language and other forms of communication, of technology, and especially of the origin and role of human forms of sex and the family. In short we need to know the animal science of the body politic as it has been and might be. I believe the result of a liberating science of animal groups would better express who the animals are as well; we might free nature in freeing ourselves. (1991: 12)

The idea of freeing nature in freeing ourselves is a radical idea that resonates with the most basic principle of Yoga. In many respects a cyborg is the embodied form of yogic practice—a kind of *jīvanmukta* as everyman. Both the yogi and the cyborg are the embodiment of mimesis and, as such, manifest profound and powerful contradictions: in Yoga experience is ignorance, but ignorance is integral to the realization of truth. In the body of the cyborg—and in the social relations produced as cyborgs engage with one another—there is both singularity and endless plurality. Focused on the present, Haraway's critically inclusive cyborg sociology seeks to liberate thought and political action from the recursive opposition of good set against evil. It does this by locating human existence in a space where nature and culture mimetically constitute a singular whole that is absolute in its inclusive, precultural singularity.

The specific relevance of this here should be unambiguous, since in most general terms anthropology has been directly concerned with, and implicated in, the relationship between nature and culture. The question of language is thought to mark, albeit with increasing ambiguity, the border between humans and nonhumans. Arguably the whole purpose of biological anthropology is to explore the evolutionary relationship between human and nonhuman species, both now and in the distant past. As recorded in popular publications and in some of the most widely read and cited professional journals, paleoarchaeology has its sights set on that illusive point in time when, with the invention of tool use and bipedalism, our species began to chart its own course "out" of nature and "into" culture. Having moved well beyond thinking in terms of evolutionary stages, social and cultural anthropology is, nevertheless, concerned with an interpretation of the complexity of human life, as this complexity is an indication of progress and development beyond the limits of our instinctive nature.

In all of this—this Anthropology with a big "A"—the figure of the animal shadows the development of a holistic science of humankind. The danger is to think of the shadow animal as a thing apart, rather than as integral to the mimetic structure of knowledge. The danger, manifest in racism, ethnic violence, sexism, and other situations that reveal the problematic of relativism, is in defining an ethics of life from the vantage point of humanism, if the term "humanism" may be used pejoratively as cognate with other "isms." Following Haraway's characterization of our cyborg selves and society, perhaps the question is not where and when that line is drawn between hominid and hominoid—animal and human—but what the implications are of founding a whole science predicated on that distinction. In most general terms, mimetic skepticism enables a further study of these implications.

How then to finally conclude, since final, definitive conclusions are meaningless? I must confess that relativism escaped me and I burst into uncontrolled laughter when I first saw a blurry, poorly reproduced photograph of Dr. Udupa's headstanding rats. Their furry bodies stuffed in glass tubes struck me as absurd and ridiculous; the antithesis of Yoga conceived of on any terms, by any stretch of the imagination, by anyone. But as I began to laugh, I also began to think, and to think not so much systematically but with sudden insight—insight of the kind that is based on uninformed general knowledge about the way in which so much science, both purely abstract and medically applied, military and commercial, chemical, biological, psychological, and astronomical (remember the chimp in the space capsule), is dependent on animal experimentation. The proverbial—and now stereotypically comical—rats in the maze are but an archetype for a whole ideology of science based on the mimesis of proxy, analogy, and metaphor: one organism refracted in another, the human reflected in the nonhuman.

After I stopped laughing, and also after I stopped thinking with the pure insight of general knowledge, I began to think backward from the headstanding rats to other rats in other laboratories and to a whole history—or a possible history—of rats and other animals, insects, organisms, and even bacteria. Once you start—into the chain of life, that is—there is no basis upon which to draw a line. Therefore Dr. Udupa's experiment is perfectly enlightening, as perfectly enlightening as the very first experiment conducted by humans on a nonhuman being—perhaps when a hapless dog, rather than somone's brother, was sent into a cave after a wounded bear—and no more or less funny or serious than the transplantation of a baboon heart into the chest of a human child. Whatever the experiment on headstanding rats was designed to show is insignificant and meaningless, except as it slips into the past and comes to constitute, in relation to other things, a fragment of Yoga's history as science. The headstanding rats are, in many ways, the shadow form of the sage lost in the Himalayas. Each makes the other possible, and in some sense they are, with reference to the past, the same—at least in terms of value. The fragmentation of meaning here is so complete that the work of reproduction—which is the fetishization of the fetish, rather than a conclusive project—will be to articulate an ethics of life that is true to nature insofar as it recognizes untruth as a condition of being human. As the author of the *Haṭhayogapradīpikā* concludes: "As long as the *Prāṇa* does not enter the flow in the middle channel and the *vindu* does not become firm by the control of the movements of the *Prāṇa;* as long as the mind does not assume the form of Brahma without any effort in contemplation, so long all the talk of knowledge and wisdom is merely the nonsensical babbling of a mad man" (IV: 113; Pancham Sinh's translation). To understand history and the history of the present one must not interpret this babbling and make sense of it, but take it seriously as babbling—babbling that obscures a perspective on Transcendent Truth, to be sure, but babbling that enables an understanding of the past, and the past's significance for the present.

NOTES

CHAPTER 1
HISTORICIZING YOGA: THE LIFE AND TIMES OF LIBERATED SOULS

1. There are numerous translations and commentaries on the *Yoga Sūtra*. In many ways the most interesting in the context of this study is B.K.S. Iyengar's *Light on the Yoga-Sūtras of Patañjali* (1993). With regard to academic works, Ian Whicher's *The Integrity of the Yoga Darśana,* though not restricted to the *Yoga Sūtra,* is extremely thorough, and situates Yoga within the context of contemporary South Asian scholarship (1998). Barbara Stoler Miller's *Yoga: Discipline of Freedom* (1996) is also a recent, comprehensive work of scholarship.

2. Clearly the key ideas in Yoga developed much earlier than this, particularly in the so-called Upaniṣadic Age (1500–1000 B.C.E.) when nescient ideas reflected in the Vedic literature (4500–2500 B.C.E.) were elaborated and refined, most significantly—at least with respect to Yoga—the ideals of world renunciation and the internalization of sacrifice. The earliest text that is explicitly "yogic" is the *Bhagavad Gītā,* which was composed in the Epic Age (1000–100 B.C.E) and is found in one of the most important texts of this period, the *Mahābhārata.*

3. Although the term "ecstasy" conveys the nature of the experience, Eliade points out that *samādhi* is an "enstatic" experience. The Greek root focuses on an external experience, whereas the orientation of the Sanskrit term is internal, though by no means personal, egocentric, or individualized.

4. Clearly commentary and textual redaction did not end when this shift took place, and there have probably been more purely textual commentaries produced since the nineteenth century than were produced before. However, it can be referred to as a paradigmatic shift insofar as it allows for what might be called meta-scholarship: the study of Yoga *through* the study of those who practice Yoga rather than just the study *of* Yoga by a yogi.

5. Sarah Strauss deals with this issue in more detail in her doctoral dissertation (1997), and points out the importance of Eliade's relationship with Dasgupta in the context of his interactions with Swami Sivananda in Rishikesh in 1929 (2000: 172).

6. To fully appreciate Eliade's interest in Yoga as well as the impact that his scholarship has had on subsequent research, it is important to note that he wrote extensively on both shamanism (1964) and alchemy (1938). It is possible to visualize Eliade's research as being concerned with the way in which embodied practice cross-cuts and unites shamanism, alchemy, and Yoga.

7. The global form of transnational Yoga is clearly a subject that deserves more careful study. The topic alone contains some of the most fantastic examples of transnational transmutation and the blurring of consumerism, holistic health, and embodied mysticism—as well as good old-fashioned Orientalism. After having read this book, readers might buy a copy of the *Yoga Journal* and also glance

at the products that can be purchased from a Gaiam *Inner Balance* catalogue. In the latter the following video and CD set is advertised as marked down from $45 to $40:

> NEW! GUIDE TO INTIMACY AND LOVING. Discover an art of loving that will forever transform lovemaking into a truly intimate, fulfilling and spiritual experience. *The Secrets of Sacred Sex* will teach you how to awaken your own natural sexual energy and experience a deeper level of connectedness with your love partner. Six engaging, real-life couples share and demonstrate over 20 magical Tantric lovemaking methods adapted for Western lovers. For adults only. (www.gaiam.com)

If nothing else, this book will help to define a possible starting point for a history of *The Secrets of Sacred Sex* and other such products.

8. Magical flight and levitation are probably among the most commonly envisioned magical powers associated with Yoga. The shaman's ability to fly and journey through time and space is explicitly embodied in this dimension of practice. In the classical literature, *laghava*—a term etymologically linked to levitation—is an experience of lightness achieved through *prāṇāyāma* breathing. As indicated in the *Tattva Vaiśāradī,* the lightness of being can also be felt by rubbing the sweat of intensive *prāṇāyāma* into the skin, in a kind of grossly mechanical reversal of flow (Feuerstein 1990: 193). Wrestlers in India rub sweat into their skin and explain that it produces a sensation of lightness. *Laghiman* denotes levitation, which is one of the eight primary magical powers.

9. Although this is obviously a kind of structured mimesis of levitation, it is interesting to note that Theos Bernard, one of the first people to write an account of the experiences associated with yogic practice (1944), points out that one of the sensations associated with deep *prāṇāyāma* is the sensation of hopping like a frog.

10. This was during the border conflict between India and Pakistan in the area of Kargil in 1998, and there was a degree of anxiety in some of the media about the possibility of war, and a high degree of jingoistic bravado in other media about the same possibility. Regardless, the idea of a "National Shield" was elaborated on Veda Vision with references to the war tactics and strategy described in the *Mahābhārata.*

11. Swami Sivananda, along with B.K.S. Iyengar, is probably most directly responsible for the phenomenal popularity of Yoga worldwide. Sarah Strauss has conducted a comprehensive study of the Divine Life Society, focusing on Yoga as part of a broader lifestyle of holistic health (1997, 2000). Many of the points she makes resonate with some of the points made here. Beyond references to some of the books written by Sivananda and his various disciples, no attempt has been made in this book to analyze Sivananda or focus on what Strauss refers to as a "transnational community of practice" based on his particular style of Yoga.

12. As a powerful trope, the sage lost in the Himalayas has become fixed in the cultural imagination of Europe and North America—and perhaps parts of Latin America, where Yoga has become very popular, largely through the influence of Indra Devi—as an index of Eastern spirituality and mysticism. It epitomizes, in

a curious way, a kind of frontier colonial ethos of self-motivated discovery, merged with and motivated by the "impenetrable mystery" of the East. In most general terms, the motif of the Himalayan sage became a central feature of the neo-Orientalism manifest in the late 1960s and early 1970s counterculture hippie movement.

13. The driving force behind the power of this motif is the spoken about but never to be revealed secret of Truth. Yoga has a vested interest in keeping this secret, but also in being able to talk about it, and reveal it—or hint about the possibility of doing so—endlessly. It is also important to note that there is a degree of congruity here between the sage and the shaman, for the spoken about but never revealed secret factors directly into the shaman's power as well, as Lévi-Strauss famously pointed out (1963) with reference to the case of Quesalid on the Northwest frontier of the United States.

14. The literature on—or related to—Sāṃkhya is, of course, extensive. I have found Larson (1969) and Larson and Bhattacharya (1987) to be most useful.

15. By far the most comprehensive and best review of the literature on alchemy and Haṭha Yoga is the chapter "Sources for the History of Tantric Alchemy" in David White's *The Alchemical Body* (1996: 78–122).

16. Sjoman's analysis is interesting and important for a number of reasons that will be taken up in this study. Here, however, the key point is the way in which his research directs attention to the need to find and analyze modern texts dating to the earliest period of modernity, as quite distinct from texts of greater antiquity that are simply reproduced during this time. To find and analyze these texts will help to clarify a key process in the history of Yoga's modern concern with health and physical fitness.

17. Jean Varenne has similarly criticized modern Yoga, calling it nothing so much as "a sort of Swedish drill interspersed with pauses for breathing" (1973: vii).

18. On this point David White's *Tantra in Practice* (2000)—beyond being a detailed study of tantra's spread throughout Asia—provides the best insight into the transmission of knowledge in an intellectual climate that self-ascribed itself as a synthesis of spirituality, philosophy, and technology that was particularly suited to the dark age of the *kāliyug*.

19. Eliade, as one of the most gifted intellectuals of the past century, takes this "problem" as an opportunity, and makes fascinating correlations between breathing in everything from the shamanistic rituals of Central Asia to Christian prayer (1990: 59–65).

20. Beyond these preliminary, thematically oriented remarks, a conscious decision has been made in this study not to engage directly with the writing and practice of B.K.S. Iyengar or his teacher, Krishnamacharya. Quite simply B.K.S. Iyengar's significance to modern Yoga is such that an adequate analysis would involve a separate and comprehensive study (see De Michelis 2001, 2004). Beyond this, Iyengar's practice evolved in the 1950s, *after* the historical period analyzed here and just before the widespread popularity of medicalized self-help Yoga in the 1970s, 1980s, and 1990s. Although Iyengar's influence in India is widespread, the impact of his teaching is even more profound in terms of Yoga's rapid globalization.

It is clearly within a transnational framework that his influence on modern Yoga should be analyzed.

21. Iyengar is not the only one who has developed a system of "forceful" Yoga. Another student of Krishnamacharya, Pittabi Jois, developed what has come to be known as Power Yoga, which has become extremely popular in the context of modern health clubs.

22. It is interesting to contrast Mahatma Gandhi's international reputation in the arena of social reform and political activism with the reputation of Vivekananda and Aurobindo. Whereas Gandhi's life and work inspired many people to produce critical scholarship on his contribution to both Indian and world history, both Vivekananda's and Aurobindo's lives and works are known primarily through the medium of hagiography. There are exceptions, to be sure. (See Jackson 1994; Rambachan 1994; Sen 2000. See also Jeffery Kripal's extraodinary analysis of Ramakrishna [1995], and, by extension, various aspects of Vivekananda's life and teaching.) And there is a vast hagiographical literature on Gandhi as well. But the broad pattern is curious, and does not only reflect the aura of sainthood. It reflects, I think, a degree of post-colonial colonialism in terms of what counts as important and also what needs to be protected—nationalistically—from close scrutiny.

23. The term Rāja Yoga—which means "Royal Yoga," but which Georg Feuerstein renders poetically as "the resplendent Yoga of spiritual kings"—seems to be a product of the sixteenth century. It was devised in order to sharpen the distinction between Haṭha Yoga and Patañjalian Yoga, which some adherents felt was being corrupted through the influence of tantrism and alchemy. However, as Elizabeth De Michelis points out (pers. comm.), it was Vivekananda who redefined Patañjalian ideas through the lens of neo-Vedānta and it is he who is responsible for giving Rāja Yoga its modern character.

24. Shri Yogendra's role in the development of modern medical yoga is as important as that of Swami Kuvalayananda. Their careers ran directly parallel to each other. Both were inspired by the same *guru*, whom they met at almost the same time. Both men changed their names, taking on titles of spiritual masters. Both founded institutes for the scientific study of Yoga, built Yoga clinics, published extensively on the subject of Yoga physiology and physical culture, established teacher-training programs, and promoted the development of Yoga as physical education. Kuvalayananda was more directly engaged with the problem of science and the institutionalization of Yoga as medicine, while Yogendra published more popular books designed as self-help guides to better health.

25. Gandhi's role was in the arena of KarmaYoga—the Yoga of action—most clearly articulated in the *Bhagavad Gītā*. It is important to point out, however, that the nature of action described and discussed in the *Gītā* is not only action that is motivated by purpose, but simply action as a natural fact of life. To live is to act. It is on this plane that the connection between Karma Yoga and Haṭha Yoga is most clearly apparent, since action is based on a sense perception of the world and by the driving force of the "qualities issuing from nature"—that is, the three *guṇa* that are integral to Sāṃkhya.

CHAPTER 2
YOGA AND THE SUPRAMENTAL BEING: MATERIALISM, METAPHYSICS, AND SOCIAL REALITY

1. Along these lines U. A. Asrani points out in *Yoga Unveiled*, part 2, that all yogis should "kindly adopt the scientific verification method" (1993: xii). In the same book, which contains a chapter on "The Scientific Vindication of Vedānta and Jñāna" and a section entitled "Science Teaches Us to Be Humble"—within a chapter called "Self-Realization Is Easy"—he writes: "Teilhard de Chardin—the famous paleontologist and anthropologist—recognized that matter and spirit are not two separate substances but only two distinct aspects of the same substance" (1993: 59).

2. Although it would be directly relevant here to go into a detailed analysis of Sri Aurobindo's Integral Yoga, to do so is beyond the scope of this book. A detailed analysis of Integral Yoga must be the subject of a separate study. Nevertheless, it should be pointed out that in developing a philosophy of *pūrṇa* Yoga, Aurobindo was struggling against what he regarded as the "refusal of asceticism" in much of the classical literature. In other words, he was critical of idealist positions wherein spirit and matter were categorically opposed to each other. As Feuerstein puts it: "Integral Yoga—which is called *pūrṇa* Yoga in Sanskrit—has the explicit purpose of bringing the 'divine consciousness' down into the human body-mind and into ordinary life" (2001: 56). Once brought down into the body-mind, divine consciousness is embodied as the Supermind. In Aurobindo's view, "the Supermind . . . powers evolution, which he understands as a steady progression towards higher forms of consciousness. As such it is also responsible for the manifestation of the human brain-mind. The mind has the innate tendency to go beyond itself and grasp the larger Whole. Yet it is destined to fail in this program as is powerfully driven home by the history of philosophy and science. The most the human mind can do is to recognize its inherent limitations and open up to the higher reality of the Supermind" (2001: 57).

3. Feuerstein provides a translation of the *Amritabindu Upaniṣad* that provides the following perspective: "The two [forms of] knowledge (*vidyā*) to be known are the Sonic Absolute (*śabda brahman*) and that which transcends it. He who is familiar with the Sonic Absolute reaches the supreme Absolute. The sage who, after studying the books, is intent on that [Absolute] through wisdom (*jñāna*) and knowledge (*vijñāna*) should discard all books, even as the husk [is discarded by a person] seeking the grain. There is but a single color for the milk of variously colored cows—thus he looks upon gnosis as on milk, and upon the [numerous] signs (*liṅgin*) as on cows. Knowledge (*vijñāna*) abides hidden in every being, as does butter in milk. By means of the mind as a churning-stick [every] being should constantly churn [this knowledge] within the mind" (2001: 35–36).

4. The principle of five sheaths or envelopes is first mentioned in the *Taittirīya Upaniṣad*, where each sheath is relatively more subtle than the preceding one. Significantly, the most subtle sheath of bliss is, in some sense, conceived of as a material manifestation of liberation. Even though Yoga texts take different positions

on this question, the idea of a hierarchy of sheaths enables the possibility of, and embodied transcendence as, an *ātivāhika deha.*

5. Yogeshwaranand's account of the embodied soul resonates most clearly with the *Taittirīya Upaniṣad* insofar as this early text provides a very visceral account of transcendence. As Feuerstein points out, from the vantage point of this text's author, everything should be regarded as food. He provides the following account of bliss, expressed several millennia ago, which in many ways echoes Yogeshwaranand's anatomically-oriented scientific discourse.

> Oh, wonderful! Oh, wonderful! Oh wonderful
> I am food! I am food! I am food!
> I am the Food-Eater! I am the Food-Eater! I am the Food-Eater!
> . . . .
> I, who am Food, eat the eater of Food!
> I have overcome the whole world!
> [My] effulgence is like the sun
> (3.10.6–7; in Feuerstein 2001: 132)

Here it should also be noted, as Whicher points out, that in the ninth century B.C.E. and earlier there were clear indications of the way in which sacrificial ritualism was being interiorized, and how this interiorization was central to the much later development of Yoga and the idea that the body could be "cooked" to perfection. In this scenario *prāṇa* replaces the sacrificial fire, and food is sacrificed to the internal breath (1998: 13).

6. Feuerstein explains this reflection as the not-quite-satisfactory yogic "solution." provided for the universal philosophical conundrum of how it is possible to know what cannot be known: "Patañjali's metaphysical dualism does not lend itself to such a solution, and yet he tries to overcome the problem by suggesting that there is some kind of connection, which he calls 'correlation' (*saṃyoga*), between the Self and Nature—that is, between pure Awareness and the complex of the body and personality" (2001: 241).

7. For an analysis of the relationship between modern scientific Yoga and the occult literature, as these two representations intersected in the early part of the nineteenth century, see Alter (n.d.b).

8. As reflected in key texts, Sri Aurobindo's (1976, 1977) and Vivekananda's (1962, 1982) teachings on Yoga are of such significance as to require a separate study. As Elizabeth De Michelis has pointed out (pers. comm.; see also 2004), Vivekananda's treatise *Rāja Yoga* is, in many ways, the first articulation of modern Yoga, if not of medicalized modern Yoga as such. It contains many references on anatomy and employs the language of science to make points about spirituality.

9. Elaborating on this point with reference to *Vyāsa-bhāṣya*, *Sāṃkhyakārikā*, and the *Bṛhadyogiyājñavalkyasmṛti*, the Philosophico-Literary Research Department of Kaivalyadhama puts it this way: "This is *mūlaprakṛti*, which is only potentiality of all kinds of change—and changing reality—and is generally known as *pradhāna*. It corresponds to Patañjali's *aliṅga* stage of differentiation in the *guṇas* and is the primeval matter of which *mahat* is the first form. It is not itself the form of any other matter" (1991: 186).

10. It is important to make a distinction here between the position of classical Yoga, which is inherently dualist, and the nondualist idealism of the *Yoga Vāsiṣṭha*. In this text the world and all things other than *citta* are simply a reflection of the Universal Mind. In other words, illusions in this formulation have no meta-material basis; they are simply figments of the imagination (see Feuerstein 2001: 304–5).

11. Significantly, there are two technical terms for this process: *sat-kārya-vāda* and *prakṛti-pariṇāma-vāda*. Although they refer to the same process, they are based on very different understandings of the ontological structure of *prakṛti*. "The former phrase implies that the effect (*kārya*) is preexistent (*sat*) in its cause, whereas the latter phrase signifies that the effect is a real transformation (*pariṇāma*) of Nature, not merely an illusory change (*vivarta*), as is thought in the idealistic schools of Vedānta and Mahāyāna Buddhism" (Feuerstein 2001: 243). It is this struggle between idealism and cosmic materialism that also seems to animate the modern discourse of meta-materialism and supramental beings.

12. The term for error is *viparyaya*, which is closely linked to, if not synonymous with, the term *kleśa*, which means affliction. In some sense ignorance is the most basic attribute of *viparyaya*, and is a term that characterizes all of the five *kleśa*. The delineation and classification of various kinds of ignorance manifest in each of the *kleśa* provide an important framework for thinking about the nature of the attachment of a person to the world in terms of levels of ignorance, ranging from spiritual ignorance to the more basic ignorance manifest in a desire for continuity through time and a fear of death.

13. *Avidyā* is, in essence, to mistake reality for what is really real—to mistake constant change and transformation for stable permanence, impure corrupt things for things that are pure, the painful suffering of existence as pleasurable, and the self for the Self. Elaborating on this, the Philosophico-Literary Research Department of Kaivalyadhama points out that "from the psychological point of view the chief importance of *avidyā* lies in its being the tendency to perceive objects as real and abiding. Whenever a sense organ is stimulated, we perceive a real lasting object, whatever the metaphysical status of the object may be" (1991: 41).

14. As reflected even in the *Yoga Sūtra*, the meta-material—rather than metaphysical—nature of this pure and perfect state cannot be emphasized enough in the context of trying to understand how a supramental being comes into being. As Feuerstein puts it: "The Undifferentiate is the transcendental core of Nature, which is pure potentiality. It is without any 'mark' (*liṅga*), or identifiable characteristic. It simply *is*. Although Patañjali does not state so explicitly, the Undifferentiate is the perfect balance of the three types of *guṇa*s" (2001: 244).

15. In this sense the *guṇa* are regarded as degrees or relative "frequencies" of movement and vibration. According to the *Varahopaniṣad*, however, the *guṇa* are believed to be three of the ninety-six *tattva*. "And according to *Gorakṣa*, they are the *prakṛti* with which *puruṣa* have *saṃyoga*. He thinks that the *kuṇḍalinī* when aroused raises upwards and the yogi is conscious of it on account of *prajivaguṇa*" (Philosophico-Literary Research Department, Kaivalyadhama 1991: 105).

16. There are a number of quite different calculations of this. For example, according to the *Varahopaniṣad* there are twenty-four *tattva*s: ten *indriya*s, five

prāṇas, five *viṣayas*, and four *antaḥkaraṇas*. This text also enumerates ninety-six. The *Brahmavidhyopaniṣad* lists fifty-one derivatives of *tattva*. In classical Sāṃkhya, however, there are twenty-four. In any case, as Georg Feuerstein notes, *tattva*, deriving from the root *tat*—meaning "that"—"can denote either Reality or a category of cosmic existence." This paradox of the manifold in the singular is expressed in the *Śivasaṃhitā* (II:54) as "when all *tattvas* have disappeared, then the *tattva* itself becomes manifest" (1990: 367). The intimate, synonymous nature of cosmic and material form is significant.

17. Here is Taimni's commentary on *sūtra* I:2:

> While *citta* may be considered as a universal medium through which consciousness functions on all the planes of the manifested Universe, the 'mind' of modern psychology is confined to the expression of only thought, volition and feeling.
>
> We should not, however, make the mistake of imagining *Citta* as a sort of material medium which is moulded into different forms when mental images of different kinds are produced. It is fundamentally of the nature of consciousness which is immaterial but affected by matter. In fact it may be called a product of both, consciousness and matter, or *Puruṣa* and *Prakṛti*, the presence of both being necessary for its functioning. (1961: 8)

18. S. K. Ramachandra Rao seems to recognize this in his concern to be clear and definitive: "Usually translated as 'vital air', 'life', 'body wind', 'respiration', 'breath' etc. [*prāṇa*] is in no sense identical with or an evolutionary product of air [*vāyu*], as it came to mean in later Indian thought. In the Sāṃkhya school, on which the basic ideas of Indian medicine are based, it is a bio-motor force, principally the action of the sense organs" (1987: 167).

19. Georg Feuerstein, who is one of a very few who have successfully walked the razor's edge between the practice of Yoga and the practice of academic scholarship, also often resorts to a discourse of hard science, though, I think, purely as metaphor: "Thus the *prāṇa* is used to stir the dormant *kuṇḍalinī* energy into action. The situation is analogous to bombarding the atomic nucleaus with high-energy particles, which destabilizes the atom and leads to a release of tremendous energy" (2001: 356).

20. U. A. Asrani describes various different degrees of *samādhi* in terms of the amplitude of brain waves, pointing out, in terms of Modern Science, what is referred to as unsupported *samādhi* in the science of Yoga: "[In] *Asamprjñāta samādhi* thoughts, emotions and the ego are left far behind; even pin pricks are not felt. The Electro-encephalograph, which records the micro-voltages constantly working in the brain called Alpha waves [shows that in] *Asamprjñāta samādhi* . . . no waves come out of the brain at all, as in the state just before death" (1993: 87).

21. According to Feuerstein, *prāṇa-dhāraṇā*, the concentration of the life force, is a technical means of projecting *prāṇa* to specific organs in order to restore health. However, in making this claim he cites the *Triśikhi Brahmana Upaniṣad* (II: 109), in which the claim seems to be rather vague, in the sense that the technique "conquers illness" (1990: 266).

CHAPTER 3
SWAMI KUVALAYANANDA: SCIENCE, YOGA, AND GLOBAL MODERNITY

1. For the profound significance of piercing as a materialized metaphor in the practice of Yoga, see David White's *The Alchemical Body* (1996: 303–34). As he puts it: "The same term, *vedha,* is employed in (1) a form of tantric initiation involving a transmission of vital fluids from teacher to disciple, (2) the haṭhayogic piercing of the *cakra*s as well as in a particular technique (called *mahāvedha,* the 'great penetration') employed to that end, and (3) the alchemical transmutation of base metals into gold" (1996: 303).

2. The idea of *jīvanmukti* has inspired a number of thinkers to imagine how this principle might provide the basis for moral and ethically based social reform. Perhaps the most clearly inspired by this ideal, and also by the embodied nature of the ideal, was Mahatmạ Gandhi. In this context, however, social reform is not so much the issue as is the body itself, and the embodiment of multiplicity and variation into the singularity of universal experience. Here it is worth keeping in mind how a *jīvanmukta* is described in the *Bhagavad Gītā:* "[He whose] mind is unagitated in suffering (*duḥkha*), devoid of longing during pleasure (*sukha*), and free from passion (*rāga*), fear (*bhaya*), and anger (*krodha*)—he is called a sage (*muni*) steadied in the vision [of the Self]" (II.56f.; Feuerstein's translation [1990: 156]).

3. Aside from postures as such, Haṭha Yoga includes a number of locks (*bandha*s) and seals (*mudrā*s). The *Gheraṇḍasaṁhitā* enumerates twenty-six. These locks and seals are of primary importance with respect to the channeled flow of *prāṇa* and the elixir of immortality that is said to pervade the body once the energy of *kuṇḍalinī* has penetrated the *Sahasrāracakra.* As Feuerstein puts it: "The locks (*bandha*) are special bodily maneuvers that are designed to confine the life force within the trunk and thereby stimulate it" (2001: 395).

4. It is a fact of some interest that Bell and Meltzer had conducted their experiments on a man by the name of Manibhai Haribhai Desai who, as Shri Yogendra, founded the Yoga Institute in the early 1920s (see chapter 5, note 22). The historical significance of the Yoga Institute is probably equal to that of Kaivalyadhamạ, but more in terms of popularization than with regard to science and medicalization as such. Here it is important to point out, however, that in disproving Bell and Meltzer's findings, Kuvalayananda was also, most likely, extending his contentious and competitive relationship with Yogendra away from a context in which they were both simply the disciples of the same *guru* and into the more global field of laboratory research.

5. As Eliade points out, the different texts enumerate different numbers of "important" or central *nāḍī*s. The *Śivasaṁhitā* counts ten, as do most texts. In the *Gorakṣa Śataka* fourteen are mentioned, and are said to terminate at the body's thirteen orifices and in the *brahmarandhra* (1990: 237).

6. Here Taimni's commentary on 2:43 of the *Yoga Sūtra* provides some insight: "It is the presence of impurity in the body and lack of control which stands in the way of its being used as a perfect instrument of consciousness. The function of the sense organs also becomes perfect because this function is really dependent upon

the currents of *Prāṇa* which are brought under the control of the *Yogi* by practices like those of *Prāṇāyāma*" (1961: 249).

7. It is noteworthy that there are deeper and deeper levels of consciousness, rather than a simple opposition of consciousness and unconsciousness or even consciousness and transcendental consciousness. The idea of bottomless or endless depths allows for the kind of shading of one kind of empirical reality into another. Along these lines Feuerstein makes reference to quantum physics to explain how a view such as this reflects a different understanding of nature: "The British physicist Harold Schilling has proposed that we look upon reality as 'a cybernetic network of circuits . . . more like a delicate fabric than an edifice of brick and mortar' [1973: 113]. But it is a network that has 'interior depth.' In fact, when we look at the inner hierarchy of reality, we perceive, as Schilling put it, 'depth within depth within depth'—an ultimately unfathomable, mysterious well of existence" (2001: 348–50).

CHAPTER 4
BIRTH OF THE ANTI-CLINIC: NATUROPATHIC YOGA IN A POST-GANDHIAN, POSTCOLONIAL STATE

1. Bradley (2002) makes the important point that hydrotherapy—and most likely other so-called marginal therapies—was practiced by mainstream "orthodox" physicians, and that it is problematic to make a sharp, binary distinction between orthodox and nonorthodox regimens of health (see also Grierson 1998; Ward 1994). Nevertheless, advocates of Nature Cure were profoundly critical of "orthodox" biomedicine, even though it is highly likely that some biomedical physicians integrated various Nature Cure therapies into their practice, especially in the early part of the nineteenth century.

2. As a point of comparison it should be noted that Homeopathy is also very popular in India, and came to India approximately thirty or forty years before Nature Cure (Arnold and Sarkar 2002). In this context it may be noted that neither Nature Cure nor Homeopathy integrated very well with Āyurveda, for a range of different reasons. Apart from being "alternative" systems of medicine, they are quite different from one another in both theory and practice. Because of this, a more systematic comparison of Nature Cure and Homeopathy in twentieth-century India would provide important insight into complex processes of "modernization" that refuse to be neatly slotted into the standard dichotomization of elite/subaltern, indigenous/foreign, colonizer/colonized, orthodox/alternative, and so on.

3. The Central Council for Research in Yoga and Naturopathy (CCRYN) was established as one of four councils under India's Union Ministry of Health and Family Welfare once the Central Council for Research in Indian Medicine and Homeopathy, which had been established in 1969, was disbanded in 1978. The CCRYN has no infrastructure for research, training, and medical care but serves as a funding body and proxy regulating agency for NGOs and academic institutions involved in the medical application of Yoga and Nature Cure. In 1997, the year for which published records are available, the CCRYN was funding seventeen

organizations involved primarily in Yoga research and twenty-one doing clinical research on Nature Cure. It also supported nine centers where one-year diploma courses are offered, two treatment-cum-propagation centers, eleven ten-bedded hospitals, and eight five-bedded institutions (1996). Funding was also provided to three institutions offering 5½-Year bachelor of naturopathy and Yogic science degrees. Beyond this, the report lists the following institutions that have active programs in the field of Nature Cure/Yoga:

Shivananda Math and Yogashram Sangha, Guwahati, Assam and Calcutta, West Bengal
Yoga Research Institute, Patmatlanka, Vijayawada, Andhra Pradesh
S. V. Institute of Yoga and Allied Sciences, Tirupati
Government Ayurvedic Hospital, Jammu, Kashmir
Government Yogic Treatment-cum-Research Center, Bapu Nagar, Rajasthan
Institute of Medical Sciences, Banaras Hindu University, Varanasi, Uttar Pradesh
Swami Dayananda Shiksha Yoga Ayurvigyan Sansthan, Fategarh, Uttar Pradesh
G. B. Pant Hospital, New Delhi
Vemana Yoga Research Institute, Secunderbad, Andhra Pradesh
All India Institute of Medical Sciences, New Delhi
Vivekananda Kendra, Yoga Research Foundation, Bangalore
National Institute of Mental Health and Neurosciences, Bangalore
Sri Choday Apparao Prakritik Chikisalayam, Pitampuram Road, Kakinada, Andhra Pradesh
Kakatiya Nature Cure Hospital, Warangal, Andhra Pradesh
Prakritik Chikitsalayam, Gandhighar, Vijaywada, Andhra Pradesh
Kasturba Nature Cure Hospital, Hyderabad, Andhra Pradesh
Nature Cure Hospital, Deoghar, Jasidhi, Bihar
Prakritik Arogyashram, Rajgir, Nalanda, Bihar
Institute of Natural Hygiene, Jammu
Shantikuti Prakritik Chikisalaya, Gopuri, Wardha, Maharashtra
Kamla Arogya Mandi, Yeotmal, Maharashtra
Nature Cure Hospital, Bapu Nagar, Rajasthan
Parmarth Nature Cure and Yoga Center, Rishikesh

4. This is particularly so since, as David Arnold and Sumit Sarkar make clear with reference to the work of a number of historians (Arnold 1993; Harrison 1994; A. Kumar 1998): "One also needs to remember that official Western medicine spread only slowly in India, due in part to the smallness of the medical service, its remoteness from the mass of the population, and the inadequacy of state investment in public health" (2002: 43).

5. Technically the term "Naturopathy" came into being in the twentieth century, and seems to be linked to the institutionalization, popularization, and discursive authorization—since the suffix "pathy" sounds scientific—of Nature Cure.

In India the terms are used interchangeably, although Naturopathy is clearly the more modern term preferred by the state.

6. As will become clear, Nature Cure is now very technology dependent, and its history is in large part defined by the invention of fabulous and ornate machines and complex regimens for the medical administration of natural elements. At base, however, it is always the natural elements that heal, and in some sense this allows for the almost "campy"—and certainly fetishistic—elaboration of more and more high-tech ways for administering sunlight, air, earth and water.

7. Here it is important to point out that Nature Cure/Yoga is not different from biomedicine in terms of its concern with prevention. Those who advocate alternative, holistic medicine often claim that biomedicine is purely reactive, forgetting that immunization, sanitation, nutrition, and many other subfields of public health are based on medical theories of disease causation and risk that are inherently preventative. What is different about biomedicine/biomedical public health and Nature Cure/Yoga is the way in which prevention is reactive and violently defensive in the former and more proactive, integrative, and symbiotic—as well as ecological—in the latter.

8. A close examination of the Nature Cure literature shows how, beneath what seems to be a rhetoric of straightforward pietistic, humanistic holism there is, in fact, a much more radical discourse concerning the way in which the body must conform to nature. Nature functions as a purely rational, ecological system, whereas the "will of man"—so to speak—is influenced by a panoply of irrational impulses and desires, even those that are constructed as rational, such as meat eating and other "normalized" abominations of civilization.

9. As Dominik Wujastyk has pointed out (pers. comm.), an environmental concept of nature as the binary opposite of everything influenced by humankind, including urbanism and agriculture most directly, is alien to Āyurveda and probably also to the philosophy of Sāṃkhya upon which Āyurveda is based. Nevertheless, the principle of *prakṛti,* as elemental nature in the structure of Āyurvedic theory, has come to be regarded as "nature" in the sense that nature is defined by culture as everything that is pure and uncontaminated in the environment. The significance of the principle of *prakṛti* in modern discourses of health is in terms of the confusion of meaning in two rather different kinds of nature, and in the place of these concepts in the structure of medical reasoning and health concerns.

10. Here Dr. Brahmachari seems to be drawing on the principle of *karma,* as *karma* is linked to rebirth. The underlining order of *karma* as "the mechanism by which conditional existence maintains itself" (Feuerstein 1990: 173) presumes that fate depends on and produces profound diversity, but that there is a logical structure to this diversity if it is understood as a process rather than as a permanent condition. One's experience of *saṁsāra* is defined by *karma,* and it is this elemental karmic consciousness that Dr. Brahmachari is concerned with.

CHAPTER 5

DR. KARANDIKAR, DR. PAL, AND THE RSS: PURIFICATION, SUBTLE GYMNASTICS, AND MAN MAKING

1. The RSS is certainly not the only organization in colonial and postcolonial India concerned with the problem of masculinity. Ashis Nandy has incisively analyzed Gandhi's ideological manipulation of gender categories (1980, 1983; see also Alter 2000a, Kakar 1990), and Kakar has indicated how masculinity and femininity factored into Vivekananda's conception of modern Hinduism (1978). It also seems clear that colonialism provokes more broad-based anxiety about masculinity, both among the colonized (Alter 1994, 2000a: 113–45) and the colonizers (Sinha 1995).

2. This concept of an invisible congregation—deployed, at least nominally, in the interest of Universal Brotherhood rather than sectarian violence—is the foundation upon which the Bharatiya Yog Sansthan has built its practice of nationalistic public health reform (Alter 1997).

3. Celibacy is a practice directly linked to the question of masculinity, though in a somewhat problematic way (see Alter 1992, 1994, 1995). There is a complex, and variously manifest, "paradox" in the embodiment of contained virility. Self-control can devolve, by proxy, into a kind of effete emasculation. This paradox is evident on a number of different levels, including in modern Āyurvedic theory and practice.

4. *Brahmacarya* (celibacy) is integral to the practice of yoga, even though, as Eliade points out, there is nothing particularly yogic about the five "restraints," of which celibacy is one kind. Nevertheless, it is possible for the RSS to draw on the logic of yogic celibacy in order to conceptualize man making. Eliade—reflecting, perhaps unconsciously, early-twentieth-century European conceptions of sexuality—makes the following point: "Sexual abstinence is practiced to the end of conserving nervous energy. Yoga attaches greatest importance to these 'secret forces of the generative faculty,' which, when they are expended, dissipate the most precious energy, debilitate mental capacity, and make concentration difficult; if, on the contrary, they are mastered and 'restrained,' they further contemplative ascent" (1990: 50). Nervous energy is directly linked to semen. As Eliade points out in his detailed discussion of Tantra and alchemy in general and *kuṇḍalinī* in particular, semen is regarded not only as the body's vital essence, but as integral to its ability to transmutate. Man making entails a similar—though less metaphysical—kind of transmutation.

5. *Prāṇa śakti* has been discussed at length in previous chapters, and so it should be clear how this rhetoric invokes the power of Yoga. It is interesting to note, however, that Seshadri's metaphor of society as a vitalized body draws on powerful images of sacrifice and Vedic orthopraxy. In being to society what *prāṇa* is to the body, the RSS is put in the position of being that to which and on which the most important sacrifice is made. Significantly, the embodiment of this sacrifice is more clearly marked in the Vedic literature than in the esoteric formulations of Patañjali. As Whicher puts it: "In the *prāṇa-agni-hotra,* the more invisible, unobvious life-force or vital energy takes the place of the visible, obvious ritual

fire. The *prāṇa* is associated with the transcendent essence—the *ātman* or spiritual Self. The more esoteric emphasis given here, however, does not as yet constitute the more fully developed form of self- or 'mental' sacrifice as is the case in yogic forms of meditation. It was enacted through one's body" (1998: 13). Whicher is probably right, although there is a "return to" the problem of *prāṇic* embodiment in the Haṭha Yoga literature where the images of self-sacrifice are both esoteric and phenomenal, and this is reflected in Seshadri's rhetoric.

6. It is important to note here that the sanskritized terminology used to designate these *āsana* evokes the idea of "timeless" authenticity, whereas in fact the terminology is often modern and simply descriptive, in the way that a push-up describes an exercise in which the arms "push up" the body. *Ardhanāvāsana* probably describes the way in which a body bent in half at the waist resembles a boat. Or "nav" may be linked to *nābhi*—navel—which is important in yogic physiology.

7. Since my research was conducted, the hostel has evolved into a degree-granting college, which is described and advertised as follows: "The Yoga College named as Navalmal Firodia Yogavaidyak Adhyasan, Pune offers a unique job-oriented opportunity for the youth!! A post-graduate course called as DIP TRY, i.e. Diploma in Therapeutic Restorative Yoga. Duration: 2 yrs. Full-time course includes theory as well as practical in yoga therapy. 3 modules: Modern medicine, Āyurveda, Yoga: theory and practical. Educational qualification: Graduate of any faculty. Age: less than 30 yrs. Starts in July every year. The college has a well-equipped library and an audio-visual centre. The teaching is done by experienced lecturers in each faculty. The college also offers residential accomodation for students outside Pune" (www.kabirbaug.com).

8. *Ākāśa* is an important and interesting concept, and Dr. Karandikar is not the only person to be inspired to "think with" the ethereal logic of Yoga. As ether, *ākāśa* denotes one of the five *bhūta* elements in the structure of Āyurvedic and yogic physiology. This is spelled out most clearly in the *Yogatattva Upaniṣad*. In the context of auto-urine therapy discussed in chapter 6 we will see how this denotation is important to the embodiment of modern health. However, *ākāśa* is also cognate with *paramātama* and *Brahman* insofar as the idea of space as such is universal and transcends the particulate nature of matter. *Ākāśa* is often referred to in terms of brilliant radiance, in the sense of being both the radiant vital force in every person's heart and the vital force of the cosmos.

9. The rationale for this is that there is a homologous relationship between *āsana* postures and the categories of all living things. According to Feuerstein, "Siva propounded 840,000 postures" (1990: 36), and in some sense this can be interpreted as a kind of "genetic" mapping of organic life in the practice of *āsanas*. This is linked to the foundational Nyāya-Vaiśeṣika idea in Āyurveda, which holds that "whatever occurs in the material world also occurs in man, and whatever is in man is also in the world" (*Carakasaṁhitā* 4:4:13, in Rao 1987).

10. In making this point Dr. Karandikar seems to be drawing on a basic, Āyurvedic understanding of physiology. In this regard it is useful to keep in mind what the Āyurvedic texts say about the relationship between *ākāśa* and other forms of embodied matter. According to Rao, "The *ākāśiya* substances are soft, subtle, light smooth and separating . . . The *ākāśiya* element is illustrated by

whatever is soft, porous, light and productive of sound; channels in the body also represent this element" (1987: 139–40). In general terms *ākāśa* is directly linked to sound and audition.

11. This idea seems to be inspired, at least in part, by key ideas in Āyurvedic theory, which in turn derive from Sāṃkhya philosophy and are thereby linked to Yoga. The three *doṣa*—*vāta, pitta,* and *kapha*—are integral, in terms of ontology, to both health and disease. The *doṣa* are the support structure for balanced, fluid health, but the term also means "corrupting agent," "vitiating factor,"and "cause of disease." Given that the *doṣa* are the precipitate material of creation, as creation is understood as a paradoxical struggle to achieve unachievable perfect balance, a concept of natural good health is difficult, if not impossible, to reconcile with Āyurveda (Alter 1999). This paradoxical struggle seems to inform Dr. Karandikar's idea of "circular causation." What he refers to as genetically based anatomical distortions can be thought of as the foundational imbalance of the *doṣa,* as this imbalance is endemic to all manifestations of disease.

12. This is interesting in that it not only allows for a hierarchical classification—and implicit critique—of biomedical procedures, but defines the relationship between psychiatry and Yoga in an intriguing way. Insofar as psychiatry is associated with words and air, Yoga manifests the most subtle element, ether. Significantly, however, this is not in terms of esoteric meditation but in terms of physical practice.

13. The idea of imbalance in *ākāśa* is linked to *Prakṛti* as a primordial, unmanifest principle that exists in a perfect state only prior to, and outside the domain of, creation. Through the dialectic of *Prakṛti/Puruṣa,* creation "corrupts" primordial *Prakṛti,* and in these terms it is possible to conceive of "empty space" as manifesting imbalance. As Whicher puts it: "*Prakṛti* is frequently defined in Sāṃkhya as the state of balance or equilibrium of the three *guṇas* (*tri-guṇa-sāmya-avasthā*). When this state of balance is disturbed or disrupted by the presence of pure consciousness (*puruṣa*), the process of the 'creation' or manifestation of the ordinary world takes place" (1998: 58).

14. To understand this it is most useful to focus on *avyakta,* which is one of the twenty-four units of the aggregate person conceived of as a physical being. It is the unit most directly linked to cognition or individualized consciousness in the frameworks of Āyurveda. As Rao puts it, "The *Carakasaṁhitā* (*sūtra* 1, 35) speaks of the 'organized person' (*rāśi-puruṣa*) involving a multiplicity of units (twenty-four of them . . .). The important unit in this organization, however, is *avyakta* (or the unmanifest *prakṛti,* including the *puruṣa*), which in fact integrates the constituents (*melaka*) and engenders experiences (*bhogasampādaka*). . . . In the psycho-physical organization that is the individual, the five primary forms of matter comprehend all the units barring *avyakta,* and consciousness alone stands out as the sixth, (*Carakasaṁhitā* 1, 16); that is, it is tantamount to *avyakta.* All the other units are inert, and, therefore, can serve only as 'tools' (*kāraṇa*) or instruments for the principle of consciousness (*Carakasaṁhitā* 1, 54); they are fields (*kṣetra*) for this unmanifest principle to operate (*jña*) (*Carakasaṁhitā* 1, 65)" (1987: 42). In this formulation *avyakta* is the materialized flow of energy that is manifest in ether according to Dr. Karandikar.

15. Although Dr. Karandikar invokes many features of Āyurvedic theory, his focus on the senses as inherently problematic and linked to pathology in the broadest sense is yogic in nature. He seems to draw on both the commonly used metaphor of the senses being like charging horses, harnessed to the mind as controlling charioteer, and a Sāṃkhyan understanding of eleven physiological sense instruments organized into three subcategories—the mind, the connotative senses, and the higher cognitive senses, as these subdivisions can be mapped out according to the familiar five-into-three mathematics of *prakṛtic* creatrix.

16. At least in part, Karandikar's novel, pluralistic theory of physiology, etiology, and therapy is enabled by the way in which a concept of the cell as central to body function does not translate at all well into the logic of either Yoga or Āyurveda. It is almost as though knowledge about cellular biochemistry on the one hand and knowledge of *prāṇa* and *paramātmic* self-realization on the other opens up a "space of knowledge" that must be filled—and must be filled with logic and logical correspondences—unless someone like Dr. Karandikar is going to renounce his world and become *either* a yogi *or* a heart surgeon.

17. As Feuerstein puts it: "As the *Yoga-Śikhā Upaniṣad* (I.27) explains, the body is ordinarily insentient (*jaḍa*) or 'uncooked' (*apakva*) and it must be 'energized' (*ranjayet*) by the yogin so that it becomes 'cooked' or 'ripe' (*pakva*)" (1990: 90).

18. In the structure of Kuṇḍalinī Yoga as it is integrated into modern medical practice, it is interesting to note that *mūlabandha*—the "root lock" that is placed on the flow of *prāṇa* through the *mūlādhāra cakra*—is regarded as particularly important, perhaps because the *mūlādhāra cakra* is regarded as a primary nexus for the flow of vital energy. Working within the neo-tantric framework of Swami Stayananda's Bihar School of Yoga, Swami Buddhananda (1996) provides a detailed analysis of *mūlabandha* that helps to make sense of Dr. Pal's statement.

19. Although the term *mahā yoga* refers to one of the "inner" tantras of *dzogchen* practice in the context of the Nyingma order of Tibetan Buddhism, where the practitioner "realizes that all phenomena are emanations of the mind, which is a combination of appearance and voidness (*śūnyatā*)" (Feuerstein 2001: 178), Dr. Pal's reference is to Mahā Yoga, one of five types of practice mentioned in the *Śiva Purāṇa*, wherein Śiva is contemplated "without any restricting conditions" (Feuerstein 2001: 299). Beyond this specificity, Mahā Yoga means simply "Great Yoga," and thus invokes a high point of final achievement in a long career of practice.

20. The embodiment of celibacy is of great importance in terms of the way in which personal, moral, and social purification is effected and affected (Alter 1994). As I have pointed out elsewhere, Gandhi came to personify the intersection of celibacy and nationalism, as both were intimately linked to questions of personal and social purification (Alter 2000a). Dr. Pal's youthful commitment to celibacy reflects similar concerns as well as what was probably a much broader pattern among young men in India; these men were inspired by Gandhi, but interpreted his teaching more broadly and adopted not just celibacy as such, but a whole lifestyle modeled on the first stage of the fourfold *āśrama dharma*. Significantly this life stage involves self-purification and submission to the will of one's

guru, even though it is not, by any means, exclusively—or even directly—linked to the practice of Yoga as such.

21. In her book *Halfway up the Mountain: The Error of Premature Claims to Enlightenment,* Mariana Caplan (1998) provides a clear perspective on the extent to which fraud factors in as a trope in the discourse of Yoga.

22. Along with Kaivalyadhama, the Yoga Institute, founded by Shri Yogendra in the 1920s, has trained thousands of Yoga physical education instructors over the years. Primarily through training camps and the publication of popular self-help books, the institute has played a very significant role in the popularization of Yoga physical culture (Alter n.d.b).

23. One way to think about this is in terms of McKim Marriott's ethnosociological approach to understanding the configuration of so-called Hindu categories (1990). In brief, what Marriott is concerned with is the structure of logic that factors into the configuration of social, moral, and physiological elements in the cultural context of South Asia. What is "Hindu" in this is not so much beliefs, practices, and expressions of culture as it is the paradigmatic cognitive structure that underlies culture. In an important way, however, the very paradigmatic structure itself refuses the separation of cognitive from material reality. On this level Dr. Pal's modern manipulation of the body is meta-materially and structurally "Hindu" in its concern with purification, among other things.

24. *Bhāratiyam,* performed on Republic Day and at various nationally important events, involves large numbers of uniformed schoolchildren performing rhythmic Yoga *āsana*s in very much the mode of mass drill.

25. During the early years of the twentieth century, the Hindu Mahasabha and other nationalist organizations sponsored so-called *śuddhi* rituals of reconversion, whereby converts to Islam and Christianity were turned back into Hindus by means of purification.

CHAPTER 6
AUTO-URINE THERAPY—THE ELIXIR OF LIFE: YOGA, ĀYURVEDA, AND SELF-PERFECTION

1. It is interesting to note, parenthetically, that if one continues to read chapter 5 of Proverbs, the reference to water, wells, and cisterns is clearly imbedded in a discussion of sex, sexuality, and both eroticism and sensuality as well as the propriety of various sexual relationships. Picking up at verse 18:

> Let your fountain be blessed,
> And rejoice in the wife of your youth.
> As a loving hind and graceful doe,
> Let her breasts satisfy you at all times;
> Be exhilarated always with her love.
> For why should you, my son, be exhilarated with an adulteress,
> And embrace the bosom of a foreigner?

2. As Feuerstein points out, the word *amarolī* is difficult to translate. Etymologically it is linked to the words *amṛta* and *amṛtatva,* which mean immortality,

and is, therefore, central to Yoga, at least conceptually if not substantively. What complicates the issue, at least in part, is the fact that *amarolī* is a *mudrā* or a seal, and although other seals involve the use of water and air as well as the reabsorption of ejaculated semen, *amarolī* is the only *mudrā* that involves ingesting and assimilating a substance for reasons that are based on the properties ascribed to that substance.

3. Enjoyment here derives from the obviously tantric nature of *amarolī* and the way in which *mudrā*s produce both *bhoga,* pleasure, and *mukti,* liberation.

4. In most of the literature, particularly the literature on Nature Cure in India, what gets rubbed in the friction sitz bath is a penis, even though the male gender of the patient is rarely if ever marked. There is, nevertheless, an implicit assumption that the therapy is as effective for women as for men. This is because of the mechanical nature of the therapy—rubbing with a wet cloth—along with the fact that the reproductive organs of both men and women are implicated in the overall health of the person in similar ways. Recognizing this, there is, nevertheless, a sense in which the link between rubbing, the organ of procreation, semen, and nerve enervation is a link that is more intimately experienced by men, and this intimate link is reflected as a bias in the literature.

5. Although having the same title, this text deals exclusively with exorcism and what can be classified as magical charms, the construction of amulets, and the concoction of potions. However, no mention of urine is made. This indicates either that Rai's text is completely different—which is most likely the case—or that the manuscript he translated did not include the *Śivambu Kalpa* section.

6. The term in the *Carakasaṁhitā* is rendered *anupāna. Anupāl* is used throughout here since that is how the term is rendered in the relevant auto-urine therapy literature.

7. As will become clear, there is some ambiguity in terminology concerning the nature of urine therapy when other substances are mixed with one's own urine. Apart from the question of *anupāna/anupāl* terminology, the description of what is mixed with urine and how it is to be mixed would seem to indicate that the mixtures described in the *Ḍāmara Tantra* should be classified as infusions within the broader framework of decoctions (*kaṣāya*).

8. Unless what is rendered *anupāl* in the *Ḍāmara Tantra* is not the same as *anupāna* in the Āyurvedic literature—which is not likely—there seems to be a degree of confusion in the auto-urine therapy literature on both the meaning and the function of *anupāl.* Strictly speaking, *anupāna/anupāl* are not decoctions of different herbs and substances. Rather they are the fluid vehicle used for the administration of medicine. The fluid itself has medicinal properties, but the property of the fluid is distinct from the medicine as such. Thus the most common "vehicles" are water, honey, ghee, butter, sugar, jaggery, buttermilk, and milk. Each vehicle is correlated both with the medicine it is used to transport and with the ailment in question. Usually the medicine is seated in—or suspended in—the vehicle, but in a number of instances the *anupāna/anupāl* is consumed shortly after the medicine is taken. In these terms it would be possible to understand urine as a vehicle of a particular kind—with more or less fixed and immutable "natural" properties—and thereby allow for a rapprochement of sorts between Nature Cure purists and Āyurvedically inclined theoreticians.

9. Although the *Ḍāmara Tantra* is a tantric text, the reference to "*kayā kalpa*"—spelled *kayā kulp*—unambiguously links it to the radical techniques of body cultivation practiced by medieval *siddhas*. As will become clear, *kayā sādhana*—the techniques used to produce an immortal body—are very similar to Āyurvedic *rasāyana* therapy.

10. As should come as no surprise to scholars familiar with Āyurveda, urine is incorporated into practice in terms of a system of extreme classification and subclassification that mirrors, in many respects, the classification and subclassification of other animal products, in particular meat. Within the broader framework of *doṣic* quality—as well as the "taste" and "property" of substances that are conceptualized as pharmaceutical—what matters is both the habitat of the animal in question and its diet, insofar as diet is a function of how an animal kills/collects its food, and the hierarchical food chain this defines (see Zimmermann 1987). Thus the urine of an animal that kills its prey with claws and lives in the hot, dry jungle is significantly different from the urine of an animal that eats vegetable matter and lives in a humid marsh. More research needs to be done on this question.

11. On the basis, it seems, purely of the logic of fluid correlation, urine can be used to replace water in the practice of such things as *jal neti kriyā* and *kunjal*. Interestingly, since Āyurveda and Yoga have many cleansing procedures in common, this may be understood as a point of functional transmutation in and between the two systems of practice.

12. The question of whether or not the time frame delineated in the text should be taken literally or read only figuratively is immaterial. Time is used here as a classificatory schema, and what matters is the logic of calibrated sequence. The text works within a framework wherein long-term drinking translates into more power over time, but it is the increments that reveal a more subtle logic of transmutation.

13. It would, of course, be possible to do an analysis of the pharmacological logic represented in this section of the *Ḍāmara Tantra*. There does not, however, seem to be any clearly apparent pattern with respect either to the drug properties of the additives in question or to their action.

14. In the Āyurvedic literature there is an important relationship between massage (*udvartana*), anointing with oil (*abhyaṅga*), and bathing (*snāna*), and to a significant degree the sharp distinction between these as they translate into English works against the logic of Āyurveda. Bathing entails oil massage. Consequently, it is important to understand what the *Ḍāmara Tantra* says about urine massage in the context of what the Āyurvedic literature says about *abhyaṇga* in general and medicated oil *abhyaṇga* in particular. Clearly *abhyaṇga* does not stand alone as a therapeutic modality. It must be understood in the context of other treatments and the patient's general condition of health. However, in most general terms, as Rao points out: "Rubbing in the form of massages (*udvartana*) relieves the aggravation of *kapha*, helps reduce fat, and invigorates the limbs of the body; the skin becomes soft, lustrous and firm. Rubbing the body with oil should be followed by a bath with hot or tepid water" (1987: 18).

15. In a clear and important way the practice of ascetic *tapas* reflects, on the plane of self-abnegation and world renunciation, the structured regimen of *kayā*

kalpa and *rasāyana*. On this plane there are countless accounts of men endowed with supernatural power by virtue of the extreme austerities they perform. Of note here is that in some instances, *tapas* is directly integrated into the *kayā kalpa* regimen, as in the case of the 185-year-old Tapasvi Maharaj, an ascetic who claimed to both do such things as stand on one leg for years at a time, and also undergo drug-based rejuvenation therapy (Murthy 1972).

16. *Kitta,* as Rao points out, is a term that means waste product. It is the undigested or undigestible part of food that is not digested or "cooked" into *sāra* in the *grahaṇī*. Most of the descriptions of *kitta* seem to indicate that it takes on a solid form, as the substantive juice of food is extracted, leaving a dry residue. In other words, liquid and the fluid character of liquids do not fit very well into the logic of *kitta* production.

17. In many ways Āyurvedic physiology is paradigmatically structured in terms of digestion. The body is "cooked" and refined by means of an endless process of metabolic transmutation. Understandably the stages of digestion that effect transmutation are carefully delineated, and the agency of digestion is clearly theorized. *Pitta* is directly implicated in digestion and the body is said to contain thirteen digestive fires. Besides the primary *jātharāgni,* there are five *bhūtāgni* elemental fires and seven *dhātavagni* constituent fires.

18. In a more general sense Rao points out that digestion is classified into two stages, the preliminary *pra-pāka* phase and the "special" or "subsequent" phase of *vipāka*. *Vipāka* is both self-contained and systemic as opposed to the constituent form and particulate function of *pra-pāka*. As Rao puts it: "The expression *vi-pāka* is explained as meaning 'the completion of the act of digestion' (*Carakasaṁhitā* 1,26,66), or the end-result of the digestive process which is the combined effect of the three phases of the *prapāka*. . . . The transformation here is special in the sense that it is not regional . . . but systemic. Whatever the taste[s] of the food that we eat, they are all changed into sweet, sour and pungent in order, during the three phases of gastro-intestinal digestion. The tastes undergo a final change in the 'subsequent' stage, and enter into the general stream of chyle (*rasa* as one of the seven body constituents) and thus conveyed to all parts of the body" (1987: 216).

19. After having laboriously worked through the logic of digestion in Āyurveda to try to understand how urine could possibly be conceptualized as an elixir—and in trying to find references to urine in both classical works and works of classical scholarship (where it does not usually rank an index entry)—I came upon David White's discussion of the relationship between nectar and ashes in the alchemical literature. As the residue of fire, ash bears a certain structural similarity to the residue of digestion. Clearly it would be possible to make much more of the congruity between urine and ash than can be done here. On a purely evocative level, however, consider White's characterization of the body "reduced to ashes" as it compares with the body "refined" through the consumption of urine, and in particular the intensive and extensive urine massages prescribed in the *Śivambu Kalpa:* "Just as the Siddha, by virtue of his having bound and pierced the volatile elements of his alchemical body, himself becomes unbindable and impenetrable

and all-binding and all-penetrating; so the same Siddha, by virtue of having calcinated and reduced his alchemical body to ashes, himself becomes uncalcinable and all-calcinating, an ashen, ash-smeared, ash-producing, alchemical touchstone" (1996: 289–90).

20. In this regard it is relevant that hair, teeth, skin, and fingernails—as well as bone—are all correlated to the most gross and earthy dimension of the body. As such they are on the opposite end of the hierarchical spectrum from the ethereal dimension of elemental sound. Their perfection is, therefore, manifest in material form.

21. This analogy is also commonly used to illustrate the relationship between semen and the body's metabolic structure (Alter 1992, 1994).

22. The logic of consuming feces is explained by Eliade, citing the work of Barrow (1893: 22), in terms of the analogy of excrement fertilizing soil (1990: 296–97). Clearly this "contrary"—but not dualistic—logic is not what is significant in the context of urine consumption, since it is said to be pure.

23. According to Caraka, pregnancy and childbirth effects are a specifically gendered transmutation of *dhātu* elements. Although often the seven *dhātu* are said to simply culminate in semen, there are clear references in a number of texts to the way in which *majjā* transmutes into *śoṇita* or menstrual blood, which is sometimes referred to as female semen. What is interesting, however, is the way in which there is a further meta-transmutation engendered by pregnancy and both the birth of a child and the agency of that child's suckling. Menstrual blood gets transformed into breast milk.

24. There is extensive discussion in the *Carakasaṁhitā* about the different ways in which the property of a drug should match—and can, by way of cultivating techniques and gathering strategies, be made to match—the *doṣic* quality of a particular disorder. Extending this logic to the person as a whole, Rao cites an interesting passage from the *Bhāva-Prakaśa-Nighantu:* "The drug will be most effective if the *bhautika*-element of the soil in which it is grown is matched with the *bhautika* element of the disorder. [The] *Bhāva-Prakāśa-Nighantu* (1,5,115) makes another classification of the soil in terms of *brāhmana* (white), *kṣattriya* (red), *vaiśya* (yellow), and *śūdra* (black); and suggests that the drug growing on these soils will be most effective when used by patients belonging to these caste-groups!" (1987: 74).

25. It is on this level that Patel's work most clearly reflects the influence of Gandhi, in terms of both the importance placed on God and devotion to God and the relative importance of nature and the truth value inherent in nature.

26. It is on this level that the ambiguity of auto-urine therapy's "fit" with Āyurveda is most clearly attenuated in the logic that Patel—following Gandhi, it seems—employs. Just as Gandhi was directly concerned with purging the body of toxins, waste, and unnatural substances, so Patel seems also to focus on a theory of health based on flushing the system out. In Āyurveda it is noteworthy that the actions of drugs fit into a rough hierarchy, with the first three being concerned with digestion and "cooking" and the next eight—*anulomana* ("carminatives"), *sraṁsana* ("laxatives"), *bhedana* ("anthracene purgatives"), *virechana* ("drastic

purgatives"), *vamana* ("emetics"), *saṁśodhana* ("eliminatives"), *chhedana* ("expectorants"), and *lekhana* ("attenuants")—being concerned with purgation. Beyond this, many of the other twenty-six drug actions seem to have purgative or purifying effects.

CHAPTER 7
MIMETIC SKEPTICISM AND YOGA: MOVING BEYOND THE PROBLEM OF CULTURE AND RELATIVISM

1. The leap from the specific domain of religion to the general framework of culture may seem rather athletic, but in an important sense culture and the process of cultural construction is like religion in terms of its fetishistic attributes vis-à-vis society.

2. It is important to note that although cultural relativism is a central problem in anthropological theory, it is a problem that is currently being explicitly debated in many different disciplines. Of course, the basic questions of truth, meaning, justice, and equality underlying cultural relativism are so general that almost all forms of knowledge have a bearing on the problem. In this regard cultural relativism may be seen less as a unique problem and more as a way of phrasing the problem of what constitutes meaning and truth. Philosophers tend to deal with it on this level of abstraction, whereas psychiatrists, social workers, nurses, lawyers, and administrators are at the other end of the spectrum, dealing with "difference on the ground," so to speak. In being concerned with many of the same broad questions as philosophers, but dealing with the everyday world of lived experience, anthropologists, among other social scientists dealing with cross-cultural comparison, are well positioned to say something about the middle ground.

3. This is not only a standard definition, but a typical one as well. See note 8 for a summary of standard definitions.

4. Empathy and sympathy are used, in this context, as value-free perspectives, such that one is able to understand how it might feel to hold the views of others.

5. Although there are several good analyses of the history of the idea of relativism, both within anthropology (Fox 1991; Hitchens 1994) and in other fields (Chase 1997; Dubow 1992; Marks 1998; R. van der Veer 1996), there is need for a comprehensive genealogy of the idea as it is linked, apparently, to German nationalism.

6. What mimetic skepticism is will become clear as the argument develops. It is based on a synthesis of Foucault's "methodological principle of neutrality or scepticism of an analysis of power, which bases itself neither on a moral philosophy nor a social ontology" (Gordon 1980: 235) and a post-Marxian understanding of fetishism as developed by Michael Taussig. Significantly, however, the principle of skepticism, manifest in a perspective of divested objectivity, is intimately linked to the epistemology of science. The point here is to radicalize skepticism and, in some sense, strategically confuse the distinction between epistemology and ontology. This prevents a retreat into the empiricism of objective social science, avoids a call for some sort of compromise, and makes it impossible to fall back on the neo-moralism of well-meaning institutions like the United Na-

tions (compare Burman 1996; Symonides 1998; B. White 1999) and the American Anthropological Association.

7. There is an unfortunate distinction between work that is "applied" and policy oriented, work that is politically "activist" in nature and intent, and work that is thought of as "purely" intellectual and therefore different in kind from the other two. The view taken here is that since power is pervasive, all intellectual work is a form of activism. It is just extremely reflexive, and thereby inconclusive work, but no less important or relevant because of that. Mimetic skepticism may be understood, by extension, as an activist intellectual critique of liberal humanism, as this perspective is reflected in many of the contributions to such journals as *Human Rights Quarterly* and *Cultural Survival.* (See, for example, Afshari 1994; Brems 1997; Marfording 1997; Pollis 1996; Tilley 2000. See also James 1994; Zechenter 1997. For an overview, see Messer 1993.)

8. Raymond Scupin provides the following gloss: "the principle that other societies must be understood through their own cultural values" (1995: 411). William Haviland and Robert Gordon provide a slightly different, nervously cautious, orientation to the subject by saying that "one cannot understand another culture without suspending judgement to see how it works on its own terms" (1996: 14). Conrad Kottak, in taking the standard view of contrasting cultural relativism with ethnocentrism, places emphasis on the problem of negative judgment by saying that it "is the argument that behavior in a particular culture should not be judged by the standards of another" (1994: 45). Carol Ember and Melvin Ember expand the perspective somewhat and link it to the problem of scientific study, calling it "the anthropological attitude that a society's customs and ideas should be described objectively and understood in the context of that society's problems and opportunities" (1996: 16; see also Bates 1996: 9; Harris 1997: 91; Rosman and Rubel 1998: 19–20). Recognizing the logical, moral, and political problems entailed in many standard definitions, Barbara D. Miller distinguishes between absolute cultural relativism, which is, essentially, the idea that anything goes because everything's legitimacy is defined by its own context, and what she calls critical cultural relativism. This latter perspective "offers an alternative view that poses questions about cultural practices and ideas in terms of who accepts them and why, and who they might be harming and helping" (1999: 12).

9. See, for example, Dirks 1998; Fox 1991; Friedrich 1992; Gupta and Ferguson 1992; Kahn 1989; Nuckolls 1998; Rodseth 1998; Rosaldo 1989; Weiner 1995.

10. My thinking here is informed by Gilles Deleuze's interpretation of Nietzsche's philosophy as it seeks to articulate a kind of creative affirmation of life that is not inhibited by a burdensome faith in being and the false affirmation of truth as real (1983: 180–86). Although deconstructionism need not be a "false affirmation" and can be creative, it seems to be encumbered by dialectical reasoning. Instead I find the principle of critical—or chronic—evaluation more useful. As Deleuze puts it: "Nietzsche's whole philosophy is opposed to the postulates of being, of man and of acceptance. . . . The world is neither true nor real but living. And the living world is will to power, will to falsehood, which is actualized in

many different powers. To actualize the will to falsehood under any quality whatever, is always to evaluate. To live is to evaluate. There is no truth of the world as it is thought, no reality of the sensible world, all is evaluation, even and above all the sensible and the real" (1983: 198).

11. The argument here picks up and develops some of the ideas first presented in *Gandhi's Body* (2000a) and *Knowing Dil Das* (2000c). In *Gandhi's Body* I was concerned with a redefinition of politics in terms of the body, and the way in which embodied politics, colonialism, and nationalism confound clear-cut distinctions. Rather than focus on the body, here I am concerned with what the implications are for anthropological knowledge that cannot rest comfortably on clear-cut, categorical distinctions. As such, this chapter is an attempt to theoretically refine—in more general and abstract terms—what is presented ethnographically in *Knowing Dil Das.*

12. There has also been significant—and very productive—discussion among those who take an interpretive, hermeneutic approach to understanding the relationship between cultural texts and contexts (Conklin 1997; Dirks 1998; Fabian 1995), and the cultural nature of scientific knowledge (Fujimura 1998; Roscoe 1995); how to integrate questions of power into textual analyses in general (Daniel 1996; Taussig 1987) and science in particular (Haraway 1991; Rabinow 1996b); what the implications are of a politics of discursive representation (Downey and Rogers 1995; Fischer 1999; Gable, Handler, and Lawson 1992); and how to account for the positionality of perspectives within interpretive frameworks (Bowlin and Stromberg 1997), for example.

13. I am making a distinction here between the past and history. People define the past selectively on the basis of various priorities and thereby make history. An unreflexive history is unaware of its selective bias. The argument being made here is that to make history requires the unmaking of unreflexive histories and the construction of new, emergent histories through a critical reexamination of the past, and of the present in terms of that past.

14. Here is Parsons: "Durkheim's important insight into the role of symbolism in religious ideas might, without further analysis, suggest that the specific patterns, hence these variations, were only of secondary importance. Indeed, there is clearly discernible in Durkheim's thinking in this field a tendency to circular reasoning in that he tends to treat religious patterns as a symbolic manifestation of 'society,' but at the same time to define the most fundamental aspect of society as a set of patterns of moral and religious sentiment" (1954: 207).

15. The idea of living subjunctively—or developing subjunctivity as a field methodology—requires further clarification. Here, however, it is sufficient to note, following the *American Heritage Dictionary,* that subjunctivity entails the enactment of "verbal" forms that express "contingent or hypothetical action" and a certain "mood of [insubordinate?] subordination."

16. The concept of agency has become a virtual mantra in contemporary anthropological theory, and I am sympathetic toward its use by some scholars to analyze the way in which humans creatively engage with the world. However, as it derives from Bourdieu's theory of practice, the idea of agency strikes me as carrying with it the problem of analytical indifference and sociological abstraction that Rabinow draws attention to in his critique: "Self interest is defined by the

complex structure of overlapping sociological fields to which the actors must be blind in order to act. Bourdieu is absolutely unequivocal that social actors, while acting in terms of their sociologically structured self-interest, can never know what that self-interest is precisely because they must believe in the illusion that they are pursuing something genuinely meaningful in order to act. Only the sociologist is capable of understanding what is really and truly going on" (1996a: 9). The concept of agency seems to acknowledge the illusion of meaning, on the one hand, but then, on the other, restores definitive meaning to the social agent in terms of an objective, disinterested—and thereby enlightened rather than deluded—scientific perspective.

17. It is surprising how much of Taussig's analysis depends on the concrete, sometimes-but-not-always reflexive, ethnographic texts of other scholars. The point is not at all to cast aspersions on Taussig's own fieldwork, or the quality of the "data" he has collected through participant observation. Rather the point is that his insightful observations on the magical reality of mimesis often depend on the reinterpretation of realist ethnography cut in a classical, modernist mold—very much as Lévi-Strauss's structuralism depended on the methods of Boasian ethnography, but was theoretically critical of historical particularism. But sooner or later the contradiction between method, data, and theory comes home to roost. This is, in part, why approaching these questions through the problem of relativism forces the issue of analytical method into the domain of field research.

18. This ripple is manifest, perhaps in its smallest, and seemingly most insignificant form, in the "difference" between skepticism and scepticism.

19. Cappai (2000) has pointed out the more general relevance of Quine's philosophy to the problem of cultural relativism.

20. In calling his imaginary field language "Jungle," Quine uncritically commits the crime of Orientalism. But, it seems to me, his thesis on the indeterminacy of translation is grounds for an acquittal.

21. A similar but more general sentiment is expressed by Roland Barthes when—caught somewhere between objectivity and subjectivity—he calls sarcasm a condition of truth (1972: 12). My sense is that this kind of sarcasm, as well as that kind of faithlessness described by Daniel, cannot be understood as a reactive principle, but only in terms of Deleuze's characterization of the Nietzschean Overman who creates through affirmation. Otherwise it becomes weak, nihilistic cynicism.

22. In this context it is important to recall, as Gregory Fields does, "that Vedic texts, particularly the *Brahmana*s, classify the human being as *pāśu*, an animal, as the preeminent animal, the ruler of all the other animals, and the only animal able to perform ritual and sacrifice" (2001: 24).

23. Keep in mind that Anthropology, "the study of humankind"—physiologically, evolutionarily, linguistically, historically, and culturally—matches, stride for stride on the sociological track, the universalist pretension of any given religion.

24. U. A. Asrani, who has written one of the most interesting—if not exactly systematic and logical—accounts of the relationship between Yoga and science gets at this question in a short section of his book *Yoga Unveiled,* part 2, entitled "Our Stupendous Dynamic Universe—Biological Sciences":

Other animals have distinct sense, distinctly sharper than ours. Still we realistically regard ourself as superior conscious beings—each separated by a skin wall, and ruling over the world outside—a world of much less conscious beings, or of unconscious matter—living in a stable earth, in an ever constant space, with time running ceaselessly independent of it all.

But science has expanded our knowledge and advanced our tools of perception immensely, beyond all such old conceptions. We are, in fact, living in a stupendous, dynamic, expanding universe. . . . Molecules of so-called dead matter are in constant, haphazard motion. . . . Each living body again, is in fact, a world unto itself—A world of living cells, millions of them dying every second, and getting replaced. The whole living world pulsates with consciousness. (1993: 208–9)

25. Although I think Haraway is right, her whole argument strains against its point of ethical and political rootedness in feminism and Marxism (1991: 160), since in a cyborg society there is no gender and no class.

26. In many interesting ways the figure of the cyborg is very much like the really magical nature of the supernatural shaman. As Taussig points out, the shaman is directly involved in a kind of politics that is factually fictional and magically real. This kind of politics clearly involves the melding of natural and supernatural, animal and human power.

27. Maryanski (1995) extends Edgerton's critique of cultural relativism into the domain of primate sociology and seeks to define what is good for humans in pan-hominoid terms.

GLOSSARY

abhyaṅga — Oil massage.
adharma — The antithesis of right conduct.
adhyātman — The innermost Self.
Aghorapanthī — Member of the Aghorī sect of ascetics.
Aghorī — Originating in the fourteenth century from the Kāpālika cult, an ascetic sect characterized by tantric practices and "countercultural" techniques for the realization of enlightenment.
agni — Fire.
agni sāra prāṇāyāma — Breathing exercise in which air is inhaled and exhaled rapidly by expanding and contracting the abdomen.
ahaṃkāra — Ego or sense of individual identity.
aindriya — Without sense; senseless.
ājñā cakra — The sixth vital center of the subtle body, located between the eyes.
ākāśa — Ether.
ākāśiya — Etheric.
akhāṛā — Gymnasium; ascetic order.
aliṅga — Without characteristics of mind or senses. Undifferentiated existence wherein there is a perfect balance of constituent categories.
amarolī — A yogic *mudrā* that involves drinking one's own urine.
amṛta — Nectar of immortality.
amṛtatva — Immortality.
anāhata cakra — The fourth vital center of the subtle body, located at the heart.
ānanda — Bliss.
ānandamaya kośa — Bliss sheath of the body.
Ananta — Infinite or endless. The name of the thousand-headed snake deity.
anna rasa — Digested food juice.
annamaya kośa — Food sheath of the body.
antaḥkaraṇa — Psyche composed of the higher mind, the mind of self-identification, and the lower mind or intellect.
anulomana — Carminatives.
anupāl — Combinations of herbs, minerals, and drugs that are mixed with urine as described in the *Ḍāmara Tantra*.
anupāna — A drink that serves as a vehicle for a particular kind of medicine.
apakva — Uncooked.
apāna — One of the five individuated *prāṇa*s. Located in the lower part of the body and responsible for evacuation and exhalation.
asamprjñāta samādhi — Supraconscious enstasy; consciousness beyond cognition wherein only the traces of subconsciousness remain. Once these traces are removed final and ultimate enlightenment is achieved.
āsana — Seat. The postures assumed in yoga practice.
asmitāmātra — Mere I-ness; self unto itself.

āśram — Hermitage. Also designates a stage, as in a particular stage in the fourfold life course.

āśrama dharma — The four life stages: *brahmacarya, garhasthya, vānaprasthya, sannyāsa.*

aṣṭāṅga yoga — The eight "limbs" of yoga: *yama, niyama, āsana, prāṇāyāma, pratyāhāra, dhāraṇā, dhyāna, samādhi.*

asteya — Nonstealing. One of the five moral practices in *yama,* the first branch of yoga practice.

asthi — Bone.

ātivāhika deha — The omnipresent body of a being who has experienced Ultimate Truth.

ātman — The self. In standard usage it can mean both the egoic self or the Universal Self, since both are—once realized as such—the same. It is used here to signify the egoic self, sometimes called the *jīvātman,* as distinct from the Universal Self, which is referred to as *paramātman.*

avidyā — Spiritual ignorance.

avyakta — Unmanifest.

Āyurveda — A South Asian medical system based on a humoral theory of physiology.

bāhyakaraṇa — External instrument.

bandha — A technique in Haṭha Yoga whereby the flow of *prāṇa* is locked and channeled.

basti — Cleaning the rectum and large intestine by means of anal suction.

bhastrikā — One of the eight primary types of breath control, in which inhalation and exhalation is modeled on the action of a blacksmith's bellows.

bhautika — Elemental or material reality.

bhāva — Emotion, mood, or feeling; disposition.

bhaya — Fear.

bhedana — Anthracene purgatives in Āyurvedic medical practice.

bhoga — Enjoyment.

bhogasampādaka — Experiences.

bhūtāgni — The five elemental fires of internal digestion.

bhūta śuddhi — Purification of the elements as this leads to the perfection of the body.

bīṛī — A small, inexpensive, cone-shaped, hand-rolled cheroot.

brahmacārī — A person who is celibate.

brahmacarya — Celibacy.

brahman — 1. The absolute. The relationship of *brahman* to *ātman* is integral to *Vedānta* and is a central theme in the *Upaniṣad*s. 2. Priestly *varṇa.*

brāhmarandhra — The opening at the top of the head through which the *suṣumṇā nāḍī* extends.

brahm tej — Supreme spiritual vitality.

buddhi — Higher mind; wisdom. The first evolute of *prakṛti* and the highest, most refined dimension of consciousness.

cakra — Wheel. Vital center of the subtle body. There are six embodied centers and a seventh which reflects transcendence.

capātī — Unleavened whole-wheat bread
celā — Disciple.
chhedana — Expectorants in Āyurvedic medical practice.
citta — Consciousness or mind.
cittavṛttinirodha — Cessation of the fluctuation of consciousness. A key principle in Yoga as expounded by Patañjali.
cutiyā — Tuft or lock of hair that is left uncut when the head is otherwise completely shaved.
ḍaṇḍa — Staff; punishment.
darśana — Vision or sight; viewpoint or perspective.
dasadik — Ten different directions.
dhāraṇā — Concentration. The sixth branch of classical yoga as expounded by Patañjali.
dharma — Right conduct.
dhātavagni — The seven constituent fires of internal digestion.
dhātu — In Āyurvedic medicine, that which supports and sustains the body.
dhauti — Washing. One of the six acts (*ṣaṭ karma*) of Haṭha Yoga, involving the cleaning of the inside of the body—throat, stomach, and intestines—as well as the teeth, heart, and rectum. Often used exclusively to refer to a technique where a strip of cloth is swallowed and then pulled out of the stomach.
dhyāna — Meditation. The seventh branch of Yoga practice.
dīkṣā — Initiation into an ascetic order.
doṣa — Physiological humor. In Āyurveda the three humors are wind, bile, and phlegm.
*doṣ*ic — Of or pertaining to *doṣa.*
duḥkha — Suffering or sorrow as a condition of existence.
gamcā — A lightweight cotton cloth wrap or towel.
gāyatrī mantra — A common prayer.
ghāṭā śuddhi — Purification of the body.
grahaṇī — Part of the abdomen between the stomach and large intestine that retains food during the process of digestion.
guṇa — Strand or quality. It defines the triad of qualities *sattva, rajas,* and *tamas* in Sāṃkhya ontology.
gurukul — A school of desciples under the preceptorship of a *guru.*
harītakī — The herb *terminalia chebula.*
Haṭha Yoga — Forceful yoga. The technique of Yoga developed by the Kānphata sect of the Nātha order. It is meant to produce self-realization by means of embodied perfection.
iḍā nāḍī — One of the three primary channels of the subtle body through which *prāṇa* flows. It is situated to the left of the *suṣumṇā.*
indriya — Sensory capacities of cognition, connotation, and mind as these are embodied.
jaḍa — The insentient body.
jal neti — A procedure to clean the nasal passages and sinuses with water.
jātharāgni — The stomach fire that is one of thirteen fires of internal digestion.
jīvanmukta — A person who is enlightened while still living in the world.

jīvanmukti — The experience or condition of a *jīvanmukta*, one who is both alive and enlightened.

jīvātman — The individuated or individual self.

jñāna — Wisdom or knowledge.

jñānendriya — Cognitive sense. The sense capacity of the eyes, ears, nose, tongue, and skin.

kāliyug — Dark age.

kapālabhāti — One of the six acts (*ṣaṭ karma*) that entails rapid breathing through the nose to "shine the skull."

Kāpālika — A tantric sect that emerged in the early centuries of this era. The name refers to the practice of using human skulls as bowls in which to collect donations of food.

kapha — Phlegm humor in Āyurvedic medicine.

kāraṇa — Cause.

kāraṇa śarīra — Causal body.

karma — Action.

karmendriya — Conative sense. The sense capacity of the voice, hands, feet, anus, and genitals.

kaśaya — A decoction boiled with various proportions of water until one quarter of the combination remains.

kayā kalpa — Transformation and perfection of the body.

khādī — Homespun rough cotton cloth.

kitta — Excreta.

kośta — A kind of fruit.

kriyā — Action or procedure.

krodha — Anger.

Kṛṣṇa — Incarnation of the god Visnu. Important to Yoga in terms of his discourse on Bhakti Yoga recounted in the *Bhagavad Gītā*.

ksatriya — Warrior *varṇa*.

ksatriya virya — The vitality and courage of warriors.

kṣetra — Region or place.

kuṇḍalinī — The serpent power. The manifest form of cosmic energy that is the agency of enlightenment as it moves up the central *suṣumṇā nāḍī* during Yoga *sādhana*.

kunjal — Internal cleansing by means of induced vomiting.

laghava — Lightness. The embodied feeling associated with the practice of *prāṇāyāma*.

laghiman — Levitation. One of the eight primary magical powers embodied through yoga practice.

laṁgot — G-string; a cloth garment that binds the genitals tightly.

lāṭhī — Stave.

lekhana — Attenuants.

liṇga — Mark; phallus. A thing with the characteristics of the three-part mind—*buddhi* (higher consciousness), *ahaṃkāra* (consciousness of the self), and *manas* (intellect)—the five cognitive senses (*jñānendriya*) and the five conative senses (*karmendriya*).

liṅga śarīra — A *Sāṃkhyan* designation meaning a body with the characteristics of the three-part mind and the ten cognitive and conative senses.
Lokāyatikas — The followers of materialist philosophy.
mahābhūta — The five primary elements: earth, water, fire, air, ether.
mahat — Higher mind; wisdom. A synonym of *buddhi,* the first evolute of *prakṛti* according to *Sāṃkhya* ontology.
mahāvedha — Great piercer. A procedure in Haṭha Yoga whereby *prāṇa* is forced into the *suṣumṇā nāḍī*—and made to pierce through the three knots—by performing a series of embodied locks (*bandha*s) and seals (*mudrā*s) and lifting and dropping the buttocks onto the ground.
Mahā Yoga — Great Yoga.
mahā yogi — Great yogi.
maithuna — Sexual intercourse. Ritualized intercourse in tantrism.
majjā — Marrow.
mala — Waste products of body metabolism.
malinīkaraṇat — Polluting agents.
māṁsa — Fat.
manas — Mind.
maṇipūra cakra — Third vital center of the subtle body, located at the navel.
manomaya kośa — Mind sheath of the body.
mastī — Energized, impassioned revery.
māyā — The web of illusion.
medagni — The cooking of fat into bone in the metabolic process of *dhātu* transformation.
medas — Flesh.
melaka — Constituents.
Mīṃāṃsā — One of the six primary schools of philosophy based on ritual practice. As a common noun it means scholarly investigation.
mokṣa — Liberation.
mṛj — To clean out or purify.
mudrā — Seals. A class of procedures and postures in Haṭha Yoga that includes *bandha*s (locks) and relates to the channeled flow of *prāṇa.*
mukti — Release.
mūla bandha — Root lock.
mūlādhāra cakra — Lowest vital center of the subtle body situated between the anus and the perineum.
mūlaprakṛti — Root or elemental nature.
muni — Sage.
mūtra — Urine.
nābhi — Navel.
nāḍī — Conduits. Channels of the subtle body.
nauli — Rolling or churning. One of the six procedures (*ṣaṭkarma*) of Yoga in which the abdominal recti are contracted and relaxed in rotating succession.
neti — Cleaning the nostrils and sinuses with water or a cotton cord.
nirvāṇa — Enlightenment.
nirvicāra — Supra-reflexion.

nirvikalpa samādhi — Enstasy without form. Synonymous with *asamprjñāta samādhi*, in which the residual traces of desire are eradicated.
niyama — Restraint. The second branch of Yoga as expounded by Patañjali, including the five practices of internal and external purification: cleanliness, contentment, asceticism, study, devotion.
Nyāya — One of the six principal schools of Indic philosophy, concerned with logic, rules, and procedural methods.
ojas — The essence of vitality.
pāka — Cooked.
pañca bhūta — The five elements: earth, water, fire, air, ether.
pañca kośa — The five sheaths of the body that mask or veil the transcendental Self.
paramātman — Ultimate Self.
pariṇāma — Transformation.
Pārvatī — Consort of Lord Śiva.
Pāśupata — An ascetic religious sect founded in the second century C.E.
Pāśupati — Another name for Lord Śiva meaning Lord of the animals.
Patañjali — The author of the *Yoga Sūtra*, who probably lived in the second century C.E. and is said to have been the incarnation of Ananta, the thousand-headed serpent.
peśāb — Urine.
pīlu-pāka — Chemical-like changes caused by the action of digestive cooking.
piṅgalā nāḍī — One of the three primary channels of the subtle body through which *prāṇa* flows. It is situated to the right of the *suṣumṇa nāḍī*.
piṭhara pāka — Physical changes caused by digestive cooking.
pitta — The humor bile in Āyurvedic medicine.
pośaṇa — The nourishment provided by the *dhātu*.
pracārak — Leadership title in the administration of the RSS. Literally, it can mean propagandist.
pradhāna — Foundation. A term used to designate the transcendental, pre-created nature of *prakṛti* apart from *puruṣa*.
prakṛti — Material, elemental nature; creation as an ongoing process.
prakṛti pariṇāma vadā — Transformations in the nature of nature.
prāṇa — The vital life force.
prāṇa agni hotra — The embodied form of the Vedic fire ritual sacrifice.
prāṇāmaya kośa — The vital force sheath of the body.
prāṇas — Individuate *prāṇa* manifest in five different aspects: *prāṇa, apāna, vyāna, udāna, samāna*.
prāṇāyāma — Breathing exercises. The fourth branch of Yoga practice.
prāṇic — Of or pertaining to *prāṇa*.
prāṇotthāna — When the inner flow of *prāṇa* produces a cold sensation and makes the hair on one's body stand on end.
prapāka — Preliminary stage of digestion.
prapañca — A spreading out of the planes of experience that involves differentiation, proliferation, and the multiplication of coordinates.
pratiloman — Brushing against the direction that the hair or fur grows.

pratimā — Icon or image of god.

pratiprasava — Involution of the *guṇa* and the dissolution of form in *prakṛtic* pre-creation.

pratyāhāra — Withdrawal. The fifth branch of Yoga practice.

pūrakā kumbhaka recaka — Inhalation, retention, and exhalation. The cycle of breathing.

pūrṇa Yoga — Yoga of the absolute.

puruṣa — The transcendental, universal Self. Also a general term for male.

rāga — Passion or attachment.

Rāja Yoga — Royal Yoga; A term used at least from the sixteenth century on to designate the classical Yoga of Patañjali. It came into common modern usage as a result of Swami Vivekananda's teachings.

rakta — Blood.

ranjayet — Energized.

rasāyana — Rejuvenation therapy in Āyurvedic medicine.

rāśi puruṣa — Conglomerate person; heap-person.

śabda brahman — The sound of absolute truth.

*sad-darśana*s. — The six classical schools of Indic philosophy, including Sāṃkhya, Vedānta, Mīṃāṃsā, Nyāya, Vaiśeṣika, and Yoga.

sādhana — Practice or procedure; the means by which self-realization is achieved.

sādhya — Object.

sahaja — Innate; spontaneous.

sahasrāra cakra — The seventh vital center of the subtle body, located at the crown of the head or above the top of the head.

śākhā — Unit.

sākśin — Witness or seer.

śakti — Power. The dynamic force of life.

sālambana samādhi — Enstasy with support.

samādhi — Enstasy; the final state of embodied enlightenment.

Sāṃkhya — One of the six classical schools of Indic philosophy, primarily concerned with ontology and the delineation of ontic categories.

saṁsāra — The perceived, sentient world of flux and impermanence.

saṁsāric — Of or pertaining to the flux of perceived reality.

saṁskāra — Ritual. The ineradicable impression left on consciousness by experience.

saṁśodhana — Eliminatives in Āyurvedic medical practice.

saṃtoṣādanuttamaḥ sukhalābhaḥ — Superlative happiness from contentment.

sāmyāvasthā — When the *guṇa* are in a state of perfect equilibrium.

saṁyoga — Combination. The correlation between *puruṣa* and *prakṛti* that is the primary cause of suffering and ignorance.

śaṅkh prakṣālan — Conch purification. A technique where water is drunk and forced through the stomach, intestines, and out the anus.

sannyāsi — World renouncer.

sāra — The essence that is left once the digestive fire separates out waste products from food.

sarvadarśanacārya — Master of all systems of Indian philosophy.

śāstra — Teaching, or spiritual and philosophical texts.

sat kārya vāda — The relationship of cause and effect wherein an effect is contained in the cause. *Prakṛti* is, in these terms, the original, pre-creation cause of creation and all manifest and unmanifest things.

sattva — Purity and radiance. One of the three *guṇa*.

sattvik — Of the nature or pertaining to *sattva*.

Śeṣa Nāga — Another name for Ananta, the thousand-headed serpent deity.

siddhi — Supernatural powers achieved through the practice of Yoga.

śītalī prāṇāyāma — Cooling breath control. One of the primary methods of *prāṇāyāma*.

Śiva — Commonly regarded as the god of destruction. Often depicted in iconography and myth as the god of yogis.

śivambu — Urine. Water of Lord Śiva.

śloka — Stanza.

snāna — Bath.

śodhana — Purification.

soma — Elixir of immortality.

śoṇita — Menstrual blood.

sraṁsana — Laxatives in Āyurvedic medical practice.

śūdra Varṇa — A group that performs what are considered to be menial services by other *varṇa* groups.

sukha — Happiness.

śukra — Semen.

sūkṣma śarīra — Subtle body.

sūkṣma vyāyām — Subtle physical exercise.

śūnyatā — Emptiness.

sūrya namaskār — Salutation to the sun. A modern Yogalike exercise routine.

suṣumṇā nāḍī — The primary medial channel of the subtle body through which the vital force of *kuṇḍalinī* ascends.

sūtra neti — A procedure to clean the nasal passages and sinuses with a cotton cord catheter.

svādhiṣṭhāna cakra — The second vital center of the subtle body, located at the genitals.

svāmī (*swāmī*) — Master of himself. A title often taken to signify the status as an adept.

tamas — Darkness and inertia. One of the three *guṇa*.

tanmātra — Subtle dimension of the material elements.

tantric — Of or pertaining to *tantra*, a religious philosophy based on the idea that *śakti* provides the motive force of liberation.

tapas — Heat or radiance derived from ascetic practices.

tattva — Thatness. The constituent categories of nature as expounded in Sāṃkhya.

tīkā — Commentary or annotation.

tridoṣa — The three humors in Āyurvedic medicine: *kapha* (phlegm), *pitta* (bile), *vāya* (wind).

uḍḍiyāna bandha — Upward lock. A procedure in which the abdomen is contracted backward toward the spine and *prāṇa* is forced upward.

udvartana — Rubbing massage.
ujāna sādhana — Going against the current; against the grain or direction of flow.
vaidya — Āyurvedic physician.
Vaiśeṣika — One of the six principal schools of Indic philosophy, concerned with understanding difference.
vaiśya — Merchant *varṇa.*
vajrolī mudrā — One of the seals, which involves sucking up, with the penis, the male and female substances that are ejaculated during sexual intercourse.
vamana — Emetics in Āyurvedic medical practice.
vamana dhauti — Washing the stomach that is done by induced vomiting.
varṇa — Color. The four social statuses: priest, warrior, merchant, and menial service.
vāsanā — Desire and the traces of desire on consciousness.
vāsanā saṃskāra — The myriad traces of desire that are permanently imprinted on the psyche.
vastra dhauti — A technique for internal cleansing of the heart whereby a strip of cloth is swallowed and then pulled out of the stomach.
vāta — Air. One of the three *doṣa.*
vāyu — Air or wind.
vāyu bhaksan kriyā — A technique whereby wind is eaten or consumed.
Vedānta — A nondualist metaphysical philosophy that is reflected in the *Upaniṣads* and is the dominant point of view in contemporary Hinduism.
vedha — Piercer.
videha — Disembodied or without corporeality. God.
vidyā — Knowledge. A term that is often translated as science.
vijñāna — Secular knowledge.
vijñānamaya kośa — Knowledge sheath of the body.
vikāra — Disease or imbalance of the *doṣa.*
vindu — Semen.
vipāka — End result of intestinal digestion.
viśuddha cakra — The fifth vital center of the subtle body, located at the throat.
vivarta — Illusory change.
vivechana — Drastic purgatives in Āyurvedic medical practice.
vṛtti — Modification. Functioning of the mind.
vyakta — Manifest.
vyāyām yoga — A modern combination of muscular exercise and Yoga training.
yama — Restraint. The first branch of Yoga as expounded by Patañjali, including five basic moral and ethical principles: nonviolence, truthfulness, nonstealing, celibacy, and covetlessness.

REFERENCES

Abhedananda, Swami. 1902. *How to Be a Yogi*. New York: Vedanta Society.

———. 1946. *The Science of Psychic Phenomenon*. Calcutta: Ramakrishna Vedanta Math.

Abu-Lughod, Lila. 1991. Writing against Culture. *Recapturing Anthropology: Working in the Present*, edited by Richard G. Fox, 137–62. Santa Fe: School of American Research Press.

———. 1993. *Writing Women's Worlds: Bedouin Stories*. Berkeley: University of California Press.

Acharya, Jagdish B., ed. 1978a. *Auto-Urine Therapy*. Bombay: Jagdish B. Acharya Publications.

———. 1978b. *Practical Guide to Auto Urine Therapy: Treatment and Diet*. Bombay: Jagdish B. Acharya Publications.

Afshari, R. 1994. An Essay on Islamic Cultural Relativism in the Discourse of Human Rights. *Human Rights Quarterly* 16, no. 2: 235–76.

Agarwal, Radheshyam. 1992. *Svāmūtra Dvāra Svasthya*. Mathura: Bhasha Bhavan.

Aicken, Frederick. 1984. *Nature of Science: A Personal View of Science and How It Has Shaped the Way We Think and Behave*. London: Heinemann.

Albertson, Edward. 1969. *Spiritual Yoga*. Los Angeles: Sherbourne Press.

Alter, Joseph S. 1992. *The Wrestler's Body: Identity and Ideology in North India*. Berkeley: University of California Press.

———. 1994. Celibacy, Sexuality, and the Transformation of Gender into Nationalism. *Journal of Asian Studies* 53, no. 1: 45–66.

———. 1995. The Celibate Wrestler: Sexual Chaos, Embodied Balance, and Competitive Politics in North India. *Contributions to Indian Sociology*, n.s., 29, nos. 1–2: 109–31.

———. 1997. A Therapy to Live By: Public Health, the Self, and Nationalism in the Practice of a North Indian Yoga Society. *Medical Anthropology* 11: 275–98.

———. 1999. Heaps of Health, Metaphysical Fitness: Ayurveda and the Ontology of Good Health in Medical Anthropology. *Current Anthropology* 40: S43–S66.

———. 2000a. *Gandhi's Body: Sex, Diet, and the Politics of Nationalism*. Philadelphia: University of Pennsylvania Press.

———. 2000b. Kabaddi, a National Sport of India: The Internationalism of Nationalism and the Foreignness of Indianness. In *Getting Into the Game: The Anthropology of Sport*, edited by Noel Dyke, 81–116. Oxford and New York: Berg.

———. 2000c. *Knowing Dil Das: Stories of a Himalayan Hunter*. Philadelphia: University of Pennsylvania Press.

———. n.d.a. Indian Clubs and Colonialism: Hindu Masculinity and Muscular Christianity. *Comparative Studies in Society and History* (forthcoming).

———. n.d.b. Yoga, Body, Fetishism: Revisiting Questions of Religion and Social Facts. Manuscript.

Altmann, Simon L. 2002. *Is Nature Supernatural?: A Philosophical Explanation of Science and Nature.* Amherst, MA: Prometheus Books.

Amin, Nanubhai. 1995. Introduction. In *Yoga: The Ultimate Attainment,* by Swami Rajarshi Muni, xix–xxii. Delhi: Jaico Publishing House.

Amritabindu Upaniṣad (as part of the *Yoga Upaniṣads*). 1938. Edited by Mahadeva Shastri. Madras: Adyar Library and Research Center.

Anand, B. K., G. S. Chhina, and B. Singh. 1961. Studies on Ramananda Yogi during His Stay in an Air-Tight Box. *Indian Journal of Medical Research* 49: 82, 89–90.

Anantharaman, T. R. 1996. *Ancient Yoga and Modern Science.* Delhi: Project in the History of Indian Science, Philosophy, and Culture.

Andersen, Walter K., and Shridhar D. Damle. 1987. *The Brotherhood in Saffron.* Boulder, CO: Westview Press.

Anonymous. 1947. To Youth. *Organizer* 8: 11.

———. 1991. Treatment of Bronchial Asthma. *Naturopathy: Bapu Nature Cure Hospital's Journal* 1, no. 3: 15–28.

———. 1992a. *Gīt Śudha.* Lucknow: Lokhit Prakashan.

———. 1992b. *Śarīrik Śikṣa, Dvitīya Varṣ.* Nagpur: Madhav Prakashan.

———. 1994a. *Śarīrik Śikṣa, Pratham Varṣ.* Nagpur: Madhav Prakashan.

———. 1994b. *Śarīrik Śikṣa, Tritiya Varṣ.* Nagpur: Madhav Prakashan.

———. n.d.a. *Deś Jagāva.* Jalandar: Apna Sahitya.

———. n.d.b. *Saral Sahāgan.* Lucknow: Lokhit Prakashan.

Appadurai, Arjun. 1991. Global Ethnoscapes: Notes and Queries for a Transnational Anthropology. In *Recapturing Anthropology: Working in the Present,* edited by Richard G. Fox, 191–210. Santa Fe: School of American Research Press.

———. 1996. *Modernity at Large.* Minneapolis: University of Minnesota Press.

Apter, Emily. 1993. Introduction. In *Fetishism as Cultural Discourse,* edited by Emily Apter and William Pietz, 1–9. Ithaca, NY: Cornell University Press.

Armstrong, John W. 1971. *The Water of Life: A Treatise on Urine Therapy.* Calcutta and Delhi: Rupa and Company.

Arnold, David. 1993. *Colonizing the Body: State Medicine and Epidemic Disease in Nineteenth-Century India.* Berkeley: University of California Press.

Arnold, David, and Sumit Sarkar. 2002. In Search of Rational Remedies: Homeopathy in Nineteenth-Century Bengal. In *Plural Medicine, Tradition, and Modernity, 1800–2000,* edited by Waltraud Ernst, 40–57. London: Routledge.

Asrani, U. A. 1993. *Yoga Unveiled,* part 2. Delhi: Motilal Banarsidass.

Aṣṭāṅgahṛdaya. 1963. Delhi: Motilal Banarsidass.

Atkinson, William Walker. 1934. *A Series of Lessons in Raja Yoga.* Chicago: Chicago Yogi Publication Society.

Atmanaṇda, Swami. 1991. *The Four Yogas: The Four Paths to Spiritual Enlightenment (in the Words of Ancient Rishis).* Bombay: Bharatiya Vidya Bhavan.

Aurobindo, Sri. 1949. On Physical Culture: A Message from Sri Aurobindo. *Advent* 6, no. 1: 13–15.

———. 1976. *The Synthesis of Yoga*. Pondicherry: Sri Aurobindo Ashram.

———. 1977. *The Life Divine*. 10th ed. Pondicherry: Sri Aurobindo Ashram.

———. n.d. *Yoga and Physical Culture According to the Integral Yoga of Sri Aurobindo and The Mother.* Pondicherry: Sri Aurobindo Ashram.

Ayyangar, T. R. Srinivasa. 1893. *Haṭhayogapradīpikā of Svātmārāma Svāmin.* Bombay: Tookaram Tatya.

———. 1952. *The Yoga Upaniṣads*. 2nd ed. Madras: Adyar Library.

Banerjee, Sikita. 1999. Warriors in Politics: Religious Nationalism, Masculine Hinduism, and the Shiv Sena in Bombay. *Women and Politics* 20, no. 3: 1–26.

———. 2000. *Warriors in Politics: Hindu Nationalism, Violence, and the Shiv Sena*. Boulder, CO: Westview.

Bapu Nature Cure Hospital and Yogashram. n.d.a. *Naturopathy Institute cum Hospital, Delhi: 100% Tax Exemption*. Delhi: Bapu Nature Cure Hospital and Yogashram.

———. n.d.b. *Promotional and Informational Brochure*. Delhi: Bapu Nature Cure Hospital and Yogashram, Center for Research and Development in Naturopathy and Yogic Sciences.

Barrow, H. W. 1893. On Aghoris and Aghorapanthis. *Proceedings of the Anthropological Society of Bombay* 3: 197–251.

Barthes, Roland. 1972. *Mythologies*. New York: Hill and Wang.

Bartnett, Beatrice. 1998. *Urine-Therapy: It May Save Your Life* . Ruidoso, NM: Lifestyle Institute.

Basu, A. 1993. Feminism Inverted—The Real Women and Gendered Imagery of Hindu Nationalism. *Bulletin of Concerned Asian Scholars* 25, no. 4: 25–36.

Basu, Shamti. 2002. *Religious Revivalism as Nationalist Discourse: Swami Vivekananda and New Hinduism in Nineteenth Century Bengal*. New Delhi: Oxford University Press.

Basu, T., et al. 1993. *Khaki Shorts and Saffron Flags*. Delhi: Orient Longman.

Bates, Daniel G. 1996. *Cultural Anthropology*. Boston: Allyn and Bacon.

Beatrix, Avivah. 1996. *My Way to Urine Therapy: The Wonder for Even Hopeless Cases; A Guide for Lasting Health*. Kooralbyn, Queensland, Australia: Self-published.

Behanan, Kovoor Thomas. 1937. *Yoga: A Scientific Evaluation*. New York: Macmillan Company.

Bernard, Theos. 1939. *Heaven Lies within Us*. New York: Scribner's and Sons.

———. 1944. *Haṭha Yoga: The Report of a Personal Experience*. New York: Columbia University Press.

Besant, Annie Wood. 1907. *An Introduction to Yoga*. Benares and London: Theosophical Publishing Society.

———. 1913. *Evolution and Occultism*. London: Theosophical Publishing Society.

Bhagavad Gītā (In *The Bhagavad Gītā in the Mahābhārata: Text and Commentary*). 1981. Edited and translated by J. A. Van Buitenen. Chicago: University of Chicago Press.

Bhagwat, J. M., S. M. Soman, and M. V. Bhole. 1981. Treatment of Bronchial Asthma: A Medical Report. *Yoga Mimamsa* 20, no. 3: 1–12.

Bhanuteja, N., Vinu Abraham, Nistula Hebbar, and Dnyanesh Jathar. 2002. Returning to Roots. *The Week* 20, no. 34: 22–27.

Bharati, Agehananda. 1965. *The Tantric Tradition*. London: Rider.

Bhardwaj, S. 1896. *Vyāyāmadīpikā*. Bangalore: Caxton Press.

Bhargava's Standard Illustrated Dictionary of the Hindi Language. 1964. Edited by R. C. Pathak. Hindi-English ed. Varanasi: Bhargava Book Depot.

Bhatt, K. G. 1992. Natural Pain Relievers. *Naturopathy: Bapu Nature Cure Hospital's Journal* 2, no. 13: 3–4.

Bhatta, Ratna Gopala. 1911. *Patāñjalayogadarśana, with the Yoga-Siddhānta-Candrikā and Sūtrārtha-Bodhinī of Nārāyaṇa Tīrtha*. Varanasi: Chowkhamba.

Bhattacarya, Santilala. 1974. *Sarbbauś adhi Śibambu: Svāmūtrakalpa-Bidhi*. Calcutta: Self-published.

Bhattacharya, Pranab Kumar. 1952. *A Scheme of Education*. Pondicherry: Sri Aurobindo Ashram.

———. 1968. The Role of Physical Education in the Sri Aurobindo Ashram. *Mother India* 20, nos. 10/11: 173–76.

Bhava Prakāśa. Bombay: Khemraj Shrikrishnadas.

Bhole, M. V., and P. V. Karambelkar. 1968. Significance of Nostrils in Breathing. *Yoga Mimamsa* 10, no. 4: 1–12.

Bhole, M. V. 1970. Yogic Treatment of Chronic Rhinitis and Sinusitis. *Maharashtra Medical Journal* 17, no. 8: 359–64.

———. 1976. Treatment of Bronchial Asthma by Yogic Methods—A Report. *Yoga Mimamsa* 9, no. 3: 33–41.

———. 1982a. Effect of Yogic Treatment on Various Lung Functions of Asthma Patients. *Yoga Mimamsa* 20, no. 4: 43–50.

———. 1982b. Fibrinolitic Activity in Blood and Three Weeks Intensive Training Program in Yogic Physical Culture. *Yoga Mimamsa* 21, nos. 1–2: 7–12.

———. 1982c. Intra-Vaginal Pressure Changes during Selected Yoga Practices. Paper presented at the National Conference on Sexology. February.

———. 1985. *Abstracts and Bibliography of Articles on Yoga: From Kaivalyadhama*. Lonavala: Kaivalyadhama SMYM Samithi.

Bhole, M. V., and R. R. Deshpande. 1982. Effect of Yogic Treatment on Total and Differential Leukocyte Counts in Asthmatics. *Yoga Mimamsa* 20, no. 4: 1–8.

Bhole, M. V., and M. L. Gharote. 1977. Effects of Yogic Treatment on Breath Holding Time in Asthmatics. *Yoga Mimamsa* 19, no. 1: 47–52.

Bhole, M. V., and P. V. Karambelkar. 1971. Effect of Yogic Treatment on Blood Picture of Asthma Patients. *Yoga Mimamsa* 14, nos. 1–2: 1–6.

Bhole, M. V., P. V. Karambelkar, and S. L. Vinekar. 1967. Underground Burial or Bhugarbha Samadhi. *Yoga Mimamsa* 10, nos. 1–2: 1–8, 2–16.

Blavatsky, H. P. 1931. *Raja-Yoga, or Occultism*. Bombay: Theosophy Company.

Bode, Maarten. 2002. Indian Indigenous Pharmaceuticals: Tradition, Modernity and Nature. In *Plural Medicine, Tradition, and Modernity, 1800–2000*, edited by Waltraud Ernst, 184–203. London: Routledge.

Bohr, Niels Henrick David. 1958. *Atomic Physics and Human Knowledge*. New York: Wiley.

———. 1972. *Collected Works*. Amsterdam: North-Holland Publishing Company.

Borofsky, Robert. 1994. Diversity and Divergence within the Anthropological Community. In *Assessing Cultural Anthropology,* edited by Robert Borofsky, 23–28. New York: McGraw-Hill.

Bosc, Ernest. 1893. *Addha-Nari; Ou, l'Occultisme dans l'Inde Antique. Védisme, Littérature Hindoue, Mythes, Religions . . . [etc.].* Paris: Librairie Galignani.

———. 1913. *Yoghisme et Fakirisme Hindous.* Paris: Librairie Internationale de la Pense Nouvelle.

Bowlin, John R., and Peter G. Stromberg. 1997. Representation and Reality in the Study of Culture. *American Anthropologist* 99, no. 1: 123–34.

Boyle, John E. Whiteford. 1983. *The Indra Web: The Renewal of Ancient Oriental Concepts in Modern Western Thought.* Washington, DC: Wheat Forders.

Bradley, James. 2002. Medicine on the Margins? Hydrotherapy and Orthodoxy in Britain, 1840–1860. In *Plural Medicine, Tradition, and Modernity, 1800–2000,* edited by Waltraud Ernst, 19–39. London: Routledge.

Brahmachari, Naresh K. 1991. Yoga—In Light of Ayurveda. *Naturopathy: Bapu Nature Cure Hospital's Journal* 1, no. 4: 9–15.

Brahmananda Baba. 1889. *Haṭhayogapradīpikā of Svātmārāma Svāmin.* Bombay.

Brahmavidyopaniṣad (as part of the *Yoga Upaniṣads*). 1938. Edited by Mahadeva Shastri. Madras: Adyar Library and Research Center.

Brass, Paul, ed. 1996. *Riots and Pogroms.* London: Macmillan.

Brems, E. 1997. Enemies or Allies? Feminism and Cultural Relativism as Dissident Voices in Human Rights Discourse. *Human Rights Quarterly* 19, no. 1: 136–64.

Bṛhadāraṇyaka Upaniṣad. 1980. In *Sixty Upaniṣads of the Veda.* Edited and translated by Paul Deussen. Translated and Edited into English by V. M. Bedekar and G. B. Palsule. Delhi: Motilal Banarsidass.

Bṛhadyogiyājñavalkyasmṛti. 1951. Lonavala: Kaivalyadhama, SMYM Samiti.

Briggs, George W. 1938. *Gorakhnāth and the Kānphata Yogīs.* Calcutta: Y.M.C.A. Publishing House.

Brightman, Robert. 1995. Forget Culture: Replacement, Transcendence, Relexification. *Cultural Anthropology* 10, no. 4: 509–46.

Brumann, Christoph. 1999. Writing for Culture: Why a Succesful Concept Should Not Be Discarded. *Current Anthropology* 40: S1–S27.

Brunton, Paul. 1939. *A Hermit in the Himalayas.* New York: E. P. Dutton and Co.

Buddhananda, Swami. 1996. *Moola Bandha: The Master Key.* Munger: Yoga Publications Trust.

Burman, E. 1996. Local, Global, or Globalized? Child Development and International Child Rights Legislation. *Childhood—A Global Journal of Child Research* 3, no. 1: 45–66.

Bynum, W. F., and R. Porter. 1987. *Medical Fringe and Medical Orthodoxy, 1750–1850.* London: Croom Helm.

Caplan, Mariana. 1999. *Halfway up the Mountain: The Error of Premature Claims to Enlightenment.* Prescott, AZ: Hohm Press.

Cappai, G. 2000. Cultural Relativism and the Translatability of the Cultural Strange in the View of Quine and Davidson: An Observation from the Point of View of Social Science. *Zeitschrift für Soziologie* 29, no. 4: 253–272.

Carakasaṃhitā. 1992. Banaras: Chowkhamba Orientalia.

Carpenter, Edward. 1911. *A Visit to a Gnani, or a Wise Man of the East.* London: G. Allen.

Carrithers, Michael. 1990. Is Anthropology Art or Science? *Current Anthropology* 31: 263–72.

Cayleff, Susan E. 1987. *Wash and Be Healed: The Water Cure Movement and Women's Health.* Philadelphia: Temple University Press.

Central Council for Research in Yoga and Naturopathy. 1996. *Activities, Achievements, and Future Programmes.* New Delhi: Ministry of Health and Family Welfare, Government of India.

Chakrabarty, B. 2001. The Emergence of Hindu Nationalism in India. *Indian Economic and Social History Review* 38, no. 3: 330–33.

Chakrabarty, Dipesh. 2000. *Provincializing Europe: Postcolonial Thought and Historical Difference.* Princeton: Princeton University Press.

Chakraborty, P. 2000. Science, Nationalism, and Colonial Contestations: P. C. Ray and His "Hindu" Chemistry. *Indian Economic and Social History Review* 37, no. 2: 185–213.

Chakravarti, Surath Chandra. 1985. *Mysterious Samadhi.* Calcutta: Firma KLM.

Chanana, P. L. Bhel. 1995. The Science of Yogic Postures (Yog Mudrās) and Their Benefits. *Naturopathy: Bapu Nature Cure Hospital's Journal* 4, no. 48: 59–61.

"Charu, Dr." 1994. Emphysema. *Naturopathy: Bapu Nature Cure Hospital's Journal* 4, no. 42: 29–33.

Chase, B. 1997. John Locke and Cultural Relativism. *Interpretation—A Journal of Political Philosophy* 25, no. 1: 59–90.

Chatterjee, Partha. 1993. *Nationalist Thought and the Colonial World: A Derivative Discourse.* Minneapolis: University of Minnesota Press.

Chattopadhyaya, D. P. 1996. Foreword. In *Ancient Yoga and Modern Science,* by T. R. Anantharaman, ix–xiii. Delhi: Project of History in Indian Science, Philosophy, and Culture.

Chingle, S. M. 1975. Sweet Reminiscences of an Inspired and an Inspiring Life. In *Kaivalyadhama, Golden Jubilee Year Souvenir, 1975,* edited by Swami Digambarji, 29–33. Lonavala: Kaivalyadhama.

Christy, Martha. 1994. *Your Own Perfect Medicine.* Scottsdale, AZ: Future Medicine.

Clifford, James, and George E. Marcus. 1986. *Writing Culture: The Poetics and Politics of Ethnography.* Berkeley: University of California Press.

Conklin, B. A. 1997. Consuming Images: Representations of Cannibalism on the Amazonian Frontier. *Anthropological Quarterly* 70, no. 2: 68–78.

Coomaraswamy, Ananda K. 1956. *The Dance of Śiva: Fourteen Indian Essays.* Bombay: Asia Publishing House.

Cooter, R. 1988. *Studies in the History of Alternative Medicine.* Basingstoke: Macmillan in association with St. Antony's College, Oxford.

Corbridge, S. 1999. "The Militarization of All Hindudom"? The Bharatiya Janata Party, the Bomb, and the Political Spaces of Hindu Nationalism. *Economy and Society* 28, no. 2: 222–55.

Ḍāmara Tantra. 1998. Translated and edited by C. P. Mishra. In *Svāmūtra Cikitsā*, by C. P. Mishra, 98–117. Varanasi: Sarva Seva Sangh.

Daniel, E. Valentine. 1984. *Fluid Signs: Being a Person the Tamil Way.* Berkeley: University of California Press.

———. 1996. *Charred Lullabies: Chapters in an Anthropography of Violence.* Princeton: Princeton University Press.

Dasgupta, Surendranath. 1920. *A Study of Patanjali.* Calcutta: Calcutta University Press.

———. 1924. *Yoga as Philosophy and Religion.* London: E.P.K. Paul, Trench, Trubner and Co.

———. 1930. *Yoga Philosophy in Relation to Other Systems of Indian Thought.* Calcutta: University of Calcutta.

de Blecourt, W., and C. Usborne. 1999. Alternative Medicine in Europe since 1800. *Medical History* 43: 283–285.

De Laurence, Lauron William. 1909. *The Mystic Test Book of "The Hindu Occult Chambers"; The Magic and Occultism of India; Hindu and Egyptian Crystal Gazing; The Hindu Magic Mirror.* Chicago: De Laurence, Scott & Co.

Deleuze, Gilles. 1983. *Nietzsche and Philosophy.* Translated by Hugh Tomlinson. New York: Columbia University Press.

De Michelis, Elizabeth. 2001. "Modern Yoga: Transmission of Theory and Practice." Ph.D. diss., University of Cambridge.

———. 2004. *A History of Modern Yoga: Patanjali and Western Esotericism.* London and New York: Continuum.

———. n.d. Notes on the Historical Development of Modern Yoga, Including Comments on the Problem of Knowledge Transmission and on Modern Yoga's Relation to Western Scientific Thought. Manuscript.

Desai, B. P., and M. V. Bhole. 1981. Gastric Responses to Vastra Dhauti as Influenced by Four Weeks Yogic Treatment in Asthmatics—A Weekwise Study. *Yoga Mimamsa* 20, no. 3: 41–50.

de Sarak, Albert. 1990. *General Treatise on Occult Science in Three Parts.* New York: New York Public Library (microfilm no. zz-30,495).

Deshmukh, Nana. 1979. *RSS, Victim of Slander: A Multi-Dimensional Study of RSS, Jana Sangh, Janata Party and the Present Political Crisis.* New Delhi: Vision Books.

Deshpande, R. R., and M. V. Bhole. 1982. Effects of Yogic Treatment on Eosinophil Count in Asthma Patients. *Yoga Mimamsa* 20, no. 4: 9–16.

Deussen, Paul. 1906. *The Philosophy of the Upaniṣads.* Edinburgh: T. & T. Clark.

———. 1920. *Allgemeine Geschichte der Philosophie.* Vol. 1, pt. 3. Leipzig: F. A. Brockhaus.

Dikshit, Rajesh. 1971. *Svāmūtra Cikitsā.* n.p.: Self-published.

Dirks, Nicholas B. 1998. *In Near Ruins: Cultural Theory at the End of the Century.* Minneapolis: University of Minnesota Press.

Downey, Gary Lee, and Juan D. Rogers. 1995. On the Politics of Theorizing in a Postmodern Academy. *American Anthropologist* 97, no. 2: 269–81.

Dubow, S. 1992. Afrikaner Nationalism, Apartheid, and the Conceptualization of Race. *Journal of African History* 33, no. 2: 209–37.

Durkheim, Emile. 1964. *The Rules of Sociological Method*. New York: Free Press.

———. 1995. *The Elementary Forms of Religious Life*. Translated by Karen E. Fields. New York: Free Press.

Dvivedi, Manilal Nabhubhai. 1992. *Raja Yoga, or The Practical Metaphysics of the Vedānta: Being a Translation of the Vākyasudhā or Drigdrishyaviveka of Bhāratitīrtha, and the Aparokshā nubhuti of Shri Shankarāchārya; With an Introduction, Appendix Containing the Sanskrit Text and Commentary of the Vākyasudhā, and Notes Explanatory and Critical*. Delhi: Antiquarian Book House.

Eliade, Mircea. 1964. *Shamanism: Archaic Techniques of Ecstasy*. Translated by Willard R. Trask. Princeton: Princeton University Press.

———. 1978. *The Forge and the Crucible*. Translated by Stephen Corrin. Chicago: University of Chicago Press.

———. 1990. *Yoga: Immortality and Freedom*. Translated by Willard R. Trask. Princeton: Princeton University Press.

Ember, Carol R., and Melvin Ember. 1996. *Cultural Anthropology*. 8th ed. Upper Saddle, NJ: Prentice Hall.

Ernst, Waltraud. 2002. Plural Medicine, Tradition, and Modernity. Historical and Contemporary Perspectives: Views from Below and from Above. In *Plural Medicine, Tradition, and Modernity, 1800–2000*, edited by Waltraud Ernst, 1–18. London: Routledge.

Ernst, Waltraud, and B. Harris. 1999. *Race, Science, and Medicine, 1700–1960*. London: Routledge.

"Experienced Physician, An." n.d. *Auto-Urine Therapy*. Ahmedabad: Navneet Publications.

Fabian, Johannes. 1995. Ethnographic Misunderstanding and the Perils of Context. *American Anthropologist* 97, no. 1: 41–50.

Feuerstein, Georg. 1980. *The Philosophy of Classical Yoga*. New York: St. Martin's Press.

———. 1989. *Yoga: The Technology of Ecstasy*. Los Angeles: J. P. Tarcher.

———. 1990. *Encyclopedic Dictionary of Yoga*. London: Unwin Paperbacks.

———. 2001. *The Yoga Tradition: Its History, Literature, Philosophy, and Practice*. Prescott, AZ: Hohm.

Feuerstein, Georg, and Larry Payne. 1999. *Yoga for Dummies*. Foster City, CA: IDGA Books Worldwide.

Feyerabend, Paul. 1978. *Against Method: Outline of an Anarchist Theory of Knowledge*. London: Verso.

Fields, Gregory P. 2001. *Religious Therapeutics*. Albany: State University of New York Press.

Fields, Karen E. 1995. Religion as an Eminently Social Thing. In *The Elementary Forms of Religious Life*, by Emile Durkheim, translated by Karen E. Fields. New York: Free Press.

Filliozat, J. 1964. *The Classical Doctrine of Indian Medicine*. Delhi: Munshi Ram Manoharlal.

Fischer, Edward F. 1999. Cultural Logic and Maya Identity: Rethinking Constructivism and Essentialism. *Current Anthropology* 40, no. 4: 473–99.

Fotedar, M. L. 1991. Messages. *Naturopathy: Bapu Nature Cure Hospital's Journal* 1, no. 3: 3–4.

Foucault, Michel. 1973. *The Birth of the Clinic: An Archaeology of Medical Perception.* New York: Pantheon Books.

———. 1980. *Power/Knowledge: Selected Interviews and Other Writings, 1972–1977.* Edited by Colin Gordon. New York: Pantheon Books.

Fox, Richard G., ed. 1991. *Recapturing Anthropology: Working in the Present.* Santa Fe, NM: School of American Research.

Friedrich, Paul. 1992. Interpretation and Vision: A Critique of Cryptopositivism. *Cultural Anthropology* 7, no. 2: 211–31.

Fujimura, Joan H. 1998. Authorizing Knowledge in Science and Anthropology. *American Anthropologist* 100, no. 2: 347–60.

Gable, E., R. Handler, and A. Lawson. 1992. On the Uses of Relativism: Fact, Conjecture, and Black-and-White Histories at Colonial Williamsburg. *American Ethnologist* 19, no. 4: 791–805.

Gandhi, Mohandas K. 1921. *The Health Guide.* Bombay: Pearl Publications.

———. 1948. *Key to Health.* Ahmedabad: Navajivan Press.

———. 1949. *Diet and Diet Reform.* Ahmedabad: Navajivan Press.

———. 1954. *Nature Cure.* Ahmedabad: Navajivan Press.

Ganguly, S. K. 1981. Effect of Short Term Yogic Training Program on Cardio-Vascular Indurance. *SNIPES Journal* 4, no. 2: 45–50.

———. 1982. Cardio-Vascular Responses to Yogic Treatment of Asthmatics. *Yoga Mimamsa* 20, no. 4: 35–42.

Ganguly, S. K., and M. L. Gharote. 1974. Cardio-Vascular Efficiency before and after Yogic Training. *Yoga Mimamsa* 17, no. 1: 89–97.

Garbe, Richard. 1894. *Die Sāṃkhya-Philosophie, eine Darstellung des Indischen Rationalismus nach den Quellen.* Leipzig: H. Haessel.

———. 1896. *Sāṃkhya und Yoga.* Strassburg: K. J. Trübner.

———. 1917. *Die Sāṃkhya Philosophie.* 2nd ed. Leipzig: H. Haessel.

Geertz, Clifford. 1973. *The Interpretation of Cultures: Selected Essays.* New York: Basic Books.

———. 1984. Distinguished Lecture: Anti Anti-Relativism. *American Anthropologist* 86: 263–78.

George, Sujatha. 1995. Mud Treatment. *Naturopathy: Bapu Nature Cure Hospital's Journal* 4, no. 48: 29–30.

Gevitz, Norman. 1988. *Other Healers: Unorthodox Medicine in America.* Baltimore: Johns Hopkins University Press.

Gharote, M. L. 1977. An Evaluation of the Effects of Yogic Treatment on Obesity. *Yoga Mimamsa* 19, no. 1: 13–37.

Gharote, M. L., and P. V. Karambelkar. 1975. Influence of Danda Dhauti on Gastric Acidity. In *Collected Papers on Yoga,* 41–47. Lonavala: Kaivalyadhama.

Gheraṇḍasaṁhitā. 1996. Edited by Rai Bahadur Srisa Chandra Vasu. New Delhi: Munshiram Manoharlal.

Ghose, J. 1930. *Sāṃkhya and Modern Thought.* Calcutta: Book Company.

Giri, Swami Hariharananda, and Ramesh Chandra Pattnaik. 1981. *Kriyā yoga:*

The Scientific Process of Soul-Culture and the Essence of All Religions. Puri: Karar Ashram.

Golwalkar, M. S. 1966. *Bunch of Thoughts*. Bangalore: Jagarana Prakashana.

Gorakṣa Śataka. 1989. In *Gorakhnāth and the Kānphata Yogis*, edited and translated by George Weston Briggs, 284–304. Delhi: Motilal Banarsidass.

Gordon, Colin. 1980. Afterword. In *Power/Knowledge: Selected Interviews and Other Writings, 1972–1977*, by Michel Foucault. New York: Pantheon Books.

Gore, M. M. 1976. Effect of Long Term Yogic Practices on Urinary Acidity. *Yoga Mimamsa* 18, no. 2: 14–21.

———. 1981. Immediate Effect of Asanas on Urinary PH; Acid Secretion and Creatinine. *Yoga Mimamsa* 20, nos. 1–2: 9–18.

———. 1982. Effect of Yogic Treatment on Some Pulmonary Functions in Asthmatics. *Yoga Mimamsa* 20, no. 4: 51–58.

Gore, M. M., and M. V. Bhole. 1982. Respiratory Responses to Vastra Dhauti in Asthmatics. *Yoga Mimamsa* 22, nos. 1–2: 47–53.

Gotham, Chamanlal. 1988. *Mūtra Cikitsā*. Barelli: Sanskrit Sansthan.

Gould, Stephen Jay. 1987. *Time's Arrow, Time's Cycle: Myth and Metaphor in the Discovery of Geological Time*. Cambridge: Harvard University Press.

———. 1999. *Rock of Ages: Science and Religion in the Fullness of Life*. New York: Ballantine Publishers.

———. 2002. *The Structure of Evolutionary Theory*. Cambridge: Harvard University Press.

Goyal, D. R. 1979. *Rashtriya Swayamsevak Sangh*. Delhi: Radha Krishna Publications.

Grierson, Janet. 1998. *Dr. Wilson and His Malvern Hydro: Park View in the Water Cure Era*. Malvern: Malvern Museum.

Gruber, Angelika. 1992. *Natürliche Heilung und Arztliche Behandlung in den Hippokratischen Epidemienbüchern*. Munich: Technische Universität München.

Gupta, Akhil, and James Ferguson. 1992. Beyond "Culture": Space, Identity, and the Politics of Difference. *Cultural Anthropology* 7: 6–23.

Haanel, C. F. 1937. *The Amazing Secrets of the Yogi*. Master Key Publishing Company.

Hampel, Petra. 1998. *Innere Medizin und Naturheilkunde: Die Auseinandersetzung in den Jahren 1882 bis 1933*. Essen: KVC Verlag.

Hancock, Mary. 1995. Hindu Culture for an Indian Nation: Gender, Politics, and Elite Identity in Urban South India. *American Ethnologist* 22, no. 4: 907–26.

Hansen, Thomas B. 1996. Recapturing Masculinity—Hindu Nationalism, Violence, and the Exorcism of the Muslim 'Other.' *Critique of Anthropology* 16, no. 2: 137–72.

———. 1999. *The Saffron Wave: Democracy and Hindu Nationalism in Modern India*. Princeton: Princeton University Press.

Haraway, Donna. 1991. *Simians, Cyborgs, and Women: The Reinvention of Nature*. New York: Routledge.

Hariharananda Giri, Swami, Ramesh Chandra Pattanaik, Raghabananda Nayak, and P. K. Goswami. 1981. *Kriyāyoga, the Scientific Process of Soul-Culture and the Essence of All Religions*. Puri: Karar Ashram.

Haritasaṁhitā. 1927. Bombay: Khemraja-Shrikrshnadas.

Harris, Iverson L. 1919. *Katherine Tingley and Her Rāja-Yoga System of Education: Its Aims and Achievements*. Point Loma, CA: Aryan Theosophical Press.

Harris, Marvin. 1997. *Culture, People, Nature: An Introduction to General Anthropology*. New York: Longman.

Harrison, Mark. 1994. *Public Health in British India: Anglo-Indian Preventative Medicine, 1859–1914*. Cambridge: Cambridge University Press.

Haṭhayogapradīpikā. 1915. Translated by Pancham Sinh. Allahabad.

Haviland, William A., and Robert J. Gordon. 1996. *Talking about People: Readings in Contemporary Cultural Anthropology*. 2nd ed. Mountain View, CA: Mayfield.

Healy, Mark. 2002. The "Bhajan Belt": Serenity in the Catskills. *New York Times*, sec. Escapes, pp. D1, 7. October 18.

Herzfeld, Michael. 1997. Anthropological Perspectives: Disturbing the Structures of Power and Knowledge. *International Social Science Journal* 49, no. 4: 453–462.

Hiralal. 1988. *Vijñānic Svāmūtra Cikitsā*. Unaw: Jan Swasthya Prakashan.

———. 1991. Śudh Śahed Kī Pehcān Aveṇ Sevan Sambandhī Sāvdhāniyan. *Naturopathy: Bapu Nature Cure Hospital's Journal* 1, no. 3: 29–31.

Hitchens, J. 1994. Critical Implications of Franz Boas' Theory and Methodology. *Dialectical Anthropology* 19, nos. 2–3: 237–53.

Humboldt, Wilhelm von. 1988. *On Language: The Diversity of Human Language Structure and Its Influence on the Mental Development of Mankind*. Cambridge: Cambridge University Press.

Iyengar, B.K.S. 1976. *Light on Yoga*. New York: Schocken Books.

———. 1993. *Light on the Yoga-Sūtras of Patañjali*. London: Aquarian/Thorsons.

Iyengar, Tirumangalum Chrishna Rajan. 1908. *The Hindu-Aryan Theory on Evolution and Involution, or, The Science of Rāja-Yoga*. New York: Funk and Wagnalls.

Jackson, Carl T. 1994. *Vedānta for the West: The Ramakrishna Movement in the United States*. Bloomington: Indiana University Press.

Jacolliot, Louis. 1971. *Occult Science in India and among the Ancients, with an Account of Their Mystic Initiations and the History of Spiritism*. New Hyde Park, England: University Books.

Jaffrelot, Christophe. 1993. Hindu Nationalism—Strategic Syncretism in Ideology Building. *Economic and Political Weekly* 28, nos. 12–13: 517–24.

———. 1996. *The Hindu Nationalist Movement in India*. New York: Columbia University Press.

Jagati, Loknatha. 1991. *Śibambu Sādhana, O, Sabuja Śudha: Sahaja Prākṛtika Cikitsā*. Cuttak: Sukhamayi Jagati.

James, S. A. 1994. Reconciling International Human Rights and Cultural Relativism: The Case of Female Circumcision. *Bioethics* 8, no. 1: 1–26.

Jeffery, Roger. 1988. *The Politics of Health in India*. Berkeley: University of California Press.

Jeyaram, S. A. 1993. Normal Natural Delivery. *Naturopathy: Bapu Nature Cure Hospital's Journal* 2, no. 20: 32–35.

Jolly, J. 1977. *Indian Medicine.* Delhi: Munshi Ram Manohar Lal.

Joshi, K. S. 1975. Place of Yoga in a Scientific Age. In *Kaivalyadhama, Golden Jubilee Year Souvenir, 1975,* edited by Swami Digambarji, 202–4. Lonavala: Kaivalyadhama.

Jussawalla, J. M. 1991. Care of the Hair. *Naturopathy: Bapu Nature Cure Hospital's Journal* 1, no. 3: 5–8.

———. 1992. Vis Medicatrix Naturae. *Naturopathy: Bapu Nature Cure Hospital's Journal* 5, no. 53: 4–7.

Just, Adolf. 1903. *Return to Nature!* New York: E. P. Dutton.

Kadir of the Monastery of Kanvallana. 1909. *L'Inde mystérieuse dévoilée.* Imprimerie Royale et Impériale.

Kahn, Joel S. 1989. Culture: Demise or Resurrection. *Critique of Anthropology* 9, no. 2: 5–25.

Kaivalyadhama and Its Activities. 1975. Lonavala: Kaivalyadhama.

Kaivalyadhama SMYM Samiti. n.d. *Platinum Jubilee, 1924–1999: Kaivalyadhama and Its Glimpses.* Lonavala: Kaivalyadhama.

Kakar, Sudhir. 1978. *The Inner World: A Psycho-analytic Study of Childhood and Society in India.* Delhi: Oxford University Press.

———. 1990. *Intimate Relations: Exploring Indian Sexuality.* Chicago: University of Chicago Press.

Kapila, Rup Chand. 1947. Compulsory Military Training for Self-Preservation. *Organizer* 21: 9.

Karambelkar, P. V. 1972. Can Yoga Cure or Prevent Cancer? *Yoga Mimamsa* 15, no. 3: 1–12.

———. 1976. Care of a Diabetic through Yogic Techniques. *Yoga Mimamsa* 18, nos. 3–4: 79–88.

Karambelkar, P. V., M. V. Bhole, and M. L. Gharote. 1969. Effect of Yogic Asanas on Uropepsin Excretion. *Indian Journal of Medical Research* 57, no. 5: 944–47.

Karambelkar, P. V., M. L. Gharote, S. K. Ganguly, and A. M. Moorthy. 1977. Effects of Short Term Yogic Training on Serum Cholesterol Level. *Yoga Mimamsa* 19, no. 1: 1–12.

Karambelkar, P. V., S. L. Vinekar, and M. V. Bhole. 1968. Studies on Human Subjects Staying in an Air Tight Pit. *Indian Journal of Medical Research* 56, no. 8: 1282–88.

Karandikar, S. V. 1997. *A Life Saver: An Illustrated Manual.* Pune: Kabir-Baug Matha Sanstha.

———. n.d.a. *The Effect of Yogasanas on Metabolism of a Cell.* Sunderraj Yoga Darshan.

———. n.d.b. *Shri Sunderraj Yoga Darshan, A Yoga Therapy Project—"A Bird's Eye View."* Sunderraj Yoga Darshan.

———. n.d.c. *Yoga Therapy in Diabetes Mellitus.* Sunderraj Yoga Darshan.

Karlekar, Ramakrishna Vasudeo. 1972. *Auto-Urine Cure.* Bombay: Shree Gajanan Book Depot.

Kaul, Narendra Nath. 1989. *Seven Steps for Simple Samadhi.* Bombay: Bharatiya Vidya Bhavan.

Kaviraj, S. 1997. Religion and Identity in India. *Ethnic and Racial Studies* 20, no. 2: 325– 44.

Keith, A. B. 1925. *Religion and Philosophy of the Veda and Upaniṣads.* Cambridge: Harvard University Press.

Kesari, M. G., P. S. Vaishawanar, and B. V. Deshkar. 1979. Effect of Yogasanas and Pranayama on Urea Clearance and Creatinine Clearance Values. *Yoga Mimamsa* 19, no. 4: 1–5.

Kirin, Ram. 1997. High Blood Pressure. *Naturopathy: Bapu Nature Cure Hospital's Journal* 7, no. 74: 3–5.

Kocher, H. C. 1973. Introverted and Extroverted Practitioners of Yoga and Their Scores on Neuroticism, Anxiety, and General Hostility. *Yoga Mimamsa* 15, no. 4: 69–74.

———. 1976. Anxiety, General Hostility, and Its Direction as a Result of Yogic Practices. *Yoga Mimamsa* 17, no. 4: 73–82.

Kocher, H. C., and V. Pratap. 1971. Anxiety Level and Yogic Practice. *Yoga Mimamsa* 15, no. 1: 11–15.

Kottak, Conrad Phillip. 1994. *Cultural Anthropology.* 6th ed. New York: McGraw-Hill.

Kripal, Jeffery John. 1995. *Kali's Child: The Mystical and the Erotic in the Life and Teaching of Ramakrishna.* Chicago: University of Chicago Press.

Krishna, Gopi. 1992. *Kundalini: Path to Higher Consciousness.* New Delhi: Orient Paperbacks.

———. n.d. *Kundalini—The Secret of Yoga.* New Delhi: UBS Publishers.

Krishnamachariya, T. N. 1935. *Yogamakaranda.* Mysore: Mysore Palace.

Krishnananda, Swami. 1997. *Yoga as a Universal Science.* Sivanandanagar: Divine Life Society.

Kroon, Coen van der. 1996. *The Golden Fountain: The Complete Guide to Urine Therapy.* Scottsdale, AZ: Wishland Publishing.

Kuhn, Thomas S. 1970. *The Structure of Scientific Revolutions.* Chicago: University of Chicago Press.

Kuhne, Louis. 1893. *The New Science of Healing; or, The Doctrine of the Unity of Disease.* Butler, NJ: Lust.

Kumar, Anil. 1998. *Medicine and the Raj: British Medical Policy in India, 1835–1911.* Delhi: Sage Publications.

Kumar, Deepak. 2001. *Disease and Medicine in India: A Historical Overview.* New Delhi: Tulika.

Kuper, A. 1994. Indigenous Ethnography, Political Correctness, and the Project of a Cosmopolitan Anthropology. *Anthropos* 89, nos. 4–6: 529–41.

Kutumbiah, P. 1962. *Ancient Indian Medicine.* Madras: Orient Longmans.

Kuvalayananda, Swami. 1924a. *Āsana.* Lonavala: Kaivalyadhama SMYM Samithi.

———. 1924b. Barometric Experiments on Nauli: "Madhavdas Vacuum." *Yoga Mimamsa* 1, no. 1: 27–28, 96–100.

———. 1925a. Madhavdas Vacuum. *Yoga Mimamsa* 1, no. 2: 96–100.

———. 1925b. X-ray Experiments on Uddiyana and Nauli in Relation to the Position of the Colon Contents. *Yoga Mimamsa* 1, no. 3: 168–89.

———. 1925c. X-ray Experiments on Uddiyana and Nauli in Relation to the Position of the Colon Contents. *Yoga Mimamsa* 1, no. 4: 250–54.

———. 1926c. X-ray Experiments on Dhauti (Uddiyana). *Yoga Mimamsa* 2, no. 3: 176–96.

———. 1926a. Blood Pressure Experiments during Sarvangasana and Matsyasana. *Yoga Mimamsa* 2, no. 1: 12–28.

———. 1926b. Blood Pressure Experiments on Shirshasana. *Yoga Mimamsa* 2, no. 2: 92–112.

———. 1928a. Experiments on Intra-Gastric Pressures. *Yoga Mimamsa* 3, no. 1: 10–17.

———. 1928b. Freedom from Emotions. *Yoga Mimamsa* 3, no. 2: 146–50.

———. 1928c. X-ray Experiments on Diaphragm and Ribs. *Yoga Mimamsa* 3, nos. 1,2,3: 18–37, 87–114, 169–209.

———. 1930. $C0_2$ Elimination in Pranayama. *Yoga Mimamsa* 4, no. 2: 95–120.

———. 1933. 0_2 Absorption and $C0_2$ Elimination in Pranayama. *Yoga Mimamsa* 4, no. 4: 267–89.

———. 1934. Alveolar Air Composition Experiments. *Yoga Mimamsa* 5, no. 1: 9–38.

———. 1963. *Yoga Therapy: Its Basic Principles and Methods.* New Delhi: Central Health Education Bureau, D.G.H.S, Ministry of Health, Government of Indian.

———. 1993. *Asanas.* Lonavala: Kaivalyadhama.

Lara, Martin J. 1999. *Uropathy: The Most Powerful Holistic Therapy.* Brooklyn, NY: Self-published.

Larson, Gerald J. 1969. *Classical Sāṃkhya: An Interpretation of Its History and Meaning.* Delhi: Motilal Banarsidass.

———. 1978. Review of Gasper M. Koelman (1970), *Pātañjala Yoga: From Related Ego to Absolute Self. East and West* 28, no. 2: 236–39.

Larson, Gerald J., and Ram S. Bhattacharya, eds. 1987. Sāṃkhya: A Dualist Tradition in Indian Philosophy. Vol. 4 of *The Encyclopedia of Indian Philosophies.* Princeton: Princeton University Press.

Latour, Bruno, and Steve Woolgar. 1979. *Laboratory Life: The Social Construction of Scientific Facts.* Beverly Hills, CA: Sage Publications.

Levi, Eliphas. 1969. *The Paradoxes of the Highest Science: In Which the Most Advanced Truths of Occultism Are for the First Time Revealed (in Order to Reconcile the Future Developments of Science and Philosophy with the Eternal Religion).* Mokelumne Hill, CA: Health Research.

Lévi-Strauss, Claude. 1963. *Structural Anthropology.* Vol. 1. New York: Basic Books.

Levinas, Emmanuel. 1987. *Collected Philosophical Papers.* Dordrecht: Martinus Nijhoff.

Lorenzen, David. 1972. *The Kāpālikas and Kālāmukhas: Two Lost Saivit Sects.* New Delhi: Motilal Banarsidass.

Ludden, David, ed. 1996. Making India Hindu. Delhi: Oxford University Press.

Mādhavācārya. 1882. *The Sarva-Darśana Saṃgraha; or, Review of the Different Systems of Hindu Philosophy.* Translated by E. B. Cowell and A. E. Gough. London: Trubner and Co.

Mahābhārata. 1933–1960. Edited by Vishnu S. Sukthankar et al. Baroda: Bhandarkar Oriental Research Institute.

Majumdar, Ashok. 1999. *Nervous System in Yoga and Tantra (Implication in Āyurveda).* Delhi: Nag Publishers.

Malik, Yogendra, and V. B. Singh. 1995. *Hindu Nationalists in India: The Rise of the Bharatiya Janata Party.* New Delhi: Vistaar Publications.

Malkani, K. R. 1980. *The R.S.S. Story.* New Delhi: Impex.

Mallapurāṇa. 1964. Edited and translated by B. J. Sandesara and R. N. Mehta. Gaekwad Oriental Series, no. 144. Baroda: Oriental Institute.

Marcus, George E. 1998. *Ethnography through Thick and Thin.* Princeton: Princton University Press.

Marcus, George E., and Michael M. J. Fischer. 1986. *Anthropology as Cultural Critique: An Experimental Moment in the Social Sciences.* Chicago: University of Chicago Press.

Marfording, A. 1997. Cultural Relativism and the Construction of Culture: An Examination of Japan. *Human Rights Quarterly* 19, no. 2: 431–48.

Marks, S. P. 1998. From the "Single Confused Page" to the "Decalogue for Six Billion Persons": The Roots of the Universal Declaration of Human Rights in the French Revolution. *Human Rights Quarterly* 20, no. 3: 459–514.

Marriott, McKim. 1990. *India through Hindu Categories.* New Delhi: Sage Publications.

Maryanski, A. R. 1995. What Is a Good Society for Hominoids? *Critical Review* 9, no. 4: 483–99.

Mathur, H. C. 1985. *Rāj Yoga as Experienced by a Scientist.* Mt. Abu: Brahma Kumaris Ishwariya Vishwa-Vidyalaya.

———. 1998. *Siddhi: The Science of Supernatural Powers.* New Delhi: Shree Publishers.

McCall, Timothy. 2003. Western Science vs. Eastern Wisdom. *Yoga Journal,* February: 88–93, 170–73.

McKean, Lise. 1996. *Divine Enterprise: Gurus and the Hindu Nationalist Movement.* Chicago: University of Chicago Press.

McKeon, Richard P. 1994. *On Knowing—The Natural Sciences.* Chicago: University of Chicago Press.

Mead, G.R.S. 1892. *Yoga: The Science of Soul.* Madras: Theosophical Publishing House.

Meade, Teresa, and Mark Walker. 1991. *Science, Medicine, and Cultural Imperialism.* New York: St. Martin's Press.

Messer, E. 1993. Anthropology and Human Rights. *Annual Review of Anthropology* 22: 221–49.

Miller, Barbara D. 1999. *Cultural Anthropology.* Boston: Allyn and Bacon.

Miller, Barbara Stoler. 1996. *Yoga: Discipline of Freedom: The Yoga Sūtra Attributed to Patañjali; A Translation of the Text, with Commentary, Introduction, and Glossary of Keywords.* Berkeley: University of California Press.

Mishra, Chandrika Prashad Shastri. 1998. *Svāmūtra Cikitsā.* Varanasi: Sarva Seva Sangh.

Misra, Amit. 2001. Public Health Issues and the Freedom Movement: Gandhi on Nutrition, Sanitation, Infectious Diseases, and Health Care. In *Disease and Medicine in India,* edited by Deepak Kumar, 249–64. New Delhi: Tulika Publications.

Misra, Shri Narayana, ed. 1971. *Pātañjalayogadarśana, with Vyāsa's Bhāśya, Vācaspati Miśra's Tattva-Vaiśāradī, and Vijñāna Bhikṣu's Yoga-Vārttika.* Varanasi: Chowkhamba.

Mithal, C. P. 1979. *Miracles of Urine Therapy.* New Delhi: Pankaj Publications.

Molinero, José Ramon. 1971. *Rāja Yoga Secreto.* Sao Paulo: Mandala.

Moorty, A. M. 1982. Relationship between Nostril Dominance and Grip Strength. *SNIPES Journal* 5, no. 1: 77–80.

Moorty, A. M., S. K. Ganguly, M. L. Gharote, and P. V. Karambelkar. 1978. Cholesterol Level and Yogic Training Program. *Journal of Research on Indian Medicine, Yoga, and Homeopathy* 13, no. 4: 1–6.

"The Mother," 1961. Physical Education and Yoga. *Mother India* 20, nos. 10/11.

———. 1979. *Health and Healing in Yoga.* Pondicherry: Sri Aurobindo Ashram.

Murthy, T. S. Anantha. 1972. *Tapasvi Maharaj: A Biography of Shriman Tapasvi Maharaj, a Mahatma Who Lived for 185 Years.* San Rafael, CA: Dawn Horse Press.

Murty, Shri Ramachandra Vayuvegula. 1979. *Neurophysiological Basis of Raja Yoga in the Light of Sahaj Marg.* Shahjahanpur: Shri Ram Candra Mission.

Nair, R. M. 1992a. *Chronic Diseases and Its Complete Cure through Naturopathy.* Delhi: Bapu Nature Cure Hospital and Yogashram.

———. 1992b. *Naturopathy: Bapu Nature Cure Hospital's Journal—Special Issue on Diseases of the Heart and Lungs.* Delhi: Bapu Nature Cure Hospital and Yogashram.

———. 1992c. *Naturopathy: Bapu Nature Cure Hospital's Journal—Special Issue on Liver and Kidneys.* Delhi: Bapu Nature Cure Hospital and Yogashram.

———. 1993. *Naturopathy: Bapu Nature Cure Hospital's Journal—Special Issue on Spinal Baths, Yoga, Pimples, and the Bad Effects of Tea.* Delhi: Bapu Nature Cure Hospital's Journal.

———. 1997. Living the Nature Cure Way. *Naturopathy: Bapu Nature Cure Hospital's Journal* 6, no. 68: 11–17.

Nair, R. M., and Rukmani Nair. 1997. Asthma—Care through Nature Cure. *Naturopathy: Bapu Nature Cure Hospital's Journal* 7, no. 73: 10–13.

Nair, Rukmani. 1994. Rheumatoid Arthritis and Naturopathy. *Naturopathy: Bapu Nature Cure Hospital's Journal* 4, no. 42: 7–14.

Nalavade, Balakrishna Lakshmana. 1974. *Śivambu (Svāmūtra) Cikitsā: Arthat, Arogyace Divyamṛta.* Pune: Nalavade.

Nanda, Serena, and Richard L. Warms. 1998. *Cultural Anthropology.* 6th ed. Belmont, CA: Wadsworth.

Nandy, Ashis. 1980. *At the Edge of Psychology: Essays in Politics and Culture.* New Delhi: Oxford University Press.

———. 1983. *The Intimate Enemy: Loss and Recovery of Self under Colonialism.* New Delhi: Oxford University Press.

———. 1995. *The Savage Freud and Other Essays on Possible and Retrievable Selves.* Princeton: Princeton University Press.

———. 1997. The Twilight of Certitudes: Secularism, Hindu Nationalism, and Other Masks of Deculturation. *Alternatives—Social Transformation and Humane Governance* 22, no. 2: 157–76.

Narayan, Kirin. 1993. Refractions of the Field at Home: American Representations of Hindu Holy Men in the 19th and 20th Centuries. *Cultural Anthropology* 8, no. 4: 476–509.

"Neelam, Shrimati." 1993. *Sex Aur Yoga.* Delhi: Sadhana Pocket Books.

Nietzsche, Friedrich. 1968. Beyond Good and Evil: Prelude to a Philosophy of the Future. In *Basic Writings of Nietzsche,* edited and translated by Walter Kaufmann, 179–435. New York: Random House.

Niraj, Nagendra K. 1995. Am. *Naturopathy: Bapu Nature Cure Hospital's Journal* 4, no. 48: 2–5.

Nuckolls, Charles W. 1998. *Culture: A Problem That Cannot Be Solved.* Madison: University of Wisconsin Press.

Oak, J. P., and M. V. Bhole. 1981a. Learning Vastra Dhauti by Asthmatics—A Preliminary Study. *Yoga Mimamsa* 20, no. 1: 19–28.

———. 1981b. Subjective Feelings and Reactions of Asthmatics While Learning Vastra Dhauti. *Yoga Mimamsa* 20, no. 3: 51–58.

———. 1982. Direction of Change in Order of Values of Asthmatics by Yogic Treatment. *Yoga Mimamsa* 20, no. 4: 25–34.

O'Flaherty, Wendy Doniger. 1984. *Dreams, Illusion, and Other Realities.* Chicago: University of Chicago Press.

Olcott, Henry Steel. 1885. *Theosophy, Religion, and Occult Science.* London: G. Redway.

Oman, John Campbell. 1903. *The Mystics, Ascetics, and Saints of India.* London: T. F. Unwin.

O'Quinn, John F. 1980. *Urine Therapy: Self-Healing through Intrinsic Medicine.* Fort Pierce, FL: Life Science Institute.

Padacandrikā (commentary on *Pātañjalayogadarśana* by Ananta-Deva Pandit). 1930. Edited by Dhundhiraja Shastri. Banaras: Chowkhamba.

Pal, Kumar. n.d.a. *Yoga International Institute for Psycho-Physical Therapy Brochure.* New Delhi: Yoga International Institute for Psycho-Physical Therapy.

———. n.d.b. *Yoga Psycho-Physical Therapy Course.* New Delhi: Yoga International Institute for Psycho-Physical Therapy.

Pandey, Gyanendra. 1990. *The Construction of Communalism in North India.* New Delhi: Oxford University Press.

———, ed. 1993. *Hindus and Others: Questions of Identity in India Today.* New York: Viking.

Paranjape, S. D., and M. V. Bhole. 1979. Resting Neuro-Muscular Activity as Influenced by Long Term Yogic Training—A Study Based on Finger Ergography. *Yoga Mimamsa* 19, no. 4: 18–26.

Parsons, Talcott. 1954. *Essay in Sociological Theory.* Glencoe, IL: Free Press.

Patel, Raojibhai Manibhai. 1991. *Manav Mootra: Auto-Urine Therapy.* Ahmedabad: Lok Seva Kendra.

Pati, Biswamoy, and Mark Harrison. 2001. *Health, Medicine and Empire: Perspectives on Colonial India.* New Delhi: Orient Longman.

Patil, Shashi. 1996. *Integrated Approach of Urine Therapy (IAUT): A Long Term Prospective Study.* Kolhapur: Samyak Publications.

Paul, N. C. 1851. *A Treatise on the Yoga Philosophy.* Banares: C. H. Voss.

———. 1888. *The Yoga Philosophy.* Bombay: Tukaram Tatya.

Pennington, B. K. 2001. Constructing Colonial Dharma: A Chronicle of Emergent Hinduism, 1830–1931. *Journal of the American Academy of Religion* 69, no. 3: 577–603.

Peschek-Böhmer, Flora. 1999. *Urine Therapy: Nature's Elixir for Good Health.* Rochester, VT: Healing Arts Press.

Philosophico-Literary Research Department of Kaivalyadhama SMYM Samiti. 1991. *Yoga Kośa.* Lonavala: Kaivalyadhama SMYM Samiti.

Pierson, Ruth Roach, and Nupur Chaudhuri. 1998. *Nation, Empire, Colony: Historicizing Gender and Race.* Bloomington: Indiana University Press.

Pietz, William. 1993. Fetishism and Materialism: The Limits of Theory in Marx. In *Fetishism as Cultural Discourse.* Edited by Emily Apter and William Pietz, 119–51. Ithaca, NY: Cornell University Press.

Pilai, M. Gnauapiakesam, and Lauron William De Laurence. 1910. *India's Hood Unveiled, Astral and Spirit Sight at Will. South India Mysteries, Hindu Hypnograph, Ancient Hindu Methods for Hindu Clairvoyance. Hindu Levitation (Raising the Human Body in the Air). Hindu Method of Burial Alive (Suspended Animation). Spirit Sight at Will.* Chicago: De Laurence, Scott & Co.

Pines, S., and T. Gelblum. 1966. Al-Biruni's Arabic Version of Patanjali's Yoga-Sutra. *Bulletin of the School of Oriental and African Studies* 29, 40: 302–25.

Pollis, A. 1996. Cultural Relativism Revisted: Through a State Prism. *Human Rights Quarterly* 18, no. 2: 316–44.

Prakash, Gyan. 1999. *Another Reason: Science and the Imagination of Modern India.* Princeton: Princeton University Press.

Prakash, Swarajya. 1996. My Experience in Bapu Nature Cure Hospital and Yogashram, Patparganj, Delhi. *Naturopathy: Bapu Nature Cure Hospital's Journal* 5, no. 57: 62.

Pranavananda, Yogi. 1992. *Pure Yoga.* Delhi: Motilal Banarsidass.

Pratap, V. 1972. Diurnal Pattern of Nostril Breathing—An Exploratory Study. *Yoga Mimamsa* 14, nos. 3–4: 1–18.

———. 1975. Kuvalayananda, a Link between East and West. In *Kaivalyadhama, Golden Jubilee Year Souvenir, 1975,* edited by Swami Digambarji, 77–80. Lonavala: Kaivalyadhama.

Price, Robin. 1981. Hydrotherapy in England, 1840–1870. *Medical History* 25.

Purani, A. B. 1950. Sri Aurobindo and Physical Culture. *Advent* 7, no. 2: 116–23.

Quine, W. V. 1992. *Pursuit of Truth.* Rev. ed. Cambridge: Harvard University Press.

———. 1995. *From Stimulus to Science.* Cambridge: Harvard University Press.

Rabinow, Paul. 1996a. *Essays on the Anthropology of Reason.* Princeton: Princeton University Press.

———. 1996b. *Making PCR: A Story of Biotechnology.* Chicago: University of Chicago Press.

Raheja, Gloria Godwin. 1988. *The Poison in the Gift: Ritual, Prestation, and the Dominant Caste in North India.* Chicago: University of Chicago Press.

Rai, Ram Kumar, ed. and trans. 1988. *Ḍāmara Tantra.* Varanasi: Prachya Prakashan.

Rajarshi Muni, Swami. 1995. *Yoga: The Ultimate Attainment.* Delhi: Jaico Publishing House.

Rama, Swami. 1972. *Perennial Psychology of the Bhagavad Gītā.* Honesdale, PA: Himalayan Institute.

———. 1976. *Lectures on Yoga: Practical Lessons on Yoga*. Honesdale, PA: Himalayan Institute.

———. 1978. *Living with the Himalayan Masters*. Honesdale, PA: Himalayan Institute.

———. 1984. *Exercise without Movement*. Honesdale, PA: Himalayan Institute.

———. 1986. *Creative Use of Emotion*. Honesdale, PA: Himalayan Institute.

———. 1999. *A Practical Guide to Holistic Health*. Honesdale, PA: Himalayan Institute.

Rama, Swami, and Swami Ajay. 1976. *Emotion without Enlightenment*. Honesdale, PA: Himalayan Institute.

Rama, Swami, and Rudolph Ballentine. 1976. *Yoga and Psychotherapy: The Evolution of Consciousness*. Glenview, IL: Himalayan Institute.

Rama, Swami, Rudolph Ballentine, and Allen Hyms. 1979. *Science of Breath: A Practical Guide*. Honesdale, PA: Himalayan Institute.

Ramacharaka, Yogi. 1904. *Haṭha Yoga*. Chicago: Yogi Publication Society.

———. 1911. *Fourteen Lessons in Yogi Philosophy and Oriental Occultism*. Chicago: Yogi Publication Society.

Rambachan, Anantanand. 1994. *The Limits of Scripture: Vivekananda's Reinterpretation of the Vedas*. Honolulu: University of Hawaii Press.

Rao, S. K. Ramachandra. 1985. *Encyclopedia of Indian Medicine*. Vol. 1: Historical Perspective. Bombay: Popular Prakashan.

———. 1987. *Encyclopedia of Indian Medicine*. Vol 2. Bombay: Popular Prakashan.

Reddy, P. N., and P. Vimladevi. 1993. S.L.E. Cured through Naturopathy. *Naturopathy: Bapu Nature Cure Hospital's Journal* 2, no. 20: 35–37.

Reddy, William M. 1997. Against Constructionism: The Historical Ethnography of Emotions. *Current Anthropology* 38, no. 3: 327–51.

Richardson, J. E., and Heinrich Hensoldt. 1911. *The Reality of Matter; a Critical Correspondence between Heinrich Hensoldt, Ph.D. of Columbia University, and a Member of the Order of the Brotherhood of India. Republished in Book Form at Request of Students and Friends of the Great Work, for the Benefit of Those Who Are Confused by the Fundamental Teachings of Christian Science and Other Cults and Schools of Mental Therapeutics*. Chicago: Indo-American Book Co.

Ritter, Helmut. 1956. Al-Biruni's Übersetzung des Yoga-Sūtra des Patañjali. *Oriens* 9, no. 2: 165–200.

Rodrigues, Santan. 1982. *The Householder Yogi: Life of Shri Yogendra*. Bombay: Yoga Institute.

Rodseth, Lars. 1998. Distributive Models of Culture: A Sapirian Alternative to Essentialism. *American Anthropologist* 100, no. 1: 55–69.

Rolls, Roger. 1988. *The Hospital of the Nation: The Story of Spa Medicine and the Mineral Water Hospital at Bath*. Bath: Bird Publications.

Rosaldo, Renato. 1989. *Culture and Truth: The Remaking of Social Analysis*. Boston.

Roscoe, Paul B. 1995. The Perils of "Positivism" in Cultural Anthropology. *American Anthropologist* 97, no. 3: 492–504.

Rosman, Abraham, and Paula G. Rubel. 1998. *The Tapistry of Culture: An Introduction to Cultural Anthropology.* 6th ed. Boston: McGraw-Hill.

Sahu, R. J., and M. V. Bhole. 1983. Effect of Two Types of Pranava (Omkar) Recitation on Psycho-Motor Performance. *Yoga Mimamsa* 22, nos. 3–4: 23–29.

Sahu, R. J., and M. L. Gharote. 1984. Effect of Short Term Yogic Training Program on Dexterity. *Yoga Mimamsa* 23, no. 2: 21–27.

Salmon, M. 1997. Ethical Considerations in Anthropology and Archaeology, or Relativism and Justice for All. *Journal of Anthropological Research* 53, no. 1: 47–63.

———. 1999. Relativist Ethics, Scientific Objectivity, and Concern for Human Rights. *Science and Engineeering Ethics* 5, no. 3: 311–18.

Sāṃkhyakārikā (of Iśvarkṛṣṇa). 1964. Edited by T. G. Mainkar. Poona: Oriental Book Agency.

Sangren, P. Steven. 1988. Rhetoric and the Authority of Ethnography: "Postmodernism" and the Social Reproduction of Texts. *Current Anthropology* 29: 405–24.

Sankaracarya, Swami Sadananda. 1888. *A Compendium of the Raja Yoga Philosophy.* Bombay: Tookaram Tatya.

Sarkar, Kishori Lal. 1902. *The Hindu System of Self-Culture of the Patanjala Yoga Shastra.* Calcutta: Sarasi Lal.

Sathe, R. V. 1975. Swami Kuvalayananda and His Mission. In *Kaivalyadhama, Golden Jubilee Year Souvenir, 1975,* edited by Swami Digambarji, 11–17. Lonavala: Kaivalyadhama.

Sathyamurty, T. V. 1997. Indian Nationalism: State of the Debate. *Economic and Political Weekly* 32, no. 14: 715–21.

Satyananda Saraswati, Swami. 1966. *Dynamics of Yoga.* Monghyr: Bihar School of Yoga.

———. 1973a. *Asan, Pranayama, Mudra, Bandha: Compiled from Lectures Given during the Nine-Month Teacher Training Course, 1970–73, at the Bihar School of Yoga.* Monghyr: Bihar School of Yoga.

———. 1973b. *Taming the Kundalini.* Monghyr: Bihar School of Yoga.

———. 1975. *Kriya Yoga: Special Anniversary Issue.* Monghyr: Bihar School of Yoga.

———. 1981. *Amaroli.* Monghyr: Bihar School of Yoga.

———. 1984. *Yoga Nidra.* Gosford, N.S.W.: Satyananda Ashram.

Savarkar, V. D. 1969. *Hindutva.* Bombay: Veer Savarkar Prakashan.

Scheper-Hughes, Nancy. 1995. The Primacy of the Ethical. *Current Anthropology* 36, no. 3: 409–40.

Schilling, Harold K. 1973. *The New Consciousness in Science and Religion.* Philadelphia: United Church Press.

Schultz, Emily A., and Robert H. Lavenda. 2001. *Cultural Anthropology: A Perspective on the Human Condition.* 5th ed. Mountain View, CA: Mayfield Publishing Co.

Scupin, Raymond. 1995. *Cultural Anthropology: A Global Perspective.* 2nd ed. Englewood Cliffs, NJ: Prentice Hall.

Sen, Amiya P. 2000. *Swami Vivekananda*. New Delhi: Oxford University Press.

Seshadri, H. V. 1992. *The Way*. New Delhi: Suruchi Prakashan.

Shaha, Jagdish, Hemant Shaha, and Haresh Dholkiya. 1997. *Mūtra Cikitsā Ka Sāthī*. Varanasi: Sarva Seva Sangh.

Sharma, S. K. 1998. *Miracles of Urine Therapy: Nature's Natural Nectar to Cure Diseases*. New Delhi: Diamond Pocket Books.

Sharma, Shiva, and Kailash Nath Sharma. 1991. *Yoga and Sex*. Bombay: B. I. Publications.

Shastri, Dhundhiraja. 1930. *Pātañjalayogadarśana, with the Rāja-Mārtaṇḍa* of Bhoja Rāja, *Pradīpikā* of Bhāvāgaṇeśa, *Vṛtti* of Nāgojī Baṭṭa, *Maṇi-Prabhā* of Rāmānanda Yati, *Pada-Candrikā* of Ananta-Deva Pandit, and *Yoga-Sudhākara* of Sadāśivendra Sarasvatī. Varanasi: Chowkhamba.

Shobhan. 1990. *Śivambu Sevana*. Ahmedabad: Ayu Prakashan.

———. 1992. *So Rogomam Śivambu-Sevana*. Ahmedabad: Ayu Prakashan.

Singh, Brajen, R. M. Nair, and Rukmani Nair. 1997. Dietary Fibre—A Kaleidoscopic Appraisal of Its Clinical Significance through Nature Cure. *Naturopathy: Bapu Nature Cure Hospital's Journal* 7, no. 73: 14–19.

Singh, Mohan. 1937. *Gorakhnāth and Mediaeval Hindu Mysticism*. Lahore: Self-published.

Singh, R. H. 1991. *The Foundations of Contemporary Yoga*. Delhi: Chaukhamba Sanskrit Pratishthan.

Sinh, Pancham. 1997. *Haṭhayogapradīpikā*. Delhi: Monshiram Manoharlal.

Sinha, Mrinalini. 1995. *Colonial Masculinity: The "Manly Englishman" and the "Effeminate Bengali" in the Late Nineteenth Century*. Manchester: Manchester University Press.

Sivananda, Swami. 1935a. *Kundalini Yoga*. Madras: P. K. Vinyagam.

———. 1935b. *Yoga Asanas*. Madras: P. K. Vinyagam.

———. 1944. *Yogic Home Exercises: Easy Course of Physical Culture for Modern Men and Women*. Bombay: D. P. Taraporevala and Sons.

———. 1950. *Haṭha Yoga: Yogic Exercises for Men and Women*. Rishikesh: Yoga Vedanta Forest Academy.

———. 1955a. *Radiant Health through Yoga: A Handbook of the Yoga-Way to Health and Long Life*. Rishikesh: Yoga Vedanta Forest Academy.

———. 1955b. *Tantra Yoga, Nada Yoga, and Kriya Yoga*. Rishikesh: Divine Life Society.

———. 1961. *Every Man's Yoga*. Rishikesh: Yoga Vedanta Forest Academy.

———. 1962a. *Essence of Yoga*. 6th ed. Rishikesh: Yoga Vedanta Forest Academy.

———. 1962b. *Science of Pranayama*. 6th ed. Rishikesh: Divine Life Society.

———. 1981. *Science of Yoga*. Shivanandanagar: Divine Life Society.

———. 1997a. *Practical Lessons in Yoga*. Rishikesh: Divine Life Society.

———. 1997b. *The Science of Prāṇāyāma*. 16th ed. Rishikesh: Divine Life Society.

Sivananda, Swami, and Swami Venkatesananda. 1986. *Raja Yoga*. Sivanandanagar: Divine Life Society.

Śiva Purāṇa. 1964. Banaras: Chaukhamba Orientalia.

Śiva Saṁhitā. 1996. Edited by Rai Bahadur Srisa Chandra Vasu. New Delhi: Munshiram Manoharlal.

Sjoman, N. E. 1996. *The Yoga Tradition of the Mysore Palace*. New Delhi: Abhinav Publications.

Spalding, Baird Thomas. 1955. *Life and Teaching of the Masters of the Far East*. Marina del Rey, CA: Devorss.

Spiro, Melford. 1992. *Anthropological Other or Burmese Brother?: Studies in Cultural Analysis*. New Brunswick: Rutgers University Press.

———. 1996. Postmodernist Anthropology, Subjectivity, and Science: A Modernist Critique. *Comparative Studies in Society and History* 38: 759–80.

Strauss, Sarah. 1997. "Re-Orienting Yoga: Transnational Flows from an Indian Center." Ph.D. diss., Department of Anthropology, University of Pennsylvania Press.

———. 2000. Locating Yoga: Ethnography and Transnational Practice. In *Constructing the Field: Ethnographic Fieldwork in the Contemporary World*. Edited by Vered Amit, 162–94. New York: Routledge.

Subramuniya, Master. 1973. *Raja Yoga*. San Francisco: Comstock House.

Surath, Shri. 1979. *Scientific Yoga for the Man of Today*. Mountain Center, CA: Ranney Publications.

Suśrutasaṁhitā. 1980. Edited by Bhaskara Govinda Ghanekar. New Delhi: Motilal Banarsidass.

Symonides, J. 1998. Cultural Rights: A Neglected Category of Human Rights. *International Social Science Journal* 50, no. 4: 559–572.

Taimni, I. K. 1961. *The Science of Yoga: A Commentary on the Yoga-Sutras of Patanjali*. Wheaton, IL: Theosophical Publishing House.

Taittirīya Upaniṣad. 1913. In *Upaniṣads: One Hundred and Eight Upaniṣads*. Bombay.

Tattva Vaiśāradī (Commentary on *Pātañjalayogadarśana* by Vācaspati Miśra). 1917. Edited by Rama Ram Bodas. Bombay: Government Central Press.

Taussig, Michael. 1987. *Shamanism, Colonialism, and the Wild Man: A Study in Terror and Healing*. Chicago: University of Chicago Press.

———. 1993a. Maleficium: State Fetishism. In *Fetishism as Cultural Discourse*. Edited by Emily S. Apter and William Pietz, 217–47. Ithaca, NY: Cornell University Press.

———. 1993b. *Memesis and Alterity: A Particular History of the Senses*. New York: Routledge.

———. 1999. *Defacement: Public Secrecy and the Labor of the Negative*. Stanford: Stanford University Press.

Thakkar, G. K. 1997. *Shivambu Geeta*. Bombay and Ahmedabad: Navneet Publications.

Tilley, J. J. 1998. Cultural Relativism, Universalism, and the Burden of Proof. *Millennium—Journal of International Studies* 27, no. 2: 275.

———. 2000. Cultural Relativism. *Human Rights Quarterly* 22, no. 2: 501–47.

Tripathi, Harihara Prasada. n.d. *Ḍāmara Tantra: Hindi Vyākya Sahita: Tantra-Sādhana Se Kāryasiddhī*. Varanasi: Kṛṣṇdasa Akadmi.

Triśikhibrāhmaṇopaniṣad (as part of the *Yoga Upaniṣads*). 1938. Edited by Mahadeva Shastri. Madras: Adyar Library and Research Center.

Turner, B. S. 1993. Outline of a Theory of Human Rights. *Journal of the British Sociological Association* 27, no. 3: 489–512.

Turner, T. 1997. Human Rights, Human Difference: Anthropology's Contribution to an Emancipatory Cultural Politics. *Journal of Anthropological Research* 53, no. 3: 273–91.

Udupa, K. N. 1989. *Stress and Its Management by Yoga*. Delhi: Motilal Banarsidass.

———. 1995. *A Manual of Science and Philosophy of Yoga*. Varanasi: Sarvodaya Sahitya Prakashana.

Upadhyaya, Deendayal. 1991. *Integral Hinduism*. Delhi: Deendayal Research Institute.

Valjavec, F. 1992. The Medium and the Message of Testimony—Self Understanding and Perspectives of a Reflective Ethnology. *Anthropos* 87, nos. 4–6: 489–509.

van Buitenen, J.A.B. 1981. *The Bhagavad Gītā in the Mahābhārata: Text and Commentary*. Chicago: University of Chicago Press.

van der Veer, Peter. 1994. *Religious Nationalism: Hindus and Muslims in India*. Berkeley: University of California Press.

van der Veer, R. 1996. On Some Historical Roots and Present Day Doubts: A Reply to Nicolopoulou and Weintraub (1996). *Culture and Psychology* 2, no. 4: 457–63.

Varadachari, K. C. 1969. *Sahaj Marg and Personality Problems and Yoga Psychology and Modern Physiological Theories*. Tirupati: Sahaj Marg Research Institute.

Varadpande, M. L. 1997. The Air outside Delhi Is a Tonic. *Pioneer,* sec. The Sunday Pioneer Pulse. May 18.

Varahopaniṣad (as part of the *Yoga Upaniṣads*). 1938. Edited by Mahadeva Shastri. Madras: Adyar Library and Research Center.

Varenne, Jean. 1973. *Yoga and the Hindu Tradition*. Delhi: Motilal Banarsidass.

Varshney, A. 1993. Contested Meanings—Indian National Identity, Hindu Nationalism, and the Politics of Anxiety. *Daedalus* 122, no. 3: 227–61.

Vasaka, Bhuvanana Chandra. 1877. *Gheraṇḍa Saṁhitā*. Calcutta.

Vasu, Rai Bahadur Srisa Chandra. 1895. *Gheraṇḍa Saṁhitā*. Bombay: Theosophical Society.

———. 1996a. *The Gheraṇḍa Saṁhitā*. Delhi: Munshiram Manoharlal.

———. 1996b. *The Śiva Saṁhitā*. Delhi: Munshiram Manoharlal.

Vinekar, S. L. 1966. Electro-Nasography (A New Approach in Neurophysiological Research). *Neurology* 14, no. 2: 75–79.

Vivekananda, Swami. 1962. *Raja-Yoga, or Conquering the Internal Nature*. Calcutta: Advaita Ashrama.

———. 1976. *Raja Yoga*. 16th ed. Pithoragarh: Advaita Ashrama.

———. 1982. *Jnana-Yoga*. New York: Ramakrishna-Vivekananda Center.

Vyāsa Bhāṣya (Commentary on *Pātañjalayogadarśana*). 1904. Edited by Kashinatha Shastri Agashe. Poona: Anandasrama.

Wakharkar, D. G. 1984. Swami Kuvalayananda—The Founder of Kaivalyadhama. In *Swami Kuvalayananda Birth Centenary, 1984*, edited by Swami Digambarji, 3–8. Lonavala: Kaivalyadhama.

Walker, Robert. 1998. Heart Saver: Critically-Ill Patients Are Extending Their Lives with Asanas Taught by an Iyengar-Trained Indian Physician. *Yoga Journal* May/June: 102–8.

Ward, Patricia Spain. 1994. *Simon Baruch: Rebel in the Ranks of Medicine, 1840–1921*. Tuscaloosa: University of Alabama Press.

Wartofsky, Marx W. 1980. Introduction. In *Science, Pseudo-Science, and Society*, edited by Robert G. Weyant, Marsha P. Hanen, and Margaret J. Osler. Waterloo, Ont.: Wilfrid Laurier University Press.

Weiner, Annette. 1995. Culture and Our Discontents. *American Anthropologist* 97, no. 1: 14–40.

Westfall, Richard S. 1998. *Never at Rest: A Biography of Isaac Newton*. Cambridge: Cambridge University Press.

Weyant, Robert G., Marsha P. Hanen, and Margaret J. Osler. 1980. *Science, Pseudo-Science, and Society*. Waterloo, Ont.: Wilfrid Laurier University Press.

Whicher, Ian. 1998. *The Integrity of the Yoga Darśana: A Reconsideration of Classical Yoga*. Albany: State University of New York Press.

White, B. 1999. Defining the Intolerable—Child Work, Global Standards, and Cultural Relativism. *Childhood—A Global Journal of Child Research* 6, no. 1: 133–44.

White, David Gordon. 1996. *The Alchemical Body: Siddha Traditions in Medieval India*. Chicago: University of Chicago Press.

———, ed. 2000. *Tantra in Practice*. Princeton: Princeton University Press.

Whorton, James C. 2002. *Nature Cures: The History of Alternative Medicine in America*. Oxford: Oxford University Press.

Williams, R. 1998. Beyond the Dominant Paradigm—Embracing the Indigenous and the Transcendental. *Futures* 30, nos. 2–3: 223–33.

Wilson, Fred. 2002. *Logic and Methodology of Science and Pseudoscience*. Toronto: Canadian Scholars Press.

Wood, Ernest. 1927. *Raja Yoga: The Occult Training of the Hindus*. Chicago: Theosophical Publishing House.

Woodroffe, Sir John. 1927. *Tantra of the Great Liberation*. Madras: Ganesh & Co.

———. 1931. *The Serpent Power; Being the Ṣaṭ-Chakranirūpaṇa and Pādukā-Pañcaka, Two Works of Laya Yoga*. Madras: Ganesh & Co.

Wrobel, Arthur. 1987. *Pseudoscience and Society in Nineteenth-Century America*. Lexington: University Press of Kentucky.

Wrong, D. H. 1997. Cultural Relativism as Ideology. *Critical Review* 11, no. 2: 291–300.

Wujastyk, Dominik. 1998. *The Roots of Āyurveda: Selections from Sanskrit Medical Writings*. New Delhi: Penguin Books.

www.apollohospdelhi.com.

www.apollohospitals.com.

www.kabirbaug.com.

www.pitt.edu/’mcenter/salute.html.

www.rss.org/mission/htm.

Yoga Bhāṣya. See *Vyāsa Bhāṣya*.

Yoga Kundālī Upaniṣad (as part of the *Yoga Upaniṣads*). 1938. Edited by Mahadeva Shastri. Madras: Adyar Library and Research Center.

Yoga Śikha Upaniṣad (as part of the *Yoga Upaniṣads*). 1938. Edited by Mahadeva Shastri. Madras: Adyar Library and Research Center.

Yoga Śudha Ākara (commentary on *Pātañjalayogadarśana* by Sadasivendra Sarsvati). 1930. Edited by Dhundhiraja Shastri. Banaras: Chowkhamba.

Yogatattva Upaniṣad (as part of the *Yoga Upaniṣads*). 1938. Edited by Mahadeva Shastri. Madras: Adyar Library and Research Center.

Yoga Upaniṣad. 1938. Edited by Mahadeva Shastri. Madras: Adyar Library and Research Center.

Yogendra, Shri. 1930. *Yoga Personal Hygiene*. Bombay: Yoga Institute.

———. 1936. *Breathing Methods*. Bombay: Yoga Institute.

———. 1991. *Yoga Asanas Simplified: Microfilmed and Preserved to Be Read after 6000 Years*. Bombay: Yoga Institute.

Yogeshwaranand, Swami. 1973. *The Science of Divinity*. Rishikesh: Yoga Niketan Trust.

———. 1978. *Prāṇa-Vijñāna—Science of Vital Forces: Prāṇa Ke Dvāra Atma Aur Paramātma Ke Sakṣatkāra Ka Naya Anusandhāna*. New Delhi: Yoga Niketan Trust.

———. 1983. *Science of Divine Light: A Latest Research on Self and God-Realization by Medium of 154 Divine Lights*. New Delhi: Yoga Niketan Trust.

———. 1984. *Science of Divine Sound—Divya Śabd Vijñāna: A Latest Research on Self and God-Realization with the Medium of Sound*. New Delhi: Yoga Niketan Trust.

———. 1987. *First Steps to Higher Yoga: An Exposition of First Five Constituents of Yoga*. New Delhi: Yoga Niketan Trust.

———. 1997. *Science of Soul*. New Delhi: Yoga Niketan Trust.

Zechenter, E. M. 1997. In the Name of Culture: Cultural Relativism and the Abuse of the Individual. *Journal of Anthropological Research* 53, no. 3: 319–47.

Ziman, John M. 1984. *Introduction to Science Studies: The Philosophical and Social Aspects of Science and Technology*. Cambridge: Cambridge University Press.

Zimmer, Heinrich Robert. 1948. *Hindu Medicine*. Baltimore: Johns Hopkins University Press.

Zimmermann, Francis. 1987. *The Jungle and the Aroma of Meats: An Ecological Theme in Hindu Medicine*. Berkeley: University of California Press.

Zukav, Gary. 1980. *The Dancing Wu Li Masters: An Overview of the New Physics*. New York: Bantam Books.

Zysk, Kenneth. 1991. *Asceticism and Healing in Ancient India: Medicine in the Buddhist Monastery*. Oxford: Oxford University Press.

INDEX

Spelling and transliteration have here been standardized to conform to the most common pattern of usage in the literature on Yoga, which typically, but not always, is the same as that which is found in the glossary. Given that many of the terms referred to here are drawn from secondary sources and not from primary Sanskrit texts, transliteration using macrons, underdots, and overdots either follows the method employed by the scholar whose work is being analyzed, or has been modified to conform to accepted Sanskrit and/or Hindi spelling. This has entailed standardization where there is variation. For example, *jātharāgni* is used as in S.K.R. Rao, rather than *jaṭharāgni* as in Wujastyk; *Carakasaṃhitā* as in Wujastyk rather than *Caraka Saṁhitā* as in White or *Caraka-saṃhitā* as in Fields; *Aghorī* as in Eliade rather than *Aghori* as in White. Variations in the spelling of text titles have been standardized usually by the removal of hyphenation and/or through conjunction as in the case of *Carakasaṃhitā*. Proper names are transliterated as they are written in English by the person in question or as they appear in the literature associated with a specific person or institution. Many of the names for specific yogic postures are transliterated in different ways by different authors, and text-to-text variation is compounded given the fact that a combination of Hindi and Sanskrit root words are used to label relatively recent, and sometimes idiosyncratic, innovations. In most instances B.K.S. Iyengar's terminology and transliteration are used as a standard, except in those instances where the *āsana* and *kriyā* appear to be distinctive and unique, as, for example, in the case of Dr. Kumar Pal's *ghāṭā śuddhi kriyā*.

BOOKS OF RELATED INTEREST FROM NAB

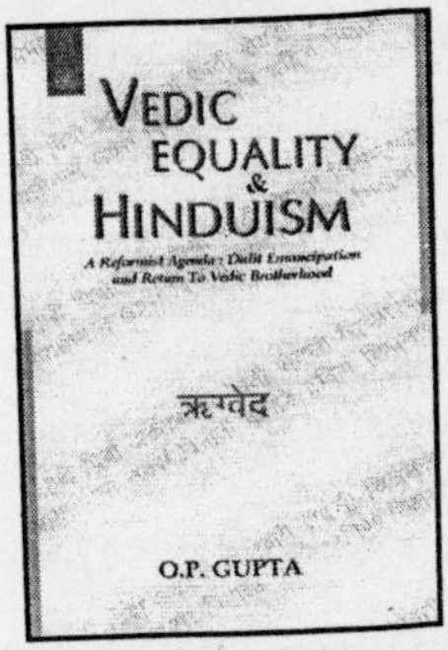

VEDIC EQUALITY AND HINDUISM: A Reformist Agenda: Dalit Emancipation and Return To Vedic Brotherhood) —*O.P. Gupta*

The author has given expression to his understanding of the original and genuine caste system, the Vedic way and approach to human life; the tradition of Sati, its misunderstanding and misrepresentation, wrong notions spread by the Manusmriti. He feels concerned about the Dalits and their emancipation as also about the ills that beset the Hindu society today and is deeply committed to their removal.

ISBN: 978-81-7822-285-1

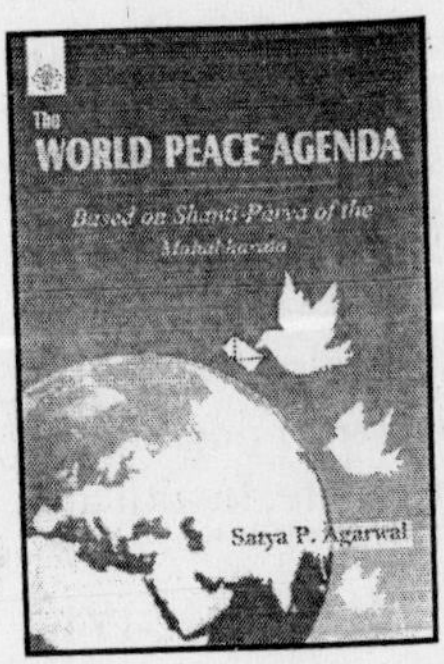

THE WORLD PEACE AGENDA: Based on Shanti-Parva of the Mahabharata —*Satya P. Agarwal*

This book presents Shanti-Parva's peace-messages for consideration by UN, UNESCO, governments, religious leaders, and by everyone else, with the hope that plenty of purposeful discussion (with an open mind) will be held, to arrive at new proposals which can help bring world peace within the reach of humankind in the twenty-first century.

ISBN: 978-81-7822-308-7

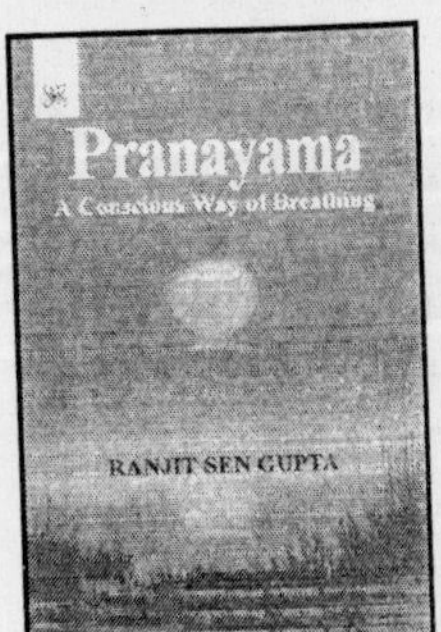

PRANAYAMA (A Conscious Way of Breathing) —*Ranjit Sen Gupta*

The present book introduces us intelligently to the basic breathing practices and describes the fundamental aspects of their psycho-physiology. This is meant for the people who are following a hectic life in the world of constant and fast changing surroundings. This will help to experience with their own breath consciously to bring a harmonious balance in their constitution of the body, mind and soul thereby getting tranquility, inner satisfaction and confidence in their life.

ISBN: 978-81-7822-083-3

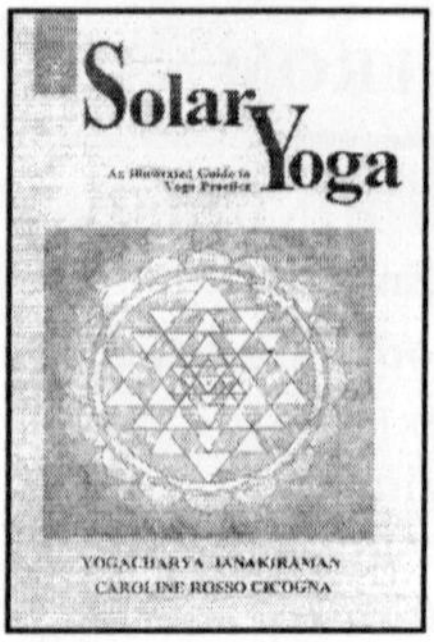

SOLAR YOGA: An Illustrated Guide to Yoga Practice—*Yogacharya Janakiraman, Caroline Rosso Cicogna*

This book offers new insights into the age-old discipline of Solar Yoga. It treats a carefully selected number of classical Yoga practices in a novel manner, integrating the use of sound vibrations with that of postures and breathing techniques at the physical, phychic and spiritual levels. Because of its clear and methodical approach, SOLAR YOGA can be enjoyed by everyone.

ISBN: 978-81-7822-247-9

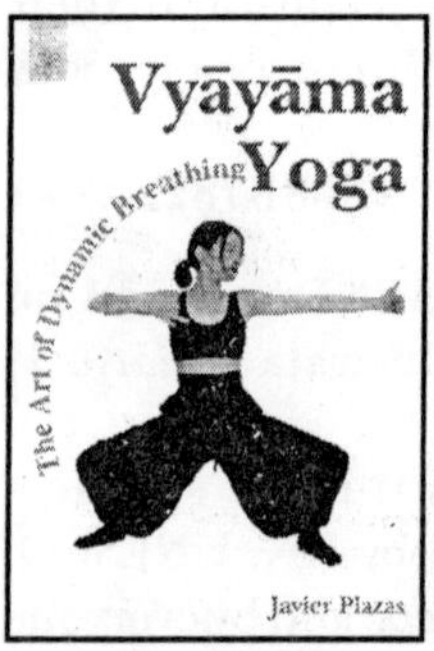

VYĀYĀMA YOGA: The Art of Dynamic Breathing—*Javier Plazas*

Vyāyāma Yoga is an energetic and curative exercise, easy to practise by any person of any age. Its exercises are easy to perform and provide great benefits, due to the continuous coordination between movement and breath. This book will become a historical document, for being the first methodological Vyāyāma book ever published, not only in Spain, but in the whole world. The book will open the door to a universe of possibilities capable of improving and transforming the quality of life, health and well-being of the practitioner.

ISBN: 978-81-7822-174-8

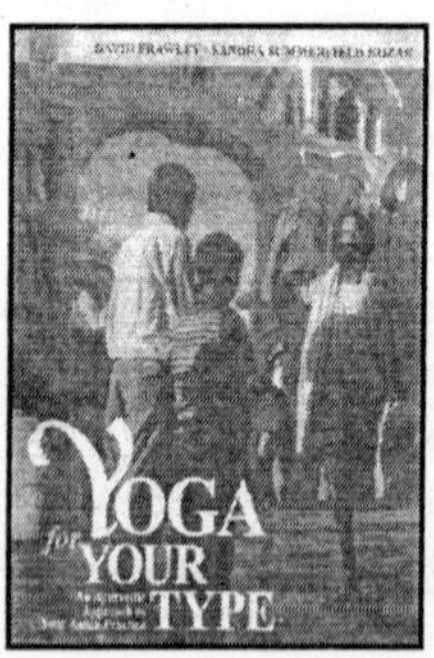

YOGA FOR YOUR TYPE: An Ayurvedic Approach to Your Asana Practice—*David Frawley, Sandra Summerfield Kozak*

Yoga is an extraordinary spiritual science of self-development and self-realization that shows us how to develop our full potential in our many-sided lives. Ayurveda is the traditional medicine healing system for body, mind and spirit. Yoga and Ayurveda have long been linked together as two complementary systems of human development. *Yoga For Your Type* presents Yoga asanas according to an ayurvedic constitutional and energetic model, with a particular regard for ayurvedic mind-body types of Vata (air), Pitta (fire) and Kapha (water).

ISBN: 978-81-7822-111-3